Learning and Intellectual Disability Nursing Practice

This well-respected core text provides a comprehensive solid foundation for students of nursing and practitioners who care for and or support people with learning/intellectual disabilities in a range of health and social care settings and scenarios.

This book addresses learning/intellectual disability nursing from various perspectives, including historical and contemporary practice, health promotion, interventions for good mental health, people with profound disabilities and complex needs, care across the lifespan, and forensics. This new edition has been comprehensively updated throughout and now includes two entirely new chapters. One covers liaison nursing, and the other explores the future for learning/intellectual disability nursing. The book includes numerous case studies and learning activities to support the reader, as well as remaining clinically relevant. Uniquely this text is linked and benchmarked to the Nursing and Midwifery Councils, UK – Future Nurse Standards of Proficiency and the Nursing and Midwifery Board of Ireland's Competencies for nursing students.

This text is essential reading for anyone studying learning/intellectual disabilities at undergraduate and post-graduate levels; it will also be a useful resource for the wider family of nursing, as well as health and social care professionals.

Kay Mafuba is a Registered Nurse (Learning Disabilities). He is Professor of Nursing (Learning Disabilities) at the University of West London, England, UK. He is also a Nursing and Midwifery Council (NMC) registrant visitor for pre-registration and post-registration programmes.

Learning and Intellectual Disability Nursing Practice

Second edition

Edited by
Kay Mafuba

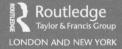

Routledge
Taylor & Francis Group

LONDON AND NEW YORK

Cover image © Getty Images

First published 2023
by Routledge
4 Park Square, Milton Park, Abingdon, Oxon OX14 4RN

and by Routledge
605 Third Avenue, New York, NY 10158

Routledge is an imprint of the Taylor & Francis Group, an informa business

© 2023 selection and editorial matter, **Kay Mafuba**; individual chapters,
the contributors

British Library Cataloguing-in-Publication Data
A catalogue record for this book is available from the British Library

ISBN: 978-1-032-28357-9 (hbk)
ISBN: 978-1-032-28276-3 (pbk)
ISBN: 978-1-003-29646-1 (ebk)

DOI: 10.4324/9781003296461

Typeset in Giovanni
by Apex CoVantage, LLC

Contents

Figures

Tables

Boxes

Contributors

Ailish McMeel is a Registered Nurse (Learning Disabilities) Lecturer in Learning Disability Nursing at Queens University Belfast, Northern Ireland, UK.

Carmel Doyle is Registered Nurse (Intellectual Disabilities, Children). Assistant Professor in Intellectual Disability Nursing at the School of Nursing and Midwifery, Trinity College, Dublin, Republic of Ireland.

Catherine Bright is a partially retired Consultant Psychiatrist in Learning Disability. Professor at Aneurin Bevan University Health Board, Wales, UK.

Chiedza Kudita is a Registered Nurse (Learning Disabilities). Senior Lecturer, and Postgraduate Diploma Course Leader (Adult, Mental Health, Learning Disabilities) at The University of West London, England, UK. She is Public Involvement Coordinator for the College of Nursing Midwifery and Healthcare (CNMH) at The University of West London.

Daniel Marsden is a Registered Nurse (Learning Disabilities). Senior Lecturer and Professional Lead for Learning Disabilities at Canterbury Christ Church University, England, UK. He is an Honorary Researcher with Kingston University and works with the Kent Surrey Sussex Learning Disability Community of Practice.

Dorothy Kupara is a Registered Nurse (Learning Disabilities), Specialist Practitioner. Senior Lecturer and Course Leader for Learning Disabilities Nursing at The University of West London, England, UK.

Eileen Carey is a Registered Nurse (Intellectual Disabilities). Lecturer in the Department of Nursing and Midwifery, Faculty of Education and Health Sciences at the University of Limerick, Republic of Ireland.

Hazel Chapman is a Registered Nurse (Learning Disabilities). Senior Lecturer in Nursing, Postgraduate Tutor, and Programme Lead for the Professional Doctorate in Health and Social Care at The University of Chester, England, UK.

James Ridley is a Registered Nurse (Learning Disabilities). Senior Lecturer, Field Advisor (Learning Disabilities), Programme Lead (B.Sc. Nursing, Learning Disabilities) at Edge Hill University, England, UK.

Jo Delrée is a Registered Nurse (Learning Disabilities). Associate Professor and Head of

Division – Mental Health and Learning Disability Nursing in the Institute of Health and Social Care at London South Bank University, England, UK.

Joann Kiernan is a Registered Nurse (Learning Disabilities) with a keen interest in supporting children, young people, and families. She is a Senior Lecturer at Edge Hill University, England, UK. She is a Consultant Learning Disability Nurse, Alder Hey Children's NHS Foundation Trust, England, UK.

Joanne Blair is a Registered Nurse (Learning Disabilities). Lecturer in the School of Nursing and Midwifery, Queen's University Belfast, Northern Ireland, UK.

Kirsty Henry is a Registered Nurse (Learning Disabilities). Lecturer in Health Sciences and the programme lead for Learning Disability Nursing at The University of East Anglia, England, UK.

Linda Hume is a Registered Nurse (Learning Disabilities). Lecturer at The University of Stirling, Scotland, UK. She is the Positive Behaviour Support (PBS) Workshop Coordinator at The Challenging Behaviour Foundation, Kent.

Linda Steven is a Registered Nurse (Learning Disabilities, Mental Health). Specialist Practitioner (Mental Health). Lecturer in the Department of Nursing and Community Health at Glasgow Caledonian University, Scotland, UK.

Lisa Oluyinka is a Registered Nurse (Learning Disabilities). is a Clinical Staff Development Facilitator, Central and North West London NHS Foundation Trust, England, UK. She is Fellow of the International Federation of National Teaching Fellows.

Louise Cogher is a Registered Nurses (Learning Disabilities). Professional Lead for Learning Disability Nursing, School of Nursing and Midwifery, Keele University, UK.

Lynette Harper is a Registered Nurse (Learning Disabilities). Senior Lecturer at Northumbria University, Newcastle, England, UK.

Michael Brown is a Registered Nurse (Adult and Learning Disabilities). Professor of Learning Disabilities and Director of Graduate Studies in the School of Nursing and Midwifery, Queen's University Belfast, Northern Ireland, UK.

Paul McAleer is a Registered Nurse (Learning Disabilities). Lecturer at Queen's University Belfast, School of Nursing and Midwifery, Northern Ireland, UK. He is chair of the Royal College of Nursing 'Nursing in Justice and Forensics' Professional Forum.

Pepsi Takawira is a Registered Nurse (Learning Disabilities and Mental Health). Senior Lecturer, Course Leader and Education Champion in the Faculty of Health, Education, Medicine and Social Care, Anglia Ruskin University, England, UK.

Rachel Morgan is a Registered Nurse (Learning Disabilities). She is a Senior Lecturer Nursing (Learning Disabilities) and Interim Head of Subject for Therapeutic Studies in the Faculty of Life Sciences and Education, University of South Wales, Wales, UK.

Rebecca Chester is a Registered Nurse (Learning Disabilities). Consultant Nurse for people with Learning Disabilities at Berkshire Health Care NHS Foundation Trust. Chair of the United Kingdom Learning Disability Consultant Nurse Network (UKLDCNN) and Clinical Advisor for Health Education England, UK.

Ruth Ryan is a Registered Nurse (Intellectual Disabilities). Lecturer in the Department of Nursing and Midwifery, Faculty of Education and Health Sciences at University of Limerick, Republic of Ireland.

Sam Abdulla is a Registered Nurse (Learning Disabilities). Lecturer Learning Disabilities Nursing at Edinburgh Napier University, Scotland, UK.

Stacey Rees is a Registered Nurse (Learning Disabilities). Course Leader for Learning Disabilities Nursing/Senior Lecturer at University of South Wales, Wales, UK.

Steven Walden is a Registered Nurse (Learning Disabilities). Certified Forensic Anthropologist. Chartered Biologist. Lecturer in Learning Disabilities Nursing and PhD supervisor at The University of South Wales, Wales, UK.

Vicky Sandy-Davis is a Registered Nurse (Learning Disabilities). Assistant Professor and Course Director in Learning Disabilities Nursing at Coventry University, England, UK. Positive Behaviour Support (PBS) Trainer, and Trainer in the assessment and management of suicide and self-harm.

Preface

In recent years, learning and intellectual[1] disability nursing has completely moved away from narrowly defined roles within long-term care to broader roles. These roles are to be found in a range of health and social settings both in the UK (United Kingdom), The Republic of Ireland and beyond. Hence, there is a pressing need for a brand-new edition of this textbook to inform students and practitioners alike as to the continued development and practice of modern-day intellectual disability nursing. These new roles span nurse practice from community support specialists, through to liaison roles between services and agencies, as well as transitional roles, and secure or forensic health settings. Intellectual disability nurses occupying these roles offer support across the age continuum. Intellectual disability nursing is a health profession supported and endorsed by many, as unique in its breadth of employment base, and located as it is among the various sectors of the health and social care economies. Uniquely to this text, the content of the book has been benchmarked against current Nursing and Midwifery Council (NMC, 2018) for the United Kingdom future nurse standards, and Nursing and Midwifery Board of Ireland (NMBI, 2016) for the Republic of Ireland standards for competence for each chapter. The nomenclature used for identifying competences, competencies and indicators adopts a numerical system that can be found in Appendices A and B, and these relate to those corresponding competencies and indicators identified at the commencement of each chapter. Also, at the commencement of each chapter the reader will find a helpful box that identifies the content that the chapter will focus on, along with further reading and further resources given at the end of each chapter.

In the first chapter, Chiedza Kudita and Kay Mafuba, both from The University of West London, explore the nature of and various manifestations of intellectual disabilities. This is explored alongside the relationship of this group of people to intellectual disability nursing. The second half of this chapter explores intellectual disability nursing, articulating its strong value base, and its long relationship in supporting people with intellectual disabilities, their families, and services, and how these nurses can contribute to the health and well-being of people with intellectual disabilities; making a valuable contribution in the improvement of the quality of lives for this group of often marginalised and vulnerable people.

In Chapter 2, Louise Cogher, Ruth Ryan and Eileen Carey, Keele and Limerick Universities explore the long and often complex historical roots and traditions of how intellectual disability nurses have offered care and support, and continue to offer support, to people with intellectual disabilities.

In Chapter 3, the nature of intellectual disability, as experienced throughout the lifespan and its relationship to intellectual disability nursing, are explored. Here Carmel Doyle, Trinity College Dublin; Daniel Marsden, Canterbury; and Eileen Carey, Limerick Universities present intellectual disability as a lifelong condition. It is not unusual for intellectual disability nurses who work with, and/or offer support to people with intellectual disabilities and their families to have a continuous presence throughout their lives, quite literally from the cradle to the grave. Holistic approaches in learning disability nursing seeking to promote interventions that adopt a whole person-centred approach are promoted. This means providing nursing that responds to the various dimensions of being, and these typically include attention to the physical, emotional, social, economic and spiritual needs of people. Therefore, this chapter focuses on the knowledge as well as the kinds of practical skills that intellectual disability nurses will need when working with people with intellectual disabilities across their lifespan. The role of the intellectual disability nurse during childhood and adolescence of people with learning disabilities is explored within the context of a diagnosis of intellectual disabilities, parenting children with intellectual disabilities, transition periods, psychological and physical changes during adolescence, and finally transition into adulthood. The lifestyle and health needs of adults and older adults with learning disabilities, employment and retirement, personal relationships, and parenting needs of adults with learning disabilities are also explored. The chapter concludes by exploring end-of-life care needs, decisions and palliative care for people with intellectual disabilities.

Chapter 4 presents key concepts and policies in public health as well as key policy 'drivers' that have refocused nursing interventions to be centrally concerned with the prevention of ill health. Lynette Harper, Northumbria; Kirsty Henry, East Anglia; Lisa Oluyinka, Central North West London Foundation NHS Trust and Louise Cogher, Keele Universities identify the role of intellectual disability nursing in helping people with intellectual disabilities plan for good health and well-being. Intellectual disability nurses' public health roles, and in particular the importance of health promotion in care planning, health facilitation and health action planning are all addressed, as well as newer roles such as health liaison nursing in primary care and acute (hospital) settings. These roles are explored in the context of some well-known health issues such as cardiovascular fitness, obesity, epilepsy, mental ill health, sexuality, diet, and smoking. It is pointed out that many of these conditions will require intellectual disability nurses to develop careful and imaginative ways of constructing nursing interventions to improve and or maintain the health status of people with intellectual disabilities.

Chapter 5 explores mental ill health in people with intellectual disabilities. In this chapter Vicky Sandy-Davis, Coventry and Linda Steven, Glasgow Caledonian Universities identify and explore the well-known challenge and implications of people with intellectual disabilities being at greater risk of developing mental health problems than the general population. And because of the higher prevalence of mental ill health in this population, there is a need to prepare intellectual disability nurses to promote good mental health and well-being, and/or its maintenance in those who are particularly vulnerable. In this chapter, the nature of, and manifestations of good mental health, as well as the manifestations of mental ill health, assessment tools used in nursing practice and how to conduct a mental state examination are all explored. A range of approaches to treatments is outlined, as well as issues related to the Care Programme Approach. Finally, relevant mental health legislation and assessment of mental capacity, Independent Mental Capacity Advocates (IMCAs), Deprivation of Liberty and safeguarding issues are all outlined.

In Chapter 6 Steven Walden, South Wales; Catherine Bright, NHS; Sam Abdulla, Napier; and Ruth Ryan, Limerick Universities outline the nature of people with profound learning disabilities and complex needs. They point out that they represent one of the most marginalised and potentially vulnerable groups of people in any society. They are at continuing risk from social exclusion, and simultaneously experience poorer health than does the rest of the population (Public Health England, 2018). Therefore, the role of the intellectual disability nurse in supporting, and where necessary providing direct care for this group of people, is particularly relevant because of the elevated levels of dependence they may have on others throughout their lives. Nursing or directed health and social care should be regarded as a way of systematically planning and documenting interventions to meet the needs of, and to support, this group of people in all aspects of their lives, when this is needed. This chapter considers both direct and indirect roles of intellectual disability nursing in supporting and/or caring for this group of people.

Chapter 7 explores the key competences, skills, knowledge, and value base required for intellectual disability nursing in forensic settings. Paul McAleer from Queens University Belfast and Pepsi Takawira, Anglia Ruskin University identify that in the intellectual disability field of nursing practice the term *forensic* is usually applied, although not always, to people who have offended and been dealt with by the courts. In relation to those who have not offended, the term *forensic* is still applied to some people with intellectual disabilities who present a significant risk to themselves or others, and who may commit an offence, as well as those who have a significant history of self-harm. Intellectual disability nursing in forensic settings is in an extraordinarily complex arena of practice, often involving the balancing of tensions between offering person-centred and therapeutic care, within a framework of a contemporary rights culture, and a need to manage risk usually within controlling systems and environments. People with intellectual disabilities and forensic histories have a diverse range of complex needs and their behaviours constitute a risk, and often result in offending that includes arson, sexually inappropriate behaviour, physical aggression, destruction of property and self-harming behaviours. It is pointed out that the causation of these behaviours is often extremely complex, with a multifactorial range of other contributory factors

including dual diagnosis of mental disorder and intellectual disabilities, the presence of Autism or Asperger syndrome, acquired brain injury and psychosocial issues such as dysfunctional family dynamics, abuse and institutionalisation.

In Chapter 8 Linda Hume, Stirling; Jo Delrée, London South Bank; and Ailish McMeel, Queens Belfast Universities explore the support of people with intellectual disabilities who present with challenging and/or distressed behaviour. The chapter promotes the unique contribution that intellectual disability nursing can provide in promoting holistic support, whilst drawing from strong professional values and an evidence base. It is pointed out that understanding challenging and or distressed behaviour in people with intellectual disabilities is problematic and managing such behaviours has been the subject of much past and recent controversy. This chapter will assert that the management and support of such individuals is of critical importance to intellectual disability nurses; this is because the collective professional integrity of this specialist field of nursing can easily be contaminated by the few who choose not to practice within an ethical and legal framework of nursing practice. Crucially, that is why this chapter will focus on the knowledge and practical skills that intellectual disability nurses need to meet the extraordinarily complex needs of this group of people.

Community intellectual nursing is presented in Chapter 9 by Stacey Rees, South Wales; Kirsty Henry, East Anglia; Rachel Morgan, South Wales; and Joanne Blair, Queens Belfast Universities. They identify how such nurses work with a wide cross section of people with intellectual disabilities and agencies. This chapter explores current and changing roles of intellectual disabilities nurses working in the community. The chapter outlines that dependent upon local configuration of services they often occupy several new and exciting roles. Many work as specialist practitioners on time limited interventions that can include personal and sexual relationships for people with intellectual disabilities, challenging behaviours, teaching direct carers, managing groups, dealing with loss and bereavement issues, working in multi-disciplinary teams, assessing

individuals, supporting clients, working as epilepsy specialists, facilitating self-advocacy groups,
as well as helping people access mainstream services. This chapter serves as a template for safe
care planning within the context of community intellectual disabilities teams and/or where
nurses are attached to Local Authorities, Clinical Commissioning Groups, and HS Boards and
(National Health Service) Trusts. Current health
and social policy, for example Clinical Commissioning, will inevitably make further demands
on the development on the everyday practice
of intellectual disabilities nurses working in the
community. The public health agenda continues
to exert its influence as central to the role of this
group of healthcare workers.

The new penultimate chapter to this text by
Dorothy Kupara and Michael Brown explores
the evidence that people with intellectual disabilities experience health inequalities and inequity; have co-morbidities and are frequent users
of acute healthcare services; and identifies that
despite this, their healthcare needs continue
to go unidentified and unmet with considerable untoward consequences. There are several
factors, including communication difficulties,
which make it difficult for them to effectively
access acute healthcare services, hence the need
for reasonable adjustments. Intellectual disability nurses now work in acute healthcare services
as a reasonable adjustment strategy to ensure
people with intellectual disabilities and their carers are supported to have good health outcomes.
This chapter explores current role of the intellectual disabilities' acute liaison nurse in acute
healthcare services. In recognition of the needs
of people with intellectual disabilities and their
carers when accessing acute healthcare services,
different hospitals have responded by appoint-
ing intellectual disability acute liaison nurses.
Most intellectual disability acute liaison nurses
undertake roles that include clinical activities,
education along with practice development,
and strategic organisational development. These

nurses also act as advocates for people with intellectual disabilities and their carers when they are
using acute healthcare services. It has been recognised that the extent of this role is varied across
the NHS. This chapter provides examples of an
intellectual disability liaison nursing models. The
chapter traces the history of how such roles were
developed and explores the future of this modern
intellectual disability nursing role in the twenty-
first century. It discusses the expectations of this
role with a focus on the skills, experience, expertise, and attitudes affecting the effectiveness of
such roles at local, national, and strategic levels.
Health and social care policy (policy frameworks
in the UK) relevant to this role are also explored.

The concluding Chapter 11 contextualises
current and future roles of intellectual disability
nursing within an arena of ever-changing health
and social care political imperatives. Here, Kay
Mafuba, West London; Rebecca Chester, NHS;
Hazel Chapman, Chester; Joann Kiernan, Edge-
hill; and Dorothy Kupara and Chiedza Kudita,
West London Universities demonstrate this can
be understood at policy level both nationally and
internationally, and it is articulated that with the
ever-growing move towards citizenship, and the
importance of human rights, intellectual disability nursing needs to place itself carefully – both
within the wider family of nursing itself – and
yet simultaneously appeal to the complex landscape of human service organisations as well as
the wider community of intellectual disabilities.
This chapter briefly reflects on the past, but most
importantly looks to the future of the modern
intellectual disability nurse practitioner. It discusses issues affecting intellectual disability nursing, such as changing professional requirements,
policy directions and ever-growing opportunities
for intellectual disability nurses to assert their
role in a widening practice arena, such as the Professional Nurse Advocate role.

We believe that *Learning and Intellectual Disability Nursing* will continue to remain a key nursing textbook – not only for the field of intellectual

disability nursing practice but also will be more widely used by many other professionals and students from wide ranging professional and academic backgrounds who have an interest in the lives of those with intellectual disabilities. We earnestly hope that all who read this book find it helpful, and that its use will assist us in helping people with intellectual disabilities enjoy health and well-being throughout their lives.

Note

1 From here on we will use the term intellectual disabilities – please refer to the note on terminology page XX.

References

Nursing and Midwifery Board of Ireland (2016) *Nurse registration programmes standards and requirements* (4th edition). Dublin: Nursing and Midwifery Board of Ireland.

Nursing and Midwifery Council (2018) *Future nurse: Standards of proficiency for registered nurses.* London: NMC.

Public Health England (2018) *Learning disabilities applying all our health: Facts health and people with a learning disability.* Available at: www.gov.uk/government/publications/learning-disability-applying-all-our-health/learning-disabilities-applying-all-our-health#facts-health-and-people-with-a-learning-disability (Accessed 9 August 2022).

A note on terminology

A note at the outset on the terminology used in this text. Within the United Kingdom of Great Britain and Northern Ireland, the term *learning disability* is used to describe a group of people who have significant developmental delay that results in arrested and or incomplete achievement of the *'normal'* milestones of human development. Other terms are more commonly used internationally, such as developmental disability and intellectual disability. Notwithstanding this wide variety of terminology, we have chosen to adopt the term *intellectual disability* throughout this book as we believe it is now more widely used, and thus will have more relevance to an international readership. Therefore, from the footnote of the preface and thereon throughout the text the term *intellectual disability* is used; save where certain Acts and/or other technical works such as citations and reports require us to use another term for accuracy.

CHAPTER 1

Chiedza Kudita and Kay Mafuba

The nature of intellectual disabilities and its relationship to intellectual disability nursing

Introduction

This chapter explores the nature and various manifestations of intellectual disabilities, along with its relationship to intellectual disability nursing. It commences by describing in some detail the term intellectual disabilities, along with some of the criteria that are used in determining its presence, and this leads us to define the term. This is sometimes difficult, as the term means different things to different people – not only in the United Kingdom, but also internationally (Gates and Mafuba, 2016). Furthermore, it will be shown that the term has different meanings between the many health and social care professionals, service agencies and other disciplines involved in supporting people with intellectual disabilities. Next, the chapter outlines some of the important issues surrounding its incidence and prevalence. Distinctions are made between pre-, peri-, and postnatal factors of causation. This is followed by an outline of causation, and some of the more common genetic and chromosomal abnormalities, and their manifestation, and the chapter will identify aspects of co-morbidity, and some of the health challenges that this group of people may experience because of these clinical manifestations. The second half of this chapter will then explore intellectual disability nursing, its strong value base, and its long relationship in supporting this group of people and their families. Also explored will be services, and how such services can contribute to the health and well-being of people with intellectual disabilities, making a small but nonetheless valuable contribution to improving the quality of lives for this often marginalised and vulnerable group of people. The content of this chapter is contextualised within the Nursing and Midwifery Council (NMC) of the United Kingdom (NMC, 2018) and Nursing and Midwifery Board of Ireland (NMBI) (NMBI, 2016) standards and requirements for competence.

DOI: 10.4324/9781003296461-1

Box 1.1 This chapter will focus on the following issues:

- Understanding intellectual disabilities: a conceptual minefield
- Legislative definitions of intellectual disability
- Adaptive ability or social (in)competence
- Defining intellectual disability
- Incidence and prevalence of intellectual disabilities
- Classification of intellectual disabilities
- Genetic causes of intellectual disabilities
- Chromosomal abnormalities
- Manifestation of autosomal abnormalities
- Manifestation of sex-chromosome abnormalities
- Genetic abnormalities
- Autosomal dominant conditions
- Autosomal recessive conditions
- X-linked recessive conditions
- Environmental factors
- Infections
- Diagnosing intellectual disabilities
- Intellectual disability nursing
- Case history 1.1: Aarav

Box 1.2 Competences

Nursing and Midwifery Council (2018) Proficiencies

Platform 1: Being an accountable professional – 1.1 1.9, 1.11, 1.12, 1.13, 1.14, 1.15, 1.16, 1.20

Platform 2: Promoting health and preventing ill health – 2.2, 2.7, 2.11, 2.12

Platform 3: Assessing needs and planning care – 3.1, 3.2, 3.3, 3.5 3.4 3.8, 3.11, 3.14

Platform 4: Providing and evaluating care – 4.1, 4.7, 4.8, 4.10, 4.12, 4.13, 4.14, 4.15

Platform 6: Improving safety and quality of care – 6.1, 6.3, 6.5, 6.6

Platform 7: Coordinating care – 7.1, 7.5

Nursing and Midwifery Board of Ireland (2016) Competences

Domain 1: Professional values and conduct of the nurse competences – 1.1, 1.3

Domain 2: Nursing practice and clinical decision-making competences – 2.1

Domain 3: Knowledge and cognitive competences – 3.1

Understanding intellectual disabilities: a conceptual minefield

In this first section, intellectual disabilities, as a concept, is explored through several different lenses of interpretation. These include intelligence, legislation, social competence, and adaptive behaviour. And this leads to an articulation of definitions about what this term means. It has been said that intelligence is an obvious indicator that may be used to judge whether someone has intellectual disabilities (Rittey, 2003). If this is so, then we must ask '*What is intelligence, and how might it be measured?*' Intelligence is concerned with logic, abstract thought, understanding, self-awareness, communication, learning, emotional knowledge, retaining, planning, and problem solving. To a lesser or greater extent, as this chapter will show, these are the things that many, if not most, people with intellectual disabilities may struggle with. Within psychology, the complexity of intelligence is evidenced by numerous schools of thought on the subject (Weinberg, 1989). But one way psychology has attempted to measure intelligence is by psychometric assessment through the well-established method of employing intelligence tests, which have been used widely since the early part of the twentieth century. These tests enable comparisons of the intellectual ability of one individual, after completing a range of standardised tests, against a large and representative sample of the wider population. Contemporary opinion about their usefulness is divided, with the view that the tests have many limitations. Some alleged limitations include failure to measure creative insight and the more practical side of intelligence, and a criticism that such tests limit people to a fixed time to complete, thus equating intelligence with speed.

Once undertaken and completed, the score attained is converted into a mental age, which is then divided by the chronological age of an individual and multiplied by 100. This process converts the score into a percentile, which is then known as an intelligence quotient (IQ) (see Figure 1.1). The IQ enables us to compare how any one individual compares with others of a similar chronological age in the wider population.

This has been (and continues to be) used as one of the principal processes for identifying intellectual disabilities. Given that intelligence is present in the general population, and that it is evenly distributed, it is possible to measure how far an individual moves away from what constitutes a '*normal*' IQ (Figure 1.2). The World Health Organisation (1992) has classified the degrees of learning disability (retardation) according to how far an individual moves away from the normal distribution of IQ for the wider population.

> ## Box 1.3
> ## Learning Activity 1.1
>
> If an individual consistently scored two standard deviations above the 'norm' of an IQ test, that is, a measured IQ of greater than 130, how do you think that might that be explained or described?

Using this system, an individual who consistently scores two standard deviations below the 'norm' of an IQ test, that is, a measured IQ of less than 70, would be defined as having an intellectual disability. Those with an IQ between 71 and 84 are said to be on the borderline of intellectual functioning, whereas those within the range 50–69 are identified as having *mild* intellectual disabilities.

The term *moderate* intellectual disabilities are used when the measured IQ is in the range of 35–49. *Severe* intellectual disabilities is reserved for people whose IQ is in the range of 20–34. Finally, the term *profound* learning disabilities is used to refer to people with complex additional disabilities, for example, sensory, physical, or behavioural. This group of people are referred to as those with profound intellectual disabilities with complex needs (see Chapter 6).

$$\frac{\text{Mental age}}{\text{Chronological age}} \times 100 = IQ$$

Figure 1.1

The intelligence quotient formula.

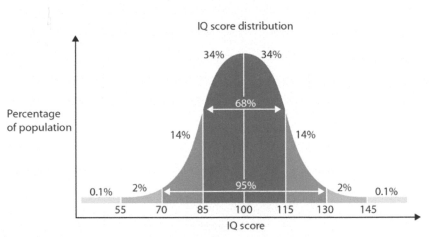

Figure 1.2

The normal distribution curve of intelligence.

Calculating an IQ in such cases can prove extremely difficult, owing to the severity of cognitive impairment and an absence of verbal communication, but there is general agreement that this is <20.

Legislative definitions of intellectual disabilities

Legislation, in both the United Kingdom and other countries, has attempted over centuries to use law to define the nature of learning disabilities. Legislation has achieved this within the framework of mental health legislation, which may explain (in part) why many people confuse intellectual disabilities with mental illness. This unfortunate conflation has resulted in people with intellectual disabilities being the subject of considerable and unnecessary legislation over many centuries. The following brief exploration considers legislation passed during the twentieth century principally in the United Kingdom, focusing upon legislation directly or indirectly related to people with intellectual disabilities. In 1904, a Royal Commission on the care and control of what was then called the *'feeble-minded'*[1] was established. The commission's report, published in 1908, was known as the Radnor Report. This report was highly influential in informing the subsequent Mental Deficiency Act 1913, which was the first specific piece of legislation by the British government to focus on people with intellectual disabilities. Up until that point historically, institutions provided care both for those who were *'feeble-minded'* and for those who were *'insane'*.

Box 1.4 Classifications of the *Mental Health Act 1959*

Sub-normality: A state of arrested or incomplete development of mind, not amounting to severe sub-normality, which includes sub-normality of intelligence, and is of such a nature or degree which requires, or is susceptible to, medical treatment or other special care or training of the patient.

Severe sub-normality: A state of arrested or incomplete development of mind that includes sub-normality of intelligence and is of such a nature or degree that the patient is incapable of living an independent life or guarding himself/herself against serious exploitation or will be so incapable when of an age to do so.

Psychopathic disorder: A persistent disorder or disability of mind, whether or not including sub-normality of intelligence, which results in abnormally aggressive or seriously irresponsible conduct on the part of the patient, and requires, or is susceptible to, medical treatment.

The Mental Deficiency Act 1913 embodied two important principles that included the separation of the feeble-minded from their communities and control. This was overseen by a regulatory body set up under the Act, the Board of Control (Cox, 1996; Thomson, 1996). This Act was to cast a long shadow over the lives of people with intellectual disabilities for many decades to come. The Act of 1913 defined what we now know as intellectual disabilities as follows:

> *Mental defectiveness means a condition of arrested or incomplete development of mind existing before the age of eighteen years, whether arising from inherent causes or induced by disease or injury.*

Following the Radnor Commission, the Mental Deficiency Act of 1913 reflected the strong eugenics (*'the science of using controlled breeding to increase the occurrence of desirable heritable characteristics in a population'* [Oxford English Dictionary, 2013]) movement of the early twentieth century. So, unsurprisingly, the Act required that *defectives* be identified and subsequently segregated from the rest of society. By 1959, terminology, and to some small extent, attitudes had changed. The Mental Health Act 1959 introduced yet more updated terms for people with intellectual disabilities (see those listed in Box 1.1).

The Mental Health Act 1959 required local authorities, for the first time, to make both day service and residential provision for people with a mental subnormality and placed a new emphasis on the reintegration of this group of people into the communities to which they belonged. However, although the terminology seems derogatory this Act should be placed and then judged in a temporal context, particularly in that it followed the implementation of the National Health Service Act 1946. The consequent medicalisation of 'mental subnormality', following the National Health Service Act, is clearly reflected in the Mental Health Act 1959, and therefore its definitions reflected this. For example, it is noteworthy that a strong emphasis in the definitions was placed on 'treatment' (Box 1.1). In addition, the Act made extensive reference to the 'Responsible Medical Officer'. And it is at this point in the history of mental health legislation that the influence of medicine in defining the nature of learning disabilities exerted its greatest impact. Notwithstanding, due to continued social reform, and continuing pressure from lobby groups, mental health legislation was again reformed in 1983–1984; but on this occasion this Act was to bring about positive outcomes for people with intellectual disabilities. Thus, the Act of 1959 was subsequently replaced with the Mental Health Act 1983; and once again old terminology was changed and replaced with new terms shown in Box 1.2.

Box 1.5 Classification of the 1983 Mental Health Act

Severe mental impairment: A state of arrested or incomplete development of mind, which includes severe impairment of intelligence and social functioning and is associated with abnormally aggressive or seriously irresponsible conduct of the person concerned.

Mental impairment: A state of arrested or incomplete development of mind (not amounting to severe mental impairment), which includes significant impairment of intelligence and social functioning and is associated with abnormally aggressive or seriously irresponsible conduct on the part of the person concerned.

Thus, the nature of these definitions at last excluded most people with intellectual disabilities; that is, unless intellectual disability (mental or severe mental impairment) coexisted with aggressive or seriously irresponsible behaviour, from mental health legislation. The 1983 Act represented a major shift in the perception of people with intellectual disabilities within mental health legislation. For the first time, this legislation distinguished and separated most people with intellectual disabilities from mental health legislation. Finally, in 2007 severe mental impairment and mental impairment were removed from mental health legislation as categories of mental health disorder (see Chapter 7).

Adaptive ability or social (in)competence

Adaptive ability or social competence is the final criterion (or indicator) used to identify intellectual disabilities that will be outlined in this chapter. It has been suggested that it is helpful to use criteria based on social competence that include the ability of an individual to adapt to the changing demands made by the society in which those individual live (British Psychological Society, 2000). These abilities are suggested to include:

- Conceptual skills: For example, the use of language, the ability to read and write, being able to use currency, understanding how to tell the time, using numbers, and being able to find one's way around a familiar environment.

- Social skills: For example, interpersonal skills, acting in a responsible manner, enjoying a positive self-esteem, avoiding being exploited, being able to solve social problems, and recognising and responding appropriately to social and cultural expectations.

- Everyday living skills: For example, activities of daily living (washing, teeth cleaning, bed-making, cooking), occupational skills, looking after yourself to maintain a healthy body, being able to use the bus and train, being able to use your own money, and being able to use a personal computer and other common electronic devices.

Thus, at one level, it may sound straightforward to identify how this criterion might be used to categorise or identify someone with intellectual disabilities. One might simply identify people who are able to adapt to their environment and demonstrate social competence and distinguish them from those who do not respond well to changing societal demands. The latter group could then be said to have intellectual disabilities. Burton (1996) has said:

> *Social competence concerns such areas as understanding and following social rules, adjusting social behaviour to the situation, social problem-solving, and understanding others. These are the areas where people typically fail independent living.*

(Burton, 1996, p. 40)

Based on an individual's performance being significantly 'below' what could be considered *normal*, for the general population one might say that some people with intellectual disabilities are socially incompetent or unable to adapt readily to their environments. However, there are several problematic issues to consider in relation to the criterion of social competence and adaptation. Firstly, social incompetence, or an inability of an individual to adapt to his or her environment, can be found in a wide cross-section of people in the population, and not just those with intellectual disabilities. Consider, for example, people with chronic mental health problems, or those with dementia, as well as those who actively choose to reject societal norms; alternatively, there may be problems of communication and cultural idiosyncrasies. Hearing and vision difficulties could cause social incompetence and may not necessarily involve intellectual disabilities. Equally, there is an issue concerning the level of expectation, and the notion of the so-called *'self-fulfilling prophecy'*. Let us imagine an individual has been identified as having an intellectual disability, because of poor adaptation, based upon some measure of social competence. Problematic is whether this should be interpreted as an intellectual disability or poor adaptation because of an environment where this individual may have spent his or her formative years. Such a finding is still not beyond the realm of credibility. In the United Kingdom and elsewhere it is still only relatively recently that the old large intellectual disability hospitals began to close. Tens of thousands of people with intellectual disabilities had been segregated from society, and consequently led to highly devalued lifestyles. Opportunities for the development of social competence were rare in such institutions. There have been many studies undertaken on the effects of people who were deprived of 'normal' nurturing environments. For example, Dennis (1973) in a classic study found that institutionalised children were delayed in basic competencies such as sitting, standing, and walking, and reported that they had no opportunity to practice these skills. He also noted that with the added lack of stimulation, there was significant delay in language acquisition, social skill development, and emotional expression:

> *. . . as babies they lay on their backs in their cribs throughout the first year and often for much of the second year. Many objects available to most children did not exist. There were no building blocks, no sandboxes, no scooters, no tricycles, no climbing apparatus, no swings. There were no pets or other animals of any sort . . . they had*

had no opportunities to learn what these objects were. They never saw persons who lived in the outside world, except for rather rare visitors.

(Dennis, 1973, pp. 22–23)

In short, the expectations of people in such environments were low; there-fore, it is reasonable to assume that their ability to develop social competence was reduced. Despite the criticisms presented in this section, the use of social competence and adaptation to identify intellectual disabilities remains a glob-ally used criterion.

Defining intellectual disabilities

In the United Kingdom, the term *learning disability is* still used and is equivalent to what other countries refer to as intellectual disabilities, and means:

a reduced intellectual ability and difficulty with everyday activities – for example house-hold tasks, socialising or managing money – which affects someone for their whole life. People with a learning disability tend to take longer to learn and may need support to develop new skills, understand complicated information and interact with other people.

(Mencap, 2022)

In Ireland, the term *intellectual disability* is used to mean:

a greater than average difficulty in learning. A person is considered to have an intellectual disability when the following factors are present: general intellectual functioning is significantly below average; significant deficits exist in adaptive skills and the condition is present from childhood (eighteen years or less).

(Inclusion Ireland, 2013)

In the United States, the American Association of Intellectual and Develop-mental Disability recently revised its definition of what was previously known as *'mental retardation'*, which was drawn up in 2002, stating:

Intellectual disability is a disability characterized by significant limitations in both intellectual functioning and in adaptive behaviour, which covers many everyday social and practical skills. This disability originates before the age of 18.

(American Association of Intellectual and Developmental Disability, 2010)

Finally, the World Health Organisation (2010) has now adopted the term *intellectual disabilities* to mean:

A significantly reduced ability to understand new or complex information and to learn and apply new skills (impaired intelligence), with a reduced ability to cope independently (impaired social functioning) which started before adulthood and has a lasting effect on development. Disability depends not only on a child's health conditions or impairments but also and crucially on the extent to which environmental factors support the child's full participation and inclusion in society. The use of the term 'intellectual disability' in this Declaration includes children with autism who have intellectual impairments. For the purposes of this Declaration, the term also encompasses children who have been institutionalized because of a perceived disability or family rejection and who acquire developmental delays and psychological problems as a result of their institutionalization.

(European Declaration on the Health of Children and Young People with
Intellectual Disabilities and their Families, WHO/Europe, 2010)

Incidence and prevalence of intellectual disabilities

Calculating the incidence of intellectual disabilities is problematic because there is no way to detect most infants who have an intellectual disability at birth. Therefore, to arrive at any estimate, one must use cumulative incidence, and this has been calculated at the age of 8 as 4.9, and for severe intellectual disabilities as 4.3 per 100 live births (Emerson *et al.*, 2001).

Nonetheless it is calculated that 2–3% of the population is likely to have learning disabilities, but it is estimated that a substantial proportion of this population will never encounter a caring agency. Therefore, it is more common to refer to *'administrative prevalence'*, which refers to the number of people provided with some form of service from caring agencies.

Historically, the consensus has been that the overall administrative prevalence of severe learning disabilities is three to four persons per 1,000 of the general population (DoH, 2001).

The Department of Health has suggested that mild intellectual disabilities are more common; the prevalence has been estimated to be in the region of 20 per 1,000 of the general population. In the United Kingdom it has been further calculated that, of the three to four persons per 1,000 of the general population with an intellectual disability, approximately 30% will present with severe or profound intellectual disabilities. Within this group it is common to find multiple disabilities, including physical or sensory impairments or disabilities, as well as behavioural difficulties.

Emerson *et al.* (2001), drawing on extensive epidemiological data, has confirmed the estimation of prevalence for severe intellectual disabilities. They have stated it to be somewhere in the region of three to four people per 1,000 of the general population. Whereas they have stated that estimating the numbers of people with *mild intellectual disabilities* are much more imprecise. It is estimated that it might be between 25 and 30 people per 1,000 of the general population. Based on these estimates, one might deduce that there are some 230,000–350,000 persons with severe intellectual disabilities, and 580,000–1,750,000 persons with mild intellectual disabilities in the United Kingdom.

More recently, Emerson *et al.* (2010) have revised these estimates and calculated that in England 1,198,000 people have intellectual disabilities. This includes

- 298,000 children (188,000 boys and 110,000 girls) ages 0–17
- 900,000 adults ages 18+ (526,000 men and 374,000 women), of whom 191,000 (21%) are known to intellectual disability services

There is a slight imbalance in the ratio of males to females in people with both mild and severe intellectual disabilities, with males having slightly higher prevalence rates. Also, there is some evidence of slightly higher prevalence rates amongst some ethnic groups, and this includes 'Black Groups in the USA and South Asian Groups in the United Kingdom' (Emerson *et al.*, 2001).

Classification of intellectual disabilities

An intellectual disability may be classified in several ways. One way is to do so by the nature of its causation. This may fall into two broad main categories: genetic or environmental. Genetic aberrations may originate prior to conception or during the very early stages of the development of a foetus. Environmental causes, on the other hand, include those external factors that can affect the development of a foetus or child in the preconceptual or pre-, peri- or postnatal periods. Where the cause of intellectual disabilities is unknown, then generally such manifestations are usually described as *idiopathic*.

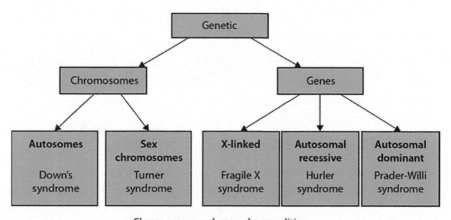

Chromosome and gene abnormalities

Figure 1.3

Simple classification system of the genetic causes of intellectual disabilities.

The following sections portray some of the clinical features associated with specific conditions or syndromes found within the population of people with intellectual disabilities. When reading each section, you may wish to reflect upon the type of healthcare support that may be required in responding to the needs of such individuals and their families.

Genetic causes of learning disabilities

Many of our physical features (phenotype) originate from our genetic makeup (genotype). The information required for the development of these characteristics exists in the form of genes passed from parents to their offspring and are shaped within a complex interaction with the environment. Genes are found located on chromosomes, of which humans have 23 pairs; 22 pairs are known as autosomes and the 23rd pair is known as the sex chromosomes. See Figure 1.4 for an example of a normal karyotype – this is the number and appearance chromosomes – of a male. These are present within the nucleus of every human cell and comprise the genetic material DNA (deoxyribonucleic acid).

It is believed that between 30% and 40% of moderate to severe intellectual disabilities are caused by changes in the genetic makeup of an individual (Knight, Regan and Nicod, 1999). Developments in genetic technology arising from the Human Genome Project have suggested that the percentage may be even higher. A study by Knight, Regan and Nicod (1999) demonstrated that several previously undiagnosed conditions in intellectual disabilities could be attributed to subtle chromosomal rearrangements. Figure 1.3 presents a simple classification system of the genetic causes of learning disabilities. An example is given for each group, and further examples are provided in the following section of this chapter.

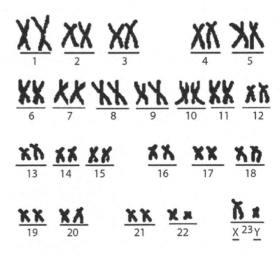

Figure 1.4

Normal metaphase karyotype of a male.

Chromosomal abnormalities

This following section provides specific examples of conditions in intellectual disabilities that result from changes in the structure or number of autosomes and sex chromosomes. Where changes in the structure of the chromosome may occur, this can include the deletion, duplication, translocation, non-disjunction, or inversion of genetic material.

Manifestation of autosomal abnormalities

Down syndrome (Trisomy 21)

Down syndrome was first described by John Langdon Down in 1866, and the condition results from the non-disjunction of chromosome 21 pair during cell division, resulting in an individual having three rather than two of chromosome 21. The incidence rate of this syndrome is between 1 in 650 and 1 in 700 (Mueller and Young, 1998), and the rate becomes higher with an increase in maternal age. Typical characteristics of individuals include short stature, small ears, ear and eye defects, heart defects, and an increased susceptibility to infections, particularly upper-respiratory tract and eye infections. In rare cases, some individuals with Down syndrome may have a mixture of cells that have either trisomy 21 or the normal number of chromosome 21 and this condition is known as *mosaicism*.

Health challenges include:
Management of weight: https://adscresources.advocatehealth.com/weight-man
    agement-in-adults-with-down-syndrome/
Congenital heart disease: http://downsyndrome.nacd.org/heart_disease.php
Hearing   challenges: www.sense.org.uk/information-and-advice/conditions/
    deafblindness/
Thyroid disorder and respiratory tract infections, www.downs-syndrome.org.uk/
Eye conditions: www.seeability.org/eye-care/eye-conditions

Cri-du-Chat

Cri-du-Chat is a rare condition with an incidence rate of approximately 1 in 37,000 live births. It was first described in 1963 by Lejeune *et al.* and given this name because affected infants are found to have high-pitched cries like those of a cat. Typical characteristics include microcephaly, low-set ears, and wide-spaced eyes. This condition is usually associated with moderate to severe learning disabilities. More often, infants present with feeding problems because of difficulty swallowing and sucking, they may have low birth weight, and they may develop challenging behaviour (Wiedemann, Kunze and Dibbern, 1992; Gilbert, 2000).

Health challenges include:

Congenital heart disease: http://pediatrics.aappublications.org/content/117/5/ e924.long

Eye abnormalities: https://rarediseases.org/rare-diseases/cri-du-chat-syndrome/

Manifestation of sex-chromosome abnormalities

Klinefelter syndrome (XXY)

Klinefelter syndrome, first described by Klinefelter and his associates in 1942, affects only males. It results from the non-disjunction of the XY chromosomes during cell division, resulting in an individual having an extra X chromosome. The incidence rate of this syndrome is between 1 in 500 and 1 in 1,000 births. Typical characteristics include a large forehead, ears, and jaw, and, following the onset of puberty, hypogonadism (small testicles) and gynecomastia (enlarged breasts). Psychosocial problems are said to be common. The degree of intellectual disability is said to be moderate, with a few cases of individuals presenting with profound intellectual disabilities (Wiedemann, Kunze and Dibbern, 1992; Gilbert, 2000).

Health challenges include:

Management of diabetes: https://pubmed.ncbi.nlm.nih.gov/31367971/

Thyroid disorder: www.nhs.uk/conditions/klinefelters-syndrome/

Turner syndrome (XO)

Turner syndrome affects only females and results from the loss of one of the two XX chromosomes. Its incidence rate is estimated to be 1 in 2,500 births. Typical characteristics include short stature, web-like neck, non-functioning ovaries, and, in some cases, intellectual disabilities. However, a normal range of intelligence is associated with this syndrome (Wiedemann, Kunze and Dibbern, 1992; Gilbert, 2000).

Health challenges include:

Management of weight: www.nhs.uk/Conditions/Turners-syndrome/Pages/ Treatment.aspx

Coarctation of the aorta: www.patient.co.uk/health/Coarctation-of-the-Aorta

Hearing challenges: www.ncbi.nlm.nih.gov/pubmed/19081146

Thyroid disorder: www.nhs.uk/Conditions/Turners-syndrome/Pages/Introduc tion.aspx

Eye abnormalities: www.nhs.uk/Conditions/Turners-syndrome/Pages/Symptoms. aspx

Genetic abnormalities

This section provides specific examples of conditions in intellectual disabilities that result from changes in the structure of the genetic material making up a gene. These changes may include the deletion, duplication, addition, inversion, and substitution of the parts of the DNA. Gene abnormalities are categorised by the mode of transmission of the defective gene. You may want to refer to the simple classification system depicted in Figure 1.4. These forms of transmission can be described as autosomal dominant, autosomal recessive, or X-linked, and are all described briefly in the following. Some conditions may also result from the interaction of various genes (polygenic), though these are not described in this book. A further reading section about specific conditions or syndromes found in the population of people with intellectual disabilities is provided at the end of this chapter.

Autosomal dominant conditions

In the case of autosomal dominant conditions, transmission is reliant upon only one parent being a carrier of the defective gene, and there is a 50% chance of the condition occurring in the offspring (Figure 1.5). The following provides examples of disorders inherited through this process.

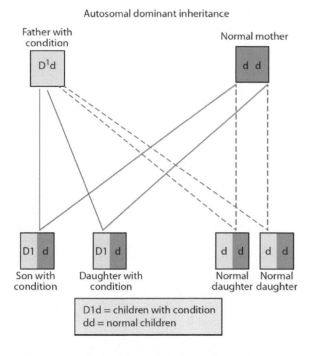

Figure 1.5

Dominant inheritance.

Prader-Willi syndrome

Prader-Willi syndrome is a condition that results from deletion of part of the genetic material on the long arm of chromosome 15 and usually originates from the father. The incidence rate is approximately 1 in 15,000 and affects both males and females. Characteristics of this condition include small hands and feet, hypogenitalism (underdeveloped testes), and cryptorchidism (undescended testes) in males. One of the most notable characteristics, however, is hyperphagia (excessive overeating). Without professional help and support, people with this syndrome commonly experience gross obesity and the related conditions of heart disease and diabetes, which may result in premature death (Wiedemann, Kunze and Dibbern, 1992; Gilbert, 2000).

Health challenges include:
Management of weight: www.nhs.uk/conditions/prader-willi-syndrome/living-with/
Scoliosis: www.nhs.uk/conditions/prader-willi-syndrome/living-with/Scoliosis:
Diabetes: http://ghr.nlm.nih.gov/condition/prader-willi-syndrome

Tuberous sclerosis (Epiloia)

First described in 1880 and estimated to affect between 1 in 30,000 to 40,000 births, tuberous sclerosis is a condition characterised by growths on the brain and major organs. A butterfly-shaped rash (adenoma sebaceum) will be present on the face. Epilepsy is common in people with this condition. Whereas normal intelligence may be present, 60% of affected people will have some degree of intellectual disabilities (Wiedemann, Kunze and Dibbern, 1992; Gilbert, 2000).

Health challenges include:
Dental care: www.nhs.uk/Conditions/Tuberous-sclerosis/Pages/Treatment.aspx
Epilepsy: www.nhs.uk/conditions/tuberous-sclerosis/Pages/Introduction.aspx
Monitoring of lesions in vital organs: https://bestpractice.bmj.com/topics/en-gb/673

Autosomal recessive condition

In the case of autosomal recessive conditions, transmission is reliant on both parents being carriers of the defective gene, and in this case, there is a 25% chance of the condition manifesting in the offspring (Figure 1.6). The following section provides examples of disorders inherited through this process.

Phenylketonuria

Described by Folling in 1934, phenylketonuria is a disorder that affects protein metabolism, resulting in raised levels of phenylalanine in the blood. If protein levels are not maintained at a normal level through diet control, they may subsequently become toxic and cause brain damage. This condition is thought to affect 1 in 12,000 live births. The condition is commonly diagnosed using the Newborn blood spot test, which is carried out 6 to 14 days (about 2 weeks) after

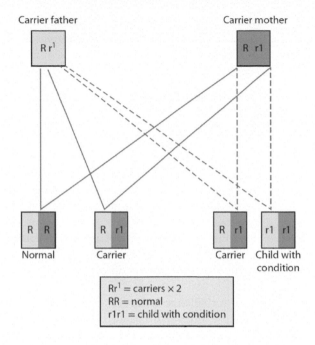

Figure 1.6

Recessive inheritance.

birth. If left untreated, typical characteristics include lack of pigmentation in the eyes, skin, and hair; hyperactivity; autistic features; epilepsy; and a severe degree of intellectual disabilities (Wiedemann, Kunze and Dibbern, 1992; Gilbert, 2000).

Health challenges include:
Management of diet: www.nhs.uk/Conditions/Phenylketonuria/Pages/Treatment. aspx

Hurler syndrome

One of several mucopolysaccharide disorders, Hurler syndrome has an esti-mated prevalence rate of 1 in 100,000 births (Defendi, 2018). It is characterised by the abnormal storage of mucopolysaccharides in connective tissue. Affected individuals are short in stature and described as having thick, coarse facial fea-tures and a low nasal bridge. Hirsutism is a common characteristic, as is the presence of heart abnormalities. Affected individuals may also have sight and hearing impairments; death normally occurs during adolescence (Wiedemann, Kunze and Dibbern, 1992; Gilbert, 2000).

Health challenges include:
Joint management, http://www.nlm.nih.gov/medlineplus/ency/article/001204.htm

Hearing and sight abnormalities, http://www.patient.co.uk/doctor/retinitis-pigmentosa

Hernias, http://www.patient.co.uk/doctor/Hurler's-Syndrome.htm

Cardiac abnormalities: https://rarediseases.info.nih.gov/diseases/12559/hurler-syndrome

X-linked recessive conditions

Fragile X syndrome

Fragile X syndrome occurs more commonly in males than in females, with a prevalence rate of 1 in 4,000 and 1 in 8,000, respectively. It is believed to be the most common cause of learning disability, next to Down syndrome. The condition arises from the bottom tip of the X chromosome breaking off, making the site fragile, hence its name. Common characteristics include an oversized head, long face, prominent ears, large jaw, language difficulties, and varying degrees of learning disability. Behavioural challenges in affected individuals are also a characteristic of this condition.

Health challenges include:
Epilepsy: https://contact.org.uk/conditions/epilepsy/
Recurrent infections: www.findresources.co.uk/the-syndromes/fragile-x/health

Environmental factors

Environmental factors have an important influence on the physical and intellectual development of individuals. Where an environment contains the positive factors necessary for healthy growth, such as food, warmth, love, safety, and sensory stimulation, normal development should occur. However, in some cases, certain environmental conditions may hinder the growth and development of an individual, which might result in intellectual disabilities. Environmental factors that may exert influence on development might occur at the preconceptual, prenatal, perinatal, and postnatal periods of human development and typically include, for example, infections, trauma, substance abuse, and social deprivation (Figure 1.7).

Preconception	Prenatal	Perinatal	Postnatal
Diet, substance abuse, pre-existing medical conditions	Infections (viral/ bacterial, e.g., congenital rubella, congenital syphilis), trauma, anoxia, x-rays	Premature birth, asphyxiation, trauma (forceps delivery)	Infection, trauma, toxic agents, nutrition, sensory/social deprivation, untreated conditions

Figure 1.7

Causation of intellectual disabilities.

Environmental causes of intellectual disabilities include trauma during the prenatal, perinatal, and postnatal phases, as well as accidental and non-accidental injury during human growth. At the prenatal stage, this could also include the delivery of a baby using forceps or suction. Restriction of the oxygen supply to the foetus during the prenatal and perinatal phases can also result in brain damage. In the latter stage, asphyxiation may occur if the umbilical cord becomes wrapped around the baby's neck for a prolonged period.

The consumption of drugs, including alcohol [substance abuse], also accounts for stunted growth and lack of brain development observed in some children. Toxic agents, lead poisoning, strontium poisoning, chemical pollutants, and hard metals, such as mercury and manganese, are also recognised causes of brain damage. In the postnatal phase of development, poor nutrition and a lack of sensory and social stimulation can impair development and result in intellectual disabilities.

Infections

Other causes of intellectual disabilities include acquired infections that can result in brain damage at the prenatal, perinatal, and the postnatal stages of development, and encompass rubella (German measles), mumps and chickenpox. In the past syphilis was also a common cause of intellectual disabilities, but this is now rare in Western countries. Viral infections may give rise to encephalitis (inflammation of the brain), and the subsequent degree of intellectual disabilities can be severe; dehydration occurs rapidly, leading to brain hemorrhage and subsequent brain damage.

Congenital rubella

First described by Gregg in 1941, congenital rubella is a condition characterised by several abnormalities that includes cataracts, deafness, congenital heart defects, and intellectual disabilities. Damage occurs when the rubella virus passes across the placenta barrier and attacks the developing nervous tissue in the unborn foetus. In recent years, the prevalence of congenital rubella has declined with the introduction of rigorous immunisation programmes.

Metal toxicity

It is believed that oxidative stress, because of environmental stressors such as heavy metals, affects sulfur metabolism. For example, prolonged exposure to Lead (Lead toxicity) has been associated with a decline of IQ. Similarly, Liu and Lewis (2013) have noted children's exposure to several metals, such as aluminum, arsenic, mercury, and lead, can cause cognitive impairment leading to intellectual and neurodevelopment disorders (Grandjean *et al.*, 2014). This risk is enhanced in children who have genetic or prenatal risk factors as well as malnutrition and they may be more vulnerable to the adverse effects of metals.

Diagnosing intellectual disabilities

This following section explores briefly how one arrives at a diagnosis of intellectual disabilities. Most parents are not aware that their child could have intellectual disabilities before birth. In most instances, only a small number of parents are given advance information, and this will come because of some form of screening investigation, such as blood tests, ultrasound scans, or diagnostic investigations such as amniocentesis, chorionic villous sampling, or other tests. These are undertaken because the parents are perceived as being at high risk. For example, increased maternal age is highly correlated with a diagnosis of Down syndrome in any offspring: age 20, 1:1,450; age 29, 1:1,050; age 39, 1:110; age 49, 1:25 (Morris *et al.*, 2003). Newer tests, such as the CytoScan Dx Assay, may help identify causation of developmental delay or intellectual disabilities, and it is believed that this test may be superior to karyotyping and chromosomal testing.

Box 1.6
Learning Activity 1.2

Research Edwards syndrome, and answer the following questions:

   What causes this syndrome?

   What potential health challenges might this condition present to individuals affected?

However, unless a definite physical abnormality or characteristic signs (as in children with Down syndrome) are present at birth, or a traumatic delivery has taken place, intellectual disabilities are seldom suspected or diagnosed at birth. A diagnosis can vary from the confirmation of the presence of a specific condition (for example, Edwards syndrome) to a much broader diagnosis of global developmental delay, with no condition being identified. Intellectual disability is generally identified during childhood, but sometimes this may not occur until early adolescence.

Children with severe or profound intellectual disabilities and with complex needs are much more likely to be noticed as having intellectual disabilities at a younger age than those with mild to moderate intellectual disabilities. Intellectual disabilities are most often diagnosed in early childhood, and usually when a child fails to reach the '*normal*' but critical developmental milestones. During this period, parents may have expressed concerns over the nature of their child's progress and suspected a problem. When this happens, a regular check should be kept on the child's progress, more frequently than the usual screening checks, and records should be kept. It will be a huge relief to both parents and professionals, after a period of observation, to be able to show that a child is reaching the normal milestones of development. Unless managed sensitively, it may be the case that active family involvement will be damaged in the short term, and possibly for many years, when a diagnosis of intellectual disabilities is finally confirmed, despite repeated concerns having been raised previously but dismissed or largely ignored. That is why it is important to identify both the nature and extent of intellectual disabilities and exclude or include other more specific developmental disorders that are sometimes present. For example, some developmental disorders include autistic spectrum conditions, attention deficit hyperactivity disorder (ADHD), and dyspraxia. Finally, identifying possible causes of intellectual disabilities, and the provision of an early diagnosis are important to:

- Limit potential feelings of self-blame that some parents may experience.
- Reduce possible challenges in the adaptation of parents to their child and hopefully avoid rejection.

Other reasons for identifying the presence of intellectual disabilities and forming a diagnosis include a need to:

- Understand the possible manifestation and trajectory of an identified condition over time
- Identify a range of therapeutic approaches that may be used to ameliorate the effects of the condition, which will include mobilising and accessing resources (Gates, 2000)
- Establish, in some cases, the degree of risk to other family members of the condition reoccurring in their siblings and offspring
- Provide parents and families with genetic counselling.

Intellectual disability nursing

Nursing has a long association of supporting or caring for people with intellectual disabilities. Currently, in the United Kingdom and Ireland, pre-registration undergraduate students of nursing choose to follow one of four fields of practice: children, adults, people with intellectual disabilities, or people with mental health challenges. These students then qualify in their chosen area of practice at the point of initial registration. Ireland and the United Kingdom are the only countries internationally to follow this approach; other countries provide a generic pre-registration education. Until 2011, all UK nurse education programmes were structured so that all students followed the same programme for the first year of their course (the Common Foundation Programme), and then focused on their chosen area for the two-year 'Branch' programme. The three-year programme comprised 50% of the time spent in the university (theory) and 50% being spent in a range of clinical placements, including schools, residential units, assessment and treatment units, hospitals, and community-based teams (practice).

In Ireland it has undergone a similar trajectory in its professional development to support people with intellectual disabilities (Doody, Slevin and Taggart, 2012; Gates *et al.*, 2020). In 2002, intellectual disabilities nursing, along with other fields of nursing practice, moved to a four-year undergraduate programme of study. Students of nursing, as do their UK counterparts, spend the practice components of the programme in a range of clinical placements that includes hospitals, schools, residential units, assessment and treatment units, day centres, recreation departments, and physiotherapy units, as well as employment settings.

Recently in the United Kingdom, the Nursing and Midwifery Council launched new standards for pre-registration nurse education in 2018 (NMC, 2018). All new programmes must now be at the undergraduate level, and students will focus on one of four 'fields of nursing practice'. However, rather than having a one-year common foundation programme, and a two-year branch programme, as was the case in the recent past, generic, and field-specific elements are now integrated throughout the programme. The programme must be a minimum of three years in length, with 2,300 hours in theoretical instruction and 2,300 hours practice learning. The programmes are competency based and require that students demonstrate competence in both generic and field-specific aspects of four domains to qualify as a registered nurse. The four domains are professional values; communication and interpersonal skills; nursing practice and decision-making; and leadership, management, and team working.

In Ireland in 2016 the NMBI published the fourth edition of its requirements and standards for nurse registration education programmes (NMBI, 2016). The theoretical and clinical instruction comprises not less than 4,600 hours. In Ireland, the academic component comprises no less than one-third of these 4,600 hours, or 1,533 hours. Time spent in practice comprises not less than one-half of these 4,600 hours, or 2,300 hours.

Nationally and internationally, the specialisation of intellectual disability nursing at a pre-registration level for this field of nursing practice has been a subject of much debate over the past three decades (Gates *et al.*, 2020). At various points, it has been proposed that there should be a generic pre-registration programme, and that intellectual disability nursing should become a post-registration specialism. However, such a model has not been effective elsewhere, such as in Australia and New Zealand (Barr and Sines, 1996), and its cessation has brought with it many challenges that need to be addressed (Barr and Sines, 1996). Subsequently, within the United Kingdom and Ireland, a specific field has been maintained, and this is further endorsed on an ongoing basis within the educational programmes that Universities offer. The new standards for pre-registration nurse education in the United Kingdom and Ireland now require newly registered nurses to be able to demonstrate specific proficiency outcomes set out in Appendix A and Appendix B. They require all registered nurses that includes intellectual disability nurses to

undertake these procedures effectively in order to provide compassionate, evidence-based person-centred nursing care.

(NMC, 2018, p. 31)

Ongoing educational and skill development for all intellectual disability nurses are essential in the context of ever-changing service configurations and the increasing complexity of client need in this population of people. Intellectual disability nurses must maintain a wide range of clinical nursing skills that enable them to assess complex needs and plan interventions in a person-centred manner (RCN, 2011; Mafuba *et al.*, 2021). This has led to some deciding to further their education by studying post-qualifying courses in diabetes, palliative care, epilepsy, challenging behaviour, and supporting older people, and they use this new knowledge and skill set to support people with intellectual disabilities, building on the knowledge and skills obtained in their pre-registration degree programme.

Today the modern practice setting for intellectual disability nursing is located in complex landscapes of service provision. This includes, for example, residential care homes, independent living homes, supported living arrangements, and people with intellectual disabilities living in their own homes, as well as family homes. There are also larger, but now much fewer than in the past, service configurations, and a range of very specialist settings, such as treatment and assessment services, challenging behaviour units, and other specialist health or social care settings. There are hospices for children with life-limiting conditions and homes for older people. In addition, intellectual disability nurses may be found supporting people with intellectual disabilities in mainstream health and social care settings, such as in general hospitals, in prison services, and in other settings (Mafuba *et al.*, 2021). Therefore, intellectual disability nurses work with people who have intellectual disabilities and their families from birth to death, and who may need a range of support throughout their lives that will range from none, or minimal support, to intensive holistic nursing aimed at meeting the multi-dimensional health needs of people with intellectual disabilities. Consequently, intellectual disability nursing is often referred to as the *'purist'* form of nursing. Unlike other fields of nursing practice, intellectual disability nurses do not concentrate on specific manifestations of physical ill health or trauma, nor do they just focus on mental health and well-being or children or childbirth. Rather, intellectual disability nurses offer all-embracing support to those with intellectual disabilities and their families that is quite literally from the cradle to the grave.

To offer comprehensive nursing interventions that meet the multi-dimensional needs of people with intellectual disabilities, it is necessary to adopt a structured approach to this field of practice. This typically consists firstly of completion of a comprehensive needs assessment (physical, psychological, social, and spiritual, emotional). If an intellectual disability nurse is required to work with someone who has intellectual disabilities, or their family, it is necessary to assess their needs and incorporate them into an individual care plan that addresses their desires, wishes, and aspirations. Clearly to do this the nurse must work closely with the client's family, with care providers, and with other professionals. Adopting this broad approach may bring important, sometimes essential, information to light for assessment. This first stage is followed by the construction of a written care plan that is then implemented and followed by ongoing review and evaluation. It is this structured approach along with partnership working, and a consideration of the multi-dimensionality of people, coupled with person-centred planning, that allows intellectual disability nursing to lay claim, which is attested by others, that they offer the purist form of nursing. In response to social and political influences, intellectual disability care models, along with that of care planning, have, over the past few years, undergone unprecedented change. Therefore, so has the practice of intellectual disability nurses (Alaszewski *et al.*, 2001; Gates, 2011; U.K. Chief Nursing Officers, 2012; Mafuba *et al.*, 2021).

During the past century, intellectual disabilities services were dominated by a medical model of care that emphasised the biological needs of people and the need to *'cure'* physical problems to allow a person to function in society (Gates *et al.*, 2020). Most people with intellectual disabilities have now long since moved out of the old long-stay hospitals, but there remain concerns that the powerful effects of the medical model continue to influence care provided in smaller community-based residences. Klotz (2004) has argued that the use of the medical model has pathologised and objectified people with intellectual disabilities, leading to them being seen as *'less human'*. Therefore, intellectual disability nurses need to consider adopting a *'nursing model'* to guide their care in practice, to counter this potentially pathologising effect, to ensure that what is offered is holistic and meets the many needs of this client group. It must be remembered that the use of any model must hold the person with intellectual disabilities as central to the care-planning process and that the nurse must be mindful that he or she uses such a model to promote what is best for that patient. Several nursing models can be adapted and used in a variety of health and social care settings. Some nursing models, such as Orem's (1991) self-care, Roper *et al.*'s (2002) activities of daily living, and Aldridge's (2004) model for practice, are well known, often cited, and used in intellectual disability nursing. It should be remembered that these models may not be seen as relevant or ideal for all people with intellectual disabilities, but such models can generally be adapted relatively easily and become ideal frameworks for assessing health and well-being as well as more general needs (Moulster *et al.*, 2019).

BOX 1.7
CASE STUDY 1.1

Aarav, an 18-year-old man, has severe learning disabilities. His General Practitioner has recently referred him to the local community team – intellectual disability (CTID). He lives at home with his parents, who worry about his future, as he has just finished school, and they are not sure what will happen to him. He is immobile, he expresses himself using nonverbal communication to express his needs, and he seemingly does not understand complex information. He depends on others to support him with all Activities of Daily living (ADL). He is at risk of chest and urine infections, and he continually develops pressure sores in the sacral area of his lower back. He needs a great deal of support to provide his basic care, and for others to understand what he is trying to communicate. Sometimes, for example, when he is upset or unhappy, he cries and bangs the back of his head against the back of his wheelchair. He is assessed as needing specialist equipment for positioning, and transfers, in maintaining posture. His parents report that he loves to get out and meet new people, who always seem to make him happy.

> ## Box 1.8
> ## Learning Activity 1.3
> Spend some time reflecting on the case history for Aarav. What do you think your role might be as his intellectual disability nurse? Consider, how you might support him to meet his needs and plans for the future? Structure your answer under two columns – one for direct support and the other for indirect support for Aarav and his family.

Temporally, intellectual disability nursing in the United Kingdom and Ireland is located within ongoing paradigm shifts in service ideologies. These ideologies have moved in recent years rapidly from an NHS (UK) dominated or congregated hospital provision (Ireland) of residential services for people with intellectual disabilities to a complex landscape of private, voluntary, and not-for-profit providers. In the United Kingdom, for example, this has resulted in nearly all NHS campuses being closed (Mair, 2009), bringing with it questions as to the need to continue commissioning a specialist intellectual disability nursing workforce. Regardless of this shift in service ideologies, some people with intellectual disabilities and their families will, arguably, always need to be supported by specialist health services, and a specialist intellectual disability nursing workforce. This is because the population of people with intellectual disabilities is increasing, owing to an increased overall life expectancy and survival into adulthood of young people with complex health needs (Parrott, Tilley and Wolstenholme, 2008).

There is now an irrefutable body of evidence showing that people with intellectual disabilities have a profile of health needs that differs from that of the health needs of the wider population (for example, Mencap, 2007, 2012; Michael, 2008; Heslop *et al.*, 2013). These needs often go unrecognised and unmet, and the health services that those with intellectual disabilities receive may not be appropriate. Intellectual disability nurses have an important role to play in addressing such deficits, and this has been articulated by the UK Chief Nursing Officers (2012).

However, intellectual disability nurse numbers have declined, and there is a need for urgent attention to workforce planning issues. Many have advocated this, because current evidence points to a potential crisis looming in the intellectual disability nursing workforce (Gates, 2011; Glover and Emerson, 2012). However, this may not yet be the case for Ireland (Gates *et al.*, 2020). In the UK this is now being addressed by the National Learning Disability Nurses' Forum. This asserts to be the '*go to*' place for the latest information about intellectual disability nursing. This forum serves as a communication resource which has been developed to support intellectual disability nurses (https://learningdis abilitynurse.co.uk/home).

Here, and as in Chapter 2, it will be shown that intellectual disability nursing has moved away from narrowly defined roles, within long-term institutionalised-based care, to much broader roles (Mafuba *et al.*, 2021). The intellectual disability nursing field spans diverse areas of practice such as community support

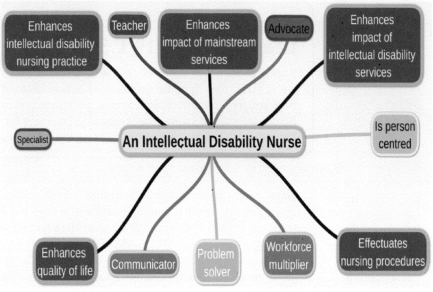

Figure 1.8

Modern-day practice of intellectual disability nursing.

specialists, liaison nurses between and within services and agencies, as well as secure or forensic health settings, and these roles offer support across the age continuum (Manthorpe, 2004). To further evidence this, more recently Mafuba *et al.* (2021) have found that intellectual disabilities nurses working within these environments undertake a complex sphere of practice. It was clear from their study that the range of interventions offered by intellectual disability nurses can adapt and engage in a wide range of roles, and that they will continue to need to be able to assimilate new and emerging roles in the future. And, as the Chief Nursing Officers have said:

> *We want to ensure that people with learning disabilities of all ages, today and tomorrow, will have access to the expert learning disabilities nursing they need, want and deserve.*

(U.K. Chief Nursing Officers, 2012, p. 4)

Conclusion

This chapter has portrayed the complexities inherent in our understanding of the nature of intellectual disabilities. Many textbooks refer to people with intellectual disabilities as a homogenous group. This is both simplistic and unhelpful, not only for people with intellectual disabilities, but also for their families and health and social professional carers.

This chapter has also examined the varying causes and manifestations of common conditions of learning disabilities. It has been demonstrated that changes in the genetic makeup of individuals result in the manifestation of specific syndromes, while environmental factors can also cause intellectual disabilities during the prenatal, perinatal, and postnatal periods. Diagnosing the cause of intellectual disabilities is important for families to allow them to adapt to, and value, their child for who he or she is, rather than for what he or she might have been. It is also important for health services, as it provides specific information about actual and potential needs of individuals, allowing the mobilisation of resources when needed. Caution, however, must be exercised, because providing diagnostic labels may reduce a approach of recognising the importance of individuality; a danger with labels is forgetting the importance of the person behind them.

As a health professional, you must ensure that you endeavour to see and value every person and their individual characteristics before any diagnosis, and to influence the approach others may adopt in the wider health and social care economies. This issue will be further developed in subsequent chapters. Reflect on the information in Figure 1.8, which depicts the complexities of the intellectual disability nurses' role in contemporary practice.

People with intellectual disabilities share a common humanity with us all. Most people desire love and a sense of connection with others to feel safe, to learn, to lead a meaningful life, to be free from ridicule and harm, and to be healthy and free from poverty. People with intellectual disabilities are no different in this respect. It is in this spirit of our collective and common humanity that this intellectual disability nursing text is presented. It is our aim that this text will, in some small part, assist intellectual disability nurses continue to make strong contributions in bringing about the inclusion of people with intellectual disabilities in their communities. It is for all intellectual disability nurses to ensure that either directly through their interventions, or indirectly through directing and leading other health and social care practitioners, that equitable healthcare and well-being is promoted to all people, regardless of their perceived differences.

Note

1   Throughout the twentieth and twenty-first centuries, terms used in the United Kingdom to describe people with intellectual disabilities have continued to change. At the beginning of the twentieth century, the term feeble-minded was in common use. Also commonly used were mentally defective, idiot, and imbecile, mental and severe mental subnormality, and then mental handicap and severe mental handicap.

References

Alaszewski, A., et al. (2001) *Diversity and change: The changing roles and education of learning disability nurses*. London: English National Board.

Aldridge, J. (2004) Intellectual disability nursing: A model for practice. In Turnbull, J. (Ed.), *Learning disability nursing*. Oxford: Blackwell Publishing.

American Association of Intellectual and Developmental Disability (2010) *Intellectual disability: Definition, classification, and systems of supports* (11th edition). Washington, DC: AAIDD.

Barr, O. and Sines, D. (1996) The development of the generalist nurse within preregistration nurse education in the UK: Some points for consideration. *Nurse Education Today*, 16(4), pp. 274–277.

British Psychological Society (2000) *Learning disability: Definitions and contexts*. www.bps.org.uk/system/files/documents/ppb_learning.pdf (Accessed 19 August 2014).

Burton, M. (1996) Intellectual disability: Developing a definition. *Journal of Learning Disabilities for Nursing, Health and Social Care*, 1(1), pp. 37–43.

Cox, P. (1996) Girls, deficiency and delinquency. In Wright, D. and Digby, A. (Eds.), *From idiocy to mental deficiency*. London: Routledge, pp. 184–206.

Defendi, G.L. (2018) Hurler syndrome, Hurler-Scheie syndrome, and Scheie syndrome (mucopolysaccharidosis type I). *Medscape*. Available at: https://emedicine.medscape.com/article/1599374-overview (Accessed 24 November 2022).

Dennis, W. (1973) *Children of the creche*. New York: Appleton Century – Crofts.

Department of Health (2001) *Valuing people: A new strategy for learning disability for the 21st century*. Cmnd 5086. London: The Stationery Office.

Doody, O.L., Slevin, E. and Taggart, L. (2012) Intellectual disability nursing: Identifying its development and future. *Journal of Intellectual Disabilities*, 16(1), pp. 7–16.

Emerson, E., *et al.* (2001) *Learning disabilities: The fundamental facts*. London: The Foundation for People with Learning Disabilities.

Emerson, E., *et al.* (2010) *People with learning disabilities in England 2010*. Lancaster: Improving Health and Lives, Learning Disabilities Observatory.

Gates, B. (2000) Knowing: The importance of diagnosing learning disabilities. *Journal of Intellectual Disabilities*, 4(1), pp. 5–6.

Gates, B. (2011) Envisioning a workforce for the 21st century. *Learning Disability Practice*, 14(1), pp. 12–18.

Gates, B. and Mafuba, K. (2016) Use of the term 'learning disabilities' in the United Kingdom: Issues for international researchers and practitioners. *Learning Disabilities: A Contemporary Journal*, 14(1), pp. 9–23.

Gates, B., *et al.* (2020) *Intellectual disability nursing: An oral history project*. Bingley: Emerald. ISBN: 9781839821554.

Gilbert, P. (2000) *A-Z of syndromes and inherited disorders* (3rd edition). Cheltenham: Stanley Thornes.

Glover, G. and Emerson, E. (2012) Patterns of decline in numbers of learning disability nurses employed by the English national health service. *Tizard Learning Disability Review*, 4(17), pp. 194–198.

Grandjean, P., *et al.* (2014) Neurotoxicity from prenatal and postnatal exposure to methylmercury. *Neurotoxicology and Teratology*, 43, pp. 39–44.

Heslop, P., *et al.* (2013) *Confidential Inquiry into premature deaths of people with learning disabilities, final report*. Bristol: Norah Fry Research Centre.

Inclusion Ireland (2013) *Intellectual disability causes and prevention: Your questions answered*. Available at: www.inclusionireland.ie/sites/default/files/documents/causesandpreventionbooklet.pdf (Accessed 19 August 2014).

Klotz, J. (2004) Sociocultural study of intellectual disability: Moving beyond labeling and social constructionist perspectives. *British Journal of Learning Disabilities*, 32(2), pp. 93–94.

Knight, S.J.L., Regan, R. and Nicod, A. (1999) Subtle chromosomal rearrangements in children with unexplained mental retardation. *The Lancet*, 345(9191), pp. 1676–1681.

Lejeune, J., *et al.* (1963) Trois casde délétion partielle du bras court d'un chromosome 5. *Comptes Rendus de l'Académie des Sciences (D)*, 257, pp. 3098–3102.

Liu, J. and Lewis, G. (2013) Environmental toxicity and poor cognitive outcomes in children and adults. *Journal of Environmental Health*, 76, pp. 130–138.

Mafuba, K., *et al.* (2021) *Understanding the contribution of intellectual disability nurses: A scoping review*. London: University of West London, RCN Foundation.

Mair, R. (2009) Trying to get it right with campus closure. *Learning Disability Today*, 9(6), pp. 10–11.

Manthorpe, J., *et al.* (2004) Learning disability nursing: A multi-method study of education and practice. *Learning in Health and Social Care*, 3(2), pp. 92–101.

Mencap (2007) *Death by indifference: Following up the Treat me right! Report*. London: Mencap.

Mencap (2012) *Death by indifference: 74 deaths and counting – a progress report 5 years on*. London: Mencap.

Mencap (2022) *What is a learning disability*. London: Mencap.

Mental deficiency act 1913. London: HMSO.

Mental health act 1959. London: HMSO.

Mental health act 1983. London: HMSO.

Michael, J. (2008) *Healthcare for all: Report of the independent inquiry into access to healthcare for people with learning disabilities*. London: HMSO.

Morris, J.K., *et al.* (2003) Comparison of models of maternal age-specific risk for down syndrome live births. *Prenatal Diagnosis*, 23(3), pp. 252–258.

Moulster, G., Ames, S., Lorizzo, J. and Kernohan, J. (2019) A flexible model to support person-centred learning disability nursing. *Nursing Times*, 115(6), pp. 56–59.

Mueller, R.F. and Young, D. (1998) *Emery's elements of medical genetics* (10th edition). Edinburgh: Churchill Livingstone.

National health service act 1946. London: HMSO.

Nursing and Midwifery Board of Ireland (2016) *Nurse registration programmes standards and requirements* (4th edition). Dublin: Nursing and Midwifery Board of Ireland.

Nursing and Midwifery Council (2018) *Future nurse: Standards of proficiency for registered nurses*. London: NMC.

Orem, D.E. (1991) *Nursing: Concepts of practice*. St Louis: Mosby.

Oxford English Dictionary (2013) Available at: http://oxforddictionaries.com/definition/english/eugenics?q=eugenics (Accessed 19 August 2014).

Parrott, R., Tilley, N. and Wolstenholme, J. (2008) Changes in demography and demand for services from people with complex needs and profound and multiple learning disabilities. *Tizard Learning Disability Review*, 13(3), pp. 26–34.

Rittey, C.D. (2003) Learning difficulties: What the neurologist needs to know. *Journal of Neurological Neurosurgery Psychiatry*, 74, pp. 130–136.

Roper, N., Logan, W. and Tierney, A. (2002) *The elements of nursing* (4th edition). Edinburgh: Churchill Livingstone.

Royal College of Nursing (2011) *Learning from the past – setting out the future: Developing learning disability nursing in the United Kingdom*. London: RCN.

Royal Commission on the Care and Control of the Feeble-Minded (1904–1908). *The Radnor report*. Cmnd 4202. London: HMSO.

Thomson, M. (1996) Family, community, and state: The micro-politics of mental deficiency. In Wright, D. and Digby, A. (Eds.), *From idiocy to mental deficiency*. London: Routledge, pp. 207–230.

U.K. Chief Nursing Officers (2012) *Strengthening the commitment: The report of the UK*. Edinburgh: Scottish Government.

Weinberg, R.A. (1989) Intelligence and IQ: Landmark issues and great debates. *American Psychologist*, 44(2), pp. 98–104.

Wiedemann, H.R., Kunze, J. and Dibbern, H. (1992) *An atlas of clinical syndromes: A visual aid to diagnosis* (2nd edition). London: Mosby-Wolfe.

World Health Organisation (1992) *ICD-10 classification of mental and behavioral disorders. Clinical descriptions and diagnostic guidelines.* Geneva: World Health Organisation.

World Health Organisation (2010) *Better health, better lives: Children and young people with intellectual disabilities and their families. European declaration on the health of children and young people with intellectual disabilities and their families.* Bucharest: World Health Organisation.

Further Reading

American Psychiatric Association (2022) *Diagnostic and statistical manual of mental disorders, DSM-5-TR.* Arlington, VA: American Psychiatric Association.

Atherton, H. and Crickmore, D. (Eds.). (2022) *Intellectual disabilities: Toward inclusion* (7th edition). Edinburgh: Elsevier.

Brown, M., Higgins, A. and MacArthur, J. (2020) Transition from child to adult health services: A qualitative study of the views and experiences of families of young adults with intellectual disabilities. *Journal of Clinical Nursing*, 29(1–2), pp. 195–207.

Bruce, A.W. and Wilmhurst, L. (2016) *Essentials of intellectual disability assessment and identification.* Hoboken, NJ: Wiley & Sons.

CIPOLD (2013) *Confidential inquiry into premature deaths of people with learning disabilities (CIPOLD).* Bristol: University of Bristol. Available at: www.bristol.ac.uk/cipold/confidential-inquiry/ (Accessed 2 August 2022).

Harris, J.C. (2006) *Intellectual disability: Understanding its development, cause, classification, evaluation and treatment.* Oxford: Oxford University Press.

Health Education England (2015) *Generic service interventions pathway: A competency framework to support development of the learning disability workforce.* Available at: www.basw.co.uk/resources/generic-service-interventions-pathway.

MacArthur, J., *et al.* (2015) Making reasonable and achievable adjustments: The contributions of learning disability liaison nurses in 'getting it right' for people with learning disabilities receiving general hospitals care. *Journal of Advanced Nursing*, 71(7), pp. 1552–1563.

Matson, J.L. (Ed.). (2019) *Handbook of intellectual disabilities – integrating theory, research, and practice.* Baton Rouge, LA: Springer.

Public Health England (2016) *Learning disabilities observatory: People with learning disabilities in England 2015.* Available at: www.gov.uk/government/publications/people-with-learning-disabilities-in-england-2015 (Accessed 2 August 2022).

Public Health England (2018) *Learning disabilities: Applying all our health.* Available at: www.gov.uk/government/publications/learning-disability-applying-all-our-health/learning-disabilities-applying-all-our-health (Accessed 2 August 2022).

University of Bristol (2021) *The learning disabilities mortality review programme (LeDeR) annual report.* Available at: www.bristol.ac.uk/sps/news/2021/leder-annual-report-2020.html (Accessed 2 August 2022).

Useful Resources

BILD: www.bild.org.uk/
Contact a Family: https://contact.org.uk/?s=home+page
Enable Scotland: www.enable.org.uk/Pages/Enable_Home.aspx

Foundation for People with Learning Disabilities: www.learningdisabilities. org.uk/
Inclusion Ireland: www.inclusionireland.ie/
Intellectual Disability Info Web Pages: www.intellectualdisability.info/
Intellectual Disability Nursing: https://learningdisabilitynurse.co.uk/home
Mencap: www.mencap.org.uk/
Mencap Northern Ireland: www.mencap.org.uk/northern-ireland
Mencap Wales: www.mencap.org.uk/wales

Policy

England: Department of Health (2009) *Valuing people now: A new three-year strategy for people with learning disabilities.* https://assets.publishing.service.gov. uk/government/uploads/system/uploads/attachment_data/file/215891/ dh_122387.pdf (Accessed 28 June 2022).
Department of Health and Social Care (2019) *Core capabilities framework for supporting autistic people.* www.skillsforhealth.org.uk/info-hub/learning-dis ability-and-autism-frameworks-2019/ (Accessed 28 June 2022).
Northern Ireland: Department of Health and Social Security (2005) *Equal lives: Review of policy and services for people with a learning disability in Northern Ireland.* www.health-ni.gov.uk/publications/bamford-published-reports (Accessed 28 June 2022).
Republic of Ireland: Health Service Executive (2011) *Time to move on from congregated settings – a strategy for community inclusion.* www.hse.ie/eng/services/list/4/ disability/congregatedsettings/timetomoveon.html (Accessed 28 June 2022).
Scotland: Scottish Government (2021) *Learning/intellectual disability and autism: Transformation plan.* www.gov.scot/publications/learning-intellectual-disabil ity-autism-towards-transformation/ (Accessed 28 June 2022).
Wales: Welsh Government (2014) *Transforming learning disability services in Wales.* https://socialcare.wales/cms_assets/file-uploads/21-Transforming-Learning-Disability-Services-in-Wales.pdf (Accessed 28 June 2022).

CHAPTER 2

Louise Cogher, Ruth Ryan and Eileen Carey

History and modern-day practice of intellectual disability nursing

Introduction

In this chapter, nursing students will explore the nature of intellectual disabilities and their relationship to intellectual disability nursing. The content of this chapter is contextualised within the Nursing and Midwifery Council (NMC) of the United Kingdom (NMC, 2018) and Nursing and Midwifery Board of Ireland (NMBI) (NMBI, 2016) standards and requirements for competence.

Intellectual disability nursing has a long and complex history and a tradition of supporting people with learning disabilities and their families. This chapter addresses the history of intellectual disability nursing, and its relationship with changing health and social policy from the 1930s to the present-day. Whilst advancements in quality, safe nursing care and service provision have contributed to enhancing the lives of people with learning disabilities, there have been instances of abuse and poor practice highlighting individual and system failures. Learning from review and analysis of these *'poor episodes of care'* has contributed to the professions' development and furthering the commitment to ensure high standards of care delivery and professional education.

This chapter demonstrates how intellectual disability nursing has evolved from a narrowly defined role in long-term care, to a broader more integrated role within health and social care services and beyond (Gates *et al.*, 2020). Modern-day intellectual disability nursing spans 'generic', 'liaison', and 'specialist' roles across health and social care services. This text is primarily aimed at undergraduate nursing students emphasising UK and Republic of Ireland health, social and community living policies shaping and framing the development of the profession.

There is a known and acknowledged history of inequity in mainstream health services for people with intellectual disabilities, and this is not acceptable (Disability Rights Commission, 2006; Mencap, 2007, 2012; Michael Report, 2008; Parliamentary and Health Ombudsmen, 2009). Further, it is internationally recognised that compared to the wider population, people with intellectual disabilities have more health and social care needs requiring additional support (Burd *et al.*, 2019). Provision of support in generalist mainstream and specialist services require many adjustments to achieve optimum health and social care entitlements. Adjustments come in many forms inclusive of universal design, alternative and augmentative communication and input from specialised services. There remains a crucial role for intellectual disability nurses to assist in meeting health and social care needs ensuring equality and a rights-based approach to enhancing the lives of people with intellectual disabilities across the lifespan. References will be made to the Nursing and Midwifery Council (NMC, 2018) and Nursing and Midwifery Board of Ireland (NMBI, 2016) standards and requirements for competence.

DOI: 10.4324/9781003296461-2

Box 2.1 This chapter will focus on the following:

- Describes intellectual disability nursing
- Outlines the origins and history of intellectual disability nursing
- Identifies health and social care policies that have enhanced intellectual disability nursing practice
- Reviews current educational standards and requirements for the profession
- Describes generic, liaison and specialist intellectual disability nursing roles
- Recognises opportunities for developing future roles to enhance safe practice and quality service delivery

Box 2.2 Competences

Nursing and Midwifery Council (2018) Proficiencies

Platform 1: Being an accountable professional – 1.9, 1.14

Platform 2: Promoting health and preventing ill health – 2.1, 2.2, 2.3, 2.4, 2.5, 2.6, 2.7, 2.10, 2.11, 2.12

Platform 3: Assessing needs and planning care – 3.6, 3.15

Platform 5: Leading and managing nursing care and working in teams – 5.12

Platform 7: Coordinating care – 7.1, 7.2, 7.3, 7.4

Nursing and Midwifery Board of Ireland (2016) Competences

Domain 1: Professional values and conduct of the nurse competences – 1.3

Domain 2: Nursing practice and clinical decision-making competences – 2.2, 2.4

Domain 3: Knowledge and cognitive competences – 3.1

Domain 6: Leadership potential and professional scholarship competences – 6.2

What is intellectual disability nursing

Intellectual disability nursing is defined as:

> *a person-centered profession with the primary aim of supporting the well-being and social inclusion of people with learning disabilities through improving or maintaining physical and mental health.*

(DH, 2007, p. 10)

Registered intellectual disability nurses provide safe and competent care from birth throughout the lifespan. This discipline of nursing offers a range of supports across the dependence to independence continuum from minimal supports through to intensive continuous nursing interventions tailored to meet individual needs within a range of settings. Describing the action of the profession, the NHS state how intellectual disability nurses provide healthcare and support to people with intellectual disabilities, as well as their families and staff teams, to help them live a fulfilling life (NHS, 2022). As a group whose educational and experiential preparation is solely focused on people with intellectual disabilities these nurses develop the knowledge, skills, attitudes, and professionalism to deliver safe, high quality, compassionate, ethical, legal and accountable practice to the individual with a learning disability across the life span and in a variety of settings (McCarron, 2018).

Intellectual disability nurses organise care and plans of care through a structured approach using the 'nursing process' of Assessment, Diagnosis, Planning, Implementation and Evaluation (further discussed in Chapter 6). Core elements of the *'nurse – person relationship'* in this discipline of nursing are therapeutic relationships, effective communication and supporting autonomy. Plans of care are written by learning and intellectual disability nurses framed within a bio-psychosocial perspective of health and well-being and centred on the person's wishes, preferences, and choices (further discussed in Chapter 6).

A guiding philosophy of intellectual nursing practice is that persons with all levels of ability have the same rights and, in so far as possible, the same responsibilities as other members of society. People with intellectual disabilities have a right to live within their community and receive services necessary to meet their needs. Intellectual disability nurses therefore have a diversity of roles and play an important part of the healthcare workforce operating in rapidly changing health and social care environments. Policies and standards within the UK (DH, DHSSPS, Welsh Government and the Scottish Government, 2012), the Republic of Ireland (McCarron, 2018) the Nursing and Midwifery Council (NMC, 2018 and the NMBI (2016) outline a vision of intellectual disability nursing within several frameworks inclusive of generalist, liaison and specialist nursing roles and practices (see Figure 2.1 and Box 2.1).

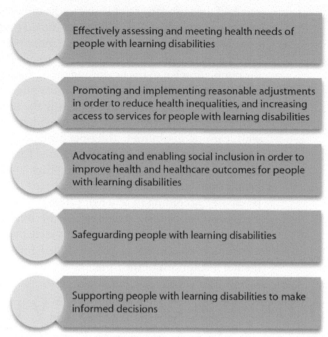

Figure 2.1 *Source:* From Strengthening the Commitment: The Report of the UK Modernising Learning Disability Nursing Review (The Scottish Government, 2012)

Key roles of intellectual disability nurses.

Box 2.3
Learning Activity 2.1

The role of learning and intellectual disability nurses

Having described intellectual disability nursing consider the following:

1. *Reflect on your knowledge and experience of intellectual disability nursing.*
2. *Identify the skills, attributes, and practices of the intellectual disability nurse.*

Origins of learning disability nursing in the United Kingdom

The introduction of asylums in the early part of the nineteenth century to accommodate the *'feeble-minded, imbeciles, or idiots'* with lifelong institutional care laid the foundations of learning disability nursing as we know it today. The purpose of this institutional care was aimed primarily at preventing sexual relations that were presumed to produce more people with mental deficiency. The fear that these people, deemed to be mentally deficient, would *'infect'* the rest of the population led to the beginning of the eugenics movement in the 1860s. The eugenics movement came to an end only after World War II, during which Nazi Germany used eugenics theory to justify the horrors of the Holocaust.

The Mental Deficiency Act 1913 provided a distinct legal identity for people with learning disabilities. The operational segregation of service provision for people with learning disabilities provided for in the Act has had a long and lasting effect on the provision of nursing care. Under the Act, service provision for people with learning disabilities was based in large asylums under the remit of psychiatry. According to Mitchell (2004), before the introduction of the Mental Deficiency Act of 1913, training for the nurses working in mental deficiency institutions was developed and provided by the Royal Medico-Psychological Association. This training was designed for the nurses who were working in mental institutions of the time.

From 'mental deficiency nursing' to 'mental handicap' nursing in the United Kingdom

The legal identity of people with *'mental deficiency'* (people with intellectual disabilities, as they were known then) introduced by the Mental Deficiency Act 1913 resulted in the development of a distinct qualification for mental deficiency nurses (as intellectual disability nurses were then known) by the Royal Medico-Psychological Association. According to Mitchell (2004), there were four distinct training courses for intellectual disability nurses (bedside nursing, occupational therapy, crafts training, and industrial therapy) designed to meet the individual needs of institutions. Following the Nurses Registration Act of 1919, the General Nursing Council created a separate Mental Nurses Supplementary Register for intellectual disability nurses. However, like mental health nurses, most intellectual disability nurses continued to register with the Royal Medico-Psychological Association rather than the General Nursing Council (GNC) until after World War II. According to Dingwall, Rafferty and Webster (1988), this was because the Royal Medico-Psychological Association examination was cheaper. In addition, medical superintendents supported the Royal Medico-Psychological Association examination. The inception of the National Health Service (NHS) in 1948 incorporated most intellectual disability institutions, and their training into the NHS (Gates *et al.*, 2020). In the early 1950s the GNC took over training for nurses working in the NHS, and that included the training of mental health nurses and learning disability nurses. The incorporation of both mental health institutions and intellectual disability institutions contributed to the medicalisation of both mental health nursing and intellectual disability nursing professions. Despite this, literature demonstrates that there was a long history of debate as to whether intellectual disability nurses should be called nurses at all (Herringham, 1926; General Nursing Council, 1926; Gates *et al.*, 2020).

The debate concerning the positionality of intellectual disability nursing within the nursing regulatory framework has existed since the Nurses Registration Act 1919 (Gates *et al.*, 2020). In the 1970s two reports were published suggesting that 'mental handicap nurses', as intellectual disability nurses were then known, should not be part of the nursing profession (Briggs, 1972; Jay, 1979). The Briggs Report (Briggs, 1972) recommended that a new profession needed to evolve and replace 'mental handicap' nursing.

To appear in the press in 1967 were serious allegations made by a nursing assistant of abuse and cruelty at the Ely Hospital in Cardiff, a unit for people with intellectual disabilities. The Howe Report (1969) confirmed longstanding abusive treatment of people with intellectual disabilities. The revelations about this scandal, and others reported in the 1960s and 1970s, presented a publicity problem for the whole nursing profession, but particularly so for intellectual disability nursing (Gates *et al.*, 2020). These scandals and discredited institutions raised further questions about the appropriateness of intellectual disability nursing being part of the wider nursing profession.

In the following decade, a long debate as to the future of mental handicap nursing did not result in a new profession, as recommended in the Briggs Report. Barbara Castle in her capacity as Secretary of State for Health in 1975 set up The Jay Committee (Jay, 1979) to review mental handicap nursing and the care these nurses provided. The Jay Report (Jay, 1979) was published just before the 1979 general election that brought Margaret Thatcher's conservative government into power. The key recommendation of the Jay Report (Jay, 1979) was that a social care profession should replace mental handicap nursing. This recommendation was rejected by the then government, which proposed joint training by the GNC and the Central Council for the Education and Training of Social Work (CCETSW) for staff working in mental handicap services (DOHSS, 1980). Whilst mental handicap nurses' roles involved working with people who were not generally physically and mentally ill, such nurses' pre-registration training was based on a medical model of sickness and intellectual disabilities (Gates *et al.*, 2020).

From mental handicap nursing to intellectual disability nursing

In 1991 Stephen Dorrell, then Health Minister, announced in the House of Commons that the term *'mentally handicapped'* would be changed to *'people with a learning disability'*. However, the United Kingdom Central Council for Nursing, Midwifery and Health Visiting (UKCC) (predecessor to the NMC) was reluctant to change the nursing qualification title to *'registered nurse for people with a learning disability'* from *'registered nurse for the mentally handicapped'* (UKCC, 1997).

Research published in the mid to late 1990s on empowerment (Sines, 1995), advocacy (Holmes, 1995), human rights issues (Carr, 1995), access to healthcare and discriminatory processes, which served to exclude individuals from receiving services on the basis of their learning disability (Bollard, 1999), and stigmatisation of people with intellectual disabilities in general hospitals (Shanley and Guest, 1995; Slevin, 1995) raised fundamental questions about the philosophical basis and values of the care of people with intellectual disabilities. Clifton, Shaw and Brown (1992) concluded that the combination of the specific and unique knowledge of the needs of people with intellectual disabilities and their nursing skills was unique to the profession. This conclusion was consistent with the observation made by Raynes *et al.* (1994), who noted a *'quality effect'* of intellectual disability nurses. Moreover, Moulster and Turnbull (2004) challenged this focus on the uniqueness of the knowledge of intellectual disability nurses, arguing that the focus on knowledge was more positivist and ignored the intuitiveness of intellectual disability nursing. A study by Turnbull (2005) noted that the uniqueness of intellectual disability nurses was inherent in their relationships with people with intellectual disabilities, which resulted in a demand for intellectual disability nurses in a wide range of services.

Whilst the academic discourse focused on the place of people with intellectual disabilities in mainstream society, and the uniqueness of the knowledge of intellectual disability nurses, the government was undecided and questioned the future role of intellectual disability nurses in the nursing profession. The publication of *Signposts for Success* (DH, 1995a) detailed the extent and complexity of the health and social care needs of people with intellectual disabilities, led to a change in the government's position. The publication of *Continuing the Commitment* (DH, 1995b) emphasised a strong future role for intellectual disability nursing.

Professional requirements of intellectual disability nurses

Educated intellectual disability nurses are essential to the delivery of high-quality health and social care for people with learning disabilities (Gates, 2011a). The changing demographics of the population with learning disabilities over the decades is multifactorial. It includes better individual health, improved living conditions, increasing longevity, increased prevalence, and recognition of specific conditions with intellectual disabilities across the lifespan through more effective assessment and timely diagnoses planning and implementation of healthcare. To achieve better outcomes for people with intellectual disabilities, intellectual disability nurses need to have the knowledge and skills to work in partnership with other nurses and a wide range of other health and social care professional. The NMC (2018) and NMBI (2016) standards require nursing graduates to be able to deliver essential support to those in their care, including people with intellectual disabilities. This emphasis places an onus on nurse education institutions to ensure that the care of people with intellectual disabilities is a key component of nurse education in the United Kingdom and in the Republic of Ireland. People with intellectual disabilities receive health and social care from a wide range of professionals and agencies. This requires inter-professional and inter-agency collaboration. An important requirement of the new pre-registration nursing education is that all nursing graduates are competent in meeting the needs of vulnerable groups, including people with intellectual disabilities, irrespective of the field of nursing practice. All registered nurses should deliver safe, effective, and compassionate immediate care for people with intellectual disabilities, where necessary, before referring them to specialist services (NMBI, 2016; NMC, 2018). Indeed, it has been mandated by the UK Government that all health and social care staff will have to undertake training in awareness and understanding of people with an intellectual disability and or autism or both (Department of Health and Social Care, 2019).

History of intellectual disability nursing in Ireland

Service provision for people with intellectual disabilities in the Republic of Ireland evolved differently from that in the United Kingdom (Robbins, 2000; Gates *et al.*, 2020). At the time of the Mental Deficiency Act 1913, the present-day Irish Republic was part of the United Kingdom. However, the Mental Deficiency Act 1913 was implemented only in England, Scotland, and Wales. In the Republic of Ireland, following the war of independence, (1919–1921) and the subsequent civil war (1922–1923), economic difficulties forced the new Irish government to rely on charitable and religious orders, county homes, and mental asylums for the provision of care for people deemed to be *'mentally deficient'* among many other poor groups of people.

Present day services in the Republic of Ireland are now delivered by the Health Service Executive (HSE) and non-statutory organisations, having developed independently and in response to local needs resulting in a wide variety of services available to disabled people throughout the country (HSE, 2022). Accounts of the development of Irish services for people with an intellectual disability and of the people who cared for them are scarce (Sweeney, 2010). Most notably, it is in the last 20 years academics and regulators have started to record this history of intellectual disability nursing development in the Republic of Ireland to articulate the philosophical underpinnings that brought about such a unique discipline of nursing (Gates *et al.*, 2020; Sweeney, 2010; Sweeney and Mitchell, 2009) and identify the focus and contribution of the role (Doody, Slevin and Taggart, 2012). A summary of these developments is presented in the following Figure 2.2.

The 1920s saw the Irish government entered into 'informal relationships' with several Catholic religious orders, whereby they were authorised and provided with funding through capitation to deliver discrete aspects of health, social care, and education on behalf of the state. Sweeney and Mitchell (2009) demonstrate the close links yet independence of both intellectual disability nursing in their *'historical review of intellectual disability nursing in the UK and Ireland'*. Both authors studied the history of the professions to attest the historical challenges of the discipline and help *'make sense of the location of their work in*

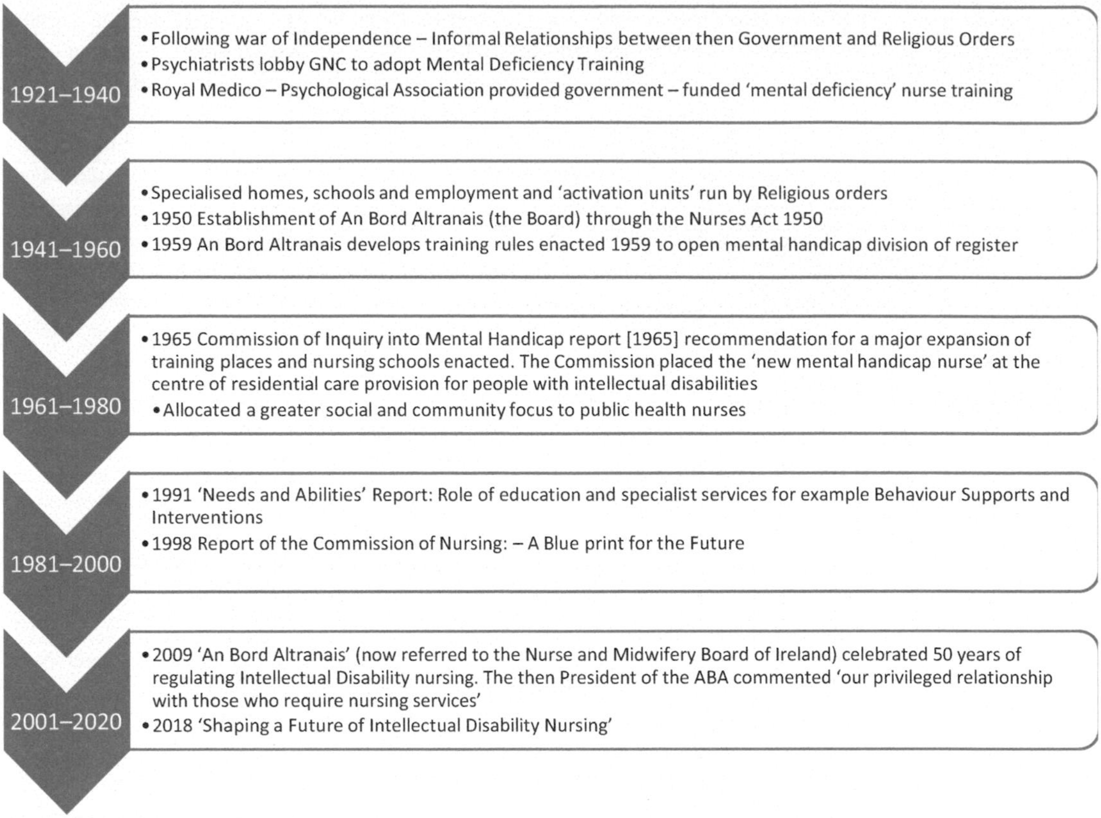

1921–1940	• Following war of Independence – Informal Relationships between then Government and Religious Orders • Psychiatrists lobby GNC to adopt Mental Deficiency Training • Royal Medico – Psychological Association provided government – funded 'mental deficiency' nurse training
1941–1960	• Specialised homes, schools and employment and 'activation units' run by Religious orders • 1950 Establishment of An Bord Altranais (the Board) through the Nurses Act 1950 • 1959 An Bord Altranais develops training rules enacted 1959 to open mental handicap division of register
1961–1980	• 1965 Commission of Inquiry into Mental Handicap report [1965] recommendation for a major expansion of training places and nursing schools enacted. The Commission placed the 'new mental handicap nurse' at the centre of residential care provision for people with intellectual disabilities • Allocated a greater social and community focus to public health nurses
1981–2000	• 1991 'Needs and Abilities' Report: Role of education and specialist services for example Behaviour Supports and Interventions • 1998 Report of the Commission of Nursing: – A Blue print for the Future
2001–2020	• 2009 'An Bord Altranais' (now referred to the Nurse and Midwifery Board of Ireland) celebrated 50 years of regulating Intellectual Disability nursing. The then President of the ABA commented 'our privileged relationship with those who require nursing services' • 2018 'Shaping a Future of Intellectual Disability Nursing'

Figure 2.2

Brief history of intellectual disability nursing development in the Republic of Ireland.

the nursing profession' contributing greatly to aiding future generations of intellectual disability nurses to understand and situate the contemporary role of the discipline of nursing. A feature of their paper outlines the early role of psychiatry and psychiatric provision in the development of intellectual disability nursing in the Republic of Ireland identifying from the 1920s how it was psychiatric nurses *'without any additional training'* who provided care for 'mental defectives' confined to 'back wards' in the district asylums under the direction of the medical superintendents, noting how psychiatrists played a key role in lobbying the first General Nursing Council to adopt *'Proficiency in the Nursing of Mental Defectives'* in the early 1920s (Sweeney and Mitchell, 2009).

The 1930s saw Catholic religious orders develop and manage specialist residential homes and schools for people with intellectual disabilities. The Royal Medico-Psychological Association provided government-funded for *'mental deficiency'* nurse training. During this era, the support of the government for mental deficiency nurse training signaled a significant shift toward people with intellectual disabilities, which resulted in distinct and separate provision for people with intellectual disabilities from generalist healthcare and mainstream psychiatric care in the late 1940s.

The emergence of An Bord Altranais (ABA, the Board) through the Nurses Act 1950 replaced the function of the Central Midwives Board (CMB) and the General Nursing Council (GNC). This brought about a nursing and midwifery regulatory body with a remit of governing nursing and midwifery practice and education, including establishing standards and requirements for nurse education. Sweeney and Mitchell note 1959 as a pinnacle point in the training for the 'mental handicap' nursing in the Republic of Ireland. With the support and funding of the Department of Health, An Bord Altranais developed training rules that were enacted in January 1959 to open a mental handicap division of its professional register. The rules not only provided for the training of new nurses, but also regularised the position of existing nurses trained under earlier schemes, allowed for reciprocal recognition of nurses trained overseas and established a post registration route for nurses qualified on other divisions of the register (Sweeney and Mitchell, 2009). ABA-registered mental handicap nurse education commenced in 1959 at two schools, Daughters of Charity at St Joseph's Clonsilla, Dublin and Brothers of Charity at St John of God Drumcar, County Louth (Gates *et al.*, 2020). The initial nursing approach was largely reflective of a custodial policy, namely congregated institutional settings (Doody, Slevin and Taggart, 2012).

The National Association for the Mentally Handicapped of Ireland (NAMHI, 1962) in Ireland were the main social and political drivers advocating for a move from a medical congregated model of support to a more inclusive social model of care. Additionally, the Commission of Inquiry on Mental Handicap (DoH, 1965) report was published which was a culmination of four years' (1961–4) examination of existing facilities for the ascertainment and treatment of intellectual disability persons and made suggestions as to how these might be improved or augmented. The report guided the developments and maturation of services for many years ahead, making some specific suggestions about nurse training. Doody, Slevin and Taggart (2012) noted how national policies and commissioned papers in addition to the role of family supporters directed developments of the discipline beyond physical and medical attention to the broader and inclusive perspective recognising the role of normalisation theories, social considerations and the concept of citizenship and equal rights as fundamental principles underpinning care approaches.

The 1990s saw the publication of the 'Needs and Abilities: A policy for the Intellectually Disabled' report of the Review Group on Mental Handicap Services in July 1990 (Government of Ireland, 1991) shaping governance. This paper commissioned by the then Minister for Health Rory O Hanlon reviewed existing services that enabled governments to plan future services and support needs across the lifespan. This report strongly recommended the importance of a multi-disciplinary approach to support and the need for ongoing and specialist training and education to meet the varying and complex needs of the intellectually disabled group. The need for ongoing education in the discipline of nursing was further supported in the Commission of Nursing report (Mella, 1998), a seminal work *'Blueprint for the Future'*, that identified an increasing demand for and proliferation of post-registration education for the nursing profession. The Commission noted the absence of a clinical career pathway in nursing and midwifery and recommended that future guidance and direction in relation to the development of specialist nursing and midwifery posts and post-registration educational programmes be offered to nurses and midwives within the parameters of professional standards and scope of practice guidelines.

In 2009, 'An Bord Altranais' [now the Nurse and Midwifery Board of Ireland] celebrated 50 years of regulating Intellectual Disability nursing. The commemoration involved an academic seminar titled, *'Early origins of the Regulation of the Registered Nurse in Intellectual Disability in Ireland 1919–2009'* by Sweeney, who detailed the developments within Intellectual Disability Nursing over the past fifty years, with an emphasis of the regulatory impact on these developments. The origins of the Registered Mental Handicap Nurse (RMHN) qualification in Ireland were outlined. He reflected on the reasons for the establishment of training for RMHNs in 1959 and the drivers for change in regulation of the profession during its first 50 years. Sweeney's presentation was later published and further details how postcolonial development in the Republic of Ireland acknowledges the role played by the Catholic Church and religious orders in developing intellectual disability services (Sweeney, 2010). In acknowledging a debt of gratitude to the Catholic Church's application of faith, moral teaching, and social action to the care of people with intellectual disabilities, important areas of social reform around, for example, the rights of adults to be regarded as sexual beings, empowerment in awareness of sexual preference and identity, safe sexual practices, pregnancy and parenting skills, have been delayed by international comparison (Sweeney, 2010).

Considering so much change in the provision of services and rights of people with intellectual disabilities, a report looking at the future role of the registered nurse in intellectual disability was completed for the Office of the Nursing and Midwifery Services Directorate (ONMSD). The report, called *'Shaping the Future of Intellectual Disability Nursing in Ireland: Supporting people with an intellectual disability to live ordinary lives in ordinary places'* (2018), later referred to as *'Shaping the Future'*, now guides Intellectual Disability Nursing in Ireland and into the future. The report and its recommendations are framed under four themes:

1. Person-Centeredness and Person-Centered Planning.
2. Supporting individuals with an Intellectual Disability with their Health, Well-being and Social Care.
3. Developing Nursing Capacity, Capability and Professional Leadership.
4. Improving the Experience and Outcome for individuals with an Intellectual Disability.

The recommendations of the report *'Shaping the Future'* are being implemented by nationally representative working groups. Recent research by Doyle (2022) report on staff of experiences during their nursing careers (a total of 31 participants, 11 from the Republic of Ireland and 20 participants from England, UK; the length of service recorded was from 31 to 47 years). These researchers noted how for both jurisdictions the underlying culture has changed over the past 30–40 years with the closing of institutions and the move to more community-based services having a positive impact on the health and well-being of people's lives. Large groups of individuals with intellectual disabilities no longer live together. Services are now person-centered and oriented around supporting the individual's preferences and wishes. Importantly, the heavily top-down quasi-military structures that used to characterise services are gone.

No longer do Matrons and Chief Nursing Officers walk the corridors of institutions. Instead, quality is monitored by the Care Quality Commission in England and HIQA in Ireland and this change has impacted on how staff feel about their work and indeed the nature of the work that they do, which has become somewhat more bureaucratic (Doyle *et al.*, 2022).

Box 2.4
Learning Activity 2.2

Origins of learning and intellectual disability nursing

Consider the origins of intellectual disability nursing and reflect on one positive and one negative lasting effect on the provision of nursing care to people with intellectual disabilities.

Current services in the United Kingdom and the republic of Ireland

Health needs

With the closure of long-stay hospitals, large residential campuses and congregated settings, primary healthcare services are now the main health and social care provider for people with intellectual disabilities. All private, independent, and public services including primary and community services and secondary and tertiary healthcare are now obligated to ensure the rights of people with intellectual disabilities are met. The population of people with intellectual disabilities is over 1.5 million in the UK and Ireland (Office for National Statistics, 2020; Hourigan *et al.*, 2018).

People with intellectual disabilities are living longer, however, co-morbidities are more common in this group relative to the general population. Comorbidity refers to a second and or multiple conditions that exist alongside the primary condition (intellectual disabilities). Therefore, a person with intellectual disabilities has a greater chance of having a second or multiple conditions by virtue of having intellectual disabilities. Comorbidities are known to have a major negative impact on quality of life, increasing functional disability and increasing the risk for suboptimal care and psychosocial milieu challenges that accompany these comorbidities (Burd *et al.*, 2019). People with severe and profound intellectual disabilities most often have multiple comorbid disorders often requiring multiple care providers. These multiple and complex needs can exist or present along the lifespan and include for example conditions such as epilepsy, sensory and communication disorders, motor disorders, nutritional complications such as constipation and gastric reflux, and age-related conditions such as sensory decline, increased frailty, cognitive decline and dementia.

Therefore, people with intellectual disabilities see multiple providers, and challenges with appointments and continuity of care have been reported by family/carers as causing major difficulties. In addition, reports following poor episodes of care have been noted throughout the years such as the *Non statutory inquiry into the transfer of Mr Peter McKenna to Leas Cross Nursing Home* (Dignam, 2000), *Treat Me Right* (Mencap, 2004), *Death by Indifference* (Mencap, 2007), the *Michael Report* (2008), *Six Lives* (Parliamentary and Health Service Ombudsman, 2009), and *Death by Indifference: 74 and Counting* (Mencap, 2012), *Winterbourne View-Time for Change* (Bubb, 2014), *What matters most* (Report of the Áras Attracta Swinford Review Group) (Áras Attracta Swinford Review Group, 2016), *Independent Review into Thomas Oliver McGowan's LeDeR Process* Phase two (Ritchie, 2020). All these reports have consistently highlighted the vulnerability of people with intellectual disabilities when accessing primary and community care services, and reveal how these services need to improve significantly on the care and treatment of people with health issues and intellectual disabilities.

The specialised knowledge base of intellectual disability nurses places them as central in healthcare professionals to promote and ensure a rights-based approach to healthcare across the lifespan. Intellectual disability nurses must continue to develop skills essential for delivering appropriate healthcare to people with intellectual disabilities in a wide range of services providing generalist and highly specialised nursing care. Furthermore, changing population demographics along with developing expertise of registered intellectual disability nurse specialists, the nature and extent of services accessible to people with intellectual disabilities is continually evolving. Intellectual disability nurses play a significant role by developing and delivering appropriate education and training, not only for their own discipline of nursing but also in the education and training for families, multi-disciplinary team members and others that provide care and support to people with intellectual disabilities.

Policy

In the United Kingdom and the Republic of Ireland, health and social care services continue to undergo significant strategic, structural, and economic changes. Recently, there has been an increased focus on equality of service provision in addition to integration of hospital and community-based services. Furthermore, and particularly in England, there have been significant changes to how intellectual disability services are commissioned and delivered. Health Services are focusing on health outcomes to ensure services are meeting individual and public needs. Intellectual disability nurses and other healthcare professionals who work with people with intellectual disabilities need to adapt to these changes to meet the increasing complexity of the health and healthcare needs of people with intellectual disabilities (Table 2.1).

Service modernisation policies in the following table represent the strategies across the United Kingdom and the Republic of Ireland:

a.   Developing person-centred health services that promote choice, independence, social inclusion, and citizenship.

Year	Author	Country	Policy Driver
1998	Carrol Department of Health	Republic of Ireland	Report of the Commission on Nursing: a blueprint for the future
2000	Scottish Executive	Scotland	The Same as You? A review of services for people with learning disabilities
2001	Department of Health	England	Valuing People: A new strategy for learning disability for the 21st century – A White Paper
2002	Department of Health	England	Action for Health, Health Action Plans and Health Facilitation: Detailed good practice guidance on implementation for learning disability partnership boards
	Scottish Executive	Scotland	Promoting Health, Supporting Inclusion: The national review of the contribution of nurses and midwives to the care and support of people with learning disabilities
	National Assembly for Wales	Wales	Inclusion, Partnership, and Innovation
2003	Department of Health/ Department for Children, Schools, and Families	England	Together from the Start: Practical guidance for professionals working with disabled children (birth to third birthday) and their families
2004	NHS Health Scotland	Scotland	Health Needs Assessment Report: People with learning disabilities in Scotland
	Welsh Assembly Government	Wales	Learning Disability Strategy. Section 7: Guidance on service principles and service responses
	National Disability Authority	Republic of Ireland	National Disability Strategy
2005	Department of Health, Social Services and Public Safety	Northern Ireland	Equal Lives: Review of policy and services for people with a learning disability in Northern Ireland: The N. I. Bamford Review
	Department of Health, Social Services and Public Safety	Northern Ireland	A Healthier Future: A twenty-year vision for health and well-being in Northern Ireland 2005–2025
2006	Department of Health, Social Services and Public Safety	Northern Ireland	The Bamford Review of Mental Health and Learning Disability (NI): Forensic services
	NHS Quality Improvement Scotland	Scotland	Best Practice Statement: Promoting access to healthcare for people with learning disabilities
2007	Department of Health	England	Good Practice in Learning Disability Nursing
	Department of Health, Social Services and Public Safety	Northern Ireland	Complex Needs: The nursing response to children and young people with complex physical healthcare needs
	Scottish Government	Scotland	Equally Well: The report of the Ministerial Task Force on Health Inequalities
	Welsh Assembly Government	Wales	Statement on Policy and Practice for Adults with Learning Disabilities
2008	Department of Health	England	Healthcare for All: Report of the independent inquiry into access to healthcare for people with learning disabilities
	Scottish Government	Scotland	Better Health, Better Care: Action plan. What it means for you
	Scottish Government	Scotland	Achieving our Potential: A framework to tackle poverty and income inequality in Scotland

Table 2.1   Policy drivers of learning and intellectual disability nursing practice in the United Kingdom and the Republic of Ireland *(Continued)*

Year	Author	Country	Policy Driver
2009	Department of Health	England	Valuing People Now: A new three-year strategy for people with learning disabilities
	Department of Health	England	World Class Commissioning for the Health and Wellbeing of People with Learning Disabilities
	Department of Health	England	The Bradley Report: Lord Bradley's review of people with mental health problems or learning disabilities in the criminal justice system
	Department of Health/ Department for Children, Schools and Families	England	Healthy Lives, Brighter Futures. The strategy for children and young people's health
	Department of Health, Social Services and Public Safety	England	Delivering the Bamford Vision. The response of the Northern Ireland Executive to the Bamford Review of Mental Health and Learning Disability action plan (2009–2011)
	Department of Health, Social Services and Public Safety	England	Integrated Care Pathway for Children and Young People with Complex Physical Healthcare Needs
	Department of Health, Social Services and Public Safety	England	Autism Spectrum Disorder (ASD) Strategic Action Plan 2008/09–2010/11
	NHS Quality Improvement Scotland	Scotland	Tackling Indifference: Healthcare services for people with learning disabilities national overview
	Welsh Assembly Government	Wales	A Community Nursing Strategy for Wales
	Welsh Assembly Government	Wales	Post Registration Career Framework for Nurses in Wales
	Welsh Assembly Government	Wales	We Are on the Way. A policy agenda to transform the lives of disabled children and young people
	Roche et al.	Republic of Ireland	Report of the Reference Group on Multidisciplinary Services for Children aged 5 to 18 Years
2010	Department of Health	England	Raising Our Sights: Services for adults with profound intellectual and multiple disabilities. A report by Professor Jim Mansell
	Nursing and Midwifery Council	England	Standards for pre-registration nursing 2010
	Department of Health, Social Services and Public Safety	Northern Ireland	Living Matters, Dying Matters: A strategy for palliative and end of life care for adults in Northern Ireland
	Department of Health, Social Services and Public Safety	Northern Ireland	A Partnership for Care: Northern Ireland strategy for nursing and midwifery 2010–2015
	Guidelines and Audit Implementation Network	Northern Ireland	Guidelines: Caring for people with a learning disability in general hospital settings
	Scottish Government	Scotland	Getting it Right for Every Child
	Scottish Government	Scotland	The Healthcare Quality Strategy for NHS Scotland
	Scottish Government	Scotland	Towards an Autism Strategy for Scotland
	Welsh Assembly Government	Wales	Setting the Direction: Primary and community services strategic delivery programme

Table 2.1   *(Continued)*

Year	Author	Country	Policy Driver
	Health Service Executive	Republic of Ireland	The National Progressing Disability Services for Children and Young People Programme
2011	Gates, B. (b).	England	Learning Disability Nursing. Task and finish group: Report for the Professional and Advisory Board for Nursing and Midwifery
	Emerson, E., *et al.*	England	Health Inequalities & People with Learning Disabilities in the UK: 2011
	Department of Health, Social Services and Public Safety	Northern Ireland	Improving Dementia Services in Northern Ireland: A regional strategy
	Department of Health, Social Services and Public Safety	Northern Ireland	Learning Disability Service Framework. Consultation document
	Learning Disability Implementation Advisory Group and Welsh Assembly Government	Wales	Practice Guidance on Developing a Commissioning Strategy for People with Learning Disabilities
	Public Health Wales and Welsh Government	Wales	Good Practice Framework for People with Learning Disabilities Requiring Planned Secondary Care
	Welsh Government	Wales	Together for Health. A five-year vision for the NHS in Wales
	Health Service Executive	Ireland	Time to Move on from Congregated Settings – A Strategy for Community Inclusion
2012	DH, DHSSPS, Welsh Government and the Scottish Government	England	Strengthening the commitment: The report of the UK Modernising Learning Disability Nursing Review
	Health Information and Quality Assurance	Ireland	National Standards for Safer Better Healthcare
	Department of Health	Ireland	Value for Money and Policy Review of Disability Services in Ireland
2013	Heslop *et al.*, 2013	England	The Confidential Inquiry into premature deaths of people with a learning disability (CIPOLD)
2014	Department of Health	Ireland	Value for Money: Implementation Framework
2015	Health Service Executive	Ireland	Interim Standards for New Directions Services and Supports for Adults with Disabilities Report
	Dept., of Justice	Ireland	The Assisted Decision Making (Capacity) Act
2016	Health Service Executive	Ireland	National Policy on Access to Services for Children & Young People with Disability & Developmental Delay
2017	Dept. of Justice	Ireland	National Disability Inclusion Strategy
2018	McCarron *et al.*	Ireland	Shaping the Future of Intellectual Disability Nursing in Ireland
	ONMSD, Health Service Executive	Ireland	National Guideline for Nursing and Midwifery Quality Care Metrics Data Measurement in Intellectual Disability Services
	Health Service Executive	Ireland	New Directions A National Framework for Person Centred Planning in Services for Persons with a Disability
	President of Ireland	Ireland	Ratification of the UN Convention on the Rights of Persons with Disabilities

(Continued)

Year	Author	Country	Policy Driver
2019	Department of Health and Social Care	UK	'Right to be heard': The Government's response to the consultation on learning disability and autism training for health and care staff
2020	Inclusion Ireland	Ireland	Progressing Disability Services for Children and Young People Programme (PDS)
2021	NHS England and NHS Improvement	UK	Learning from lives and deaths – people with a learning disability and autistic people (LeDeR) policy

Table 2.1   *(Continued)*

b. Progressing integration of health and social care services.
c. Promoting community-based primary care services.
d. Ensuring access to health and healthcare services.
e. Developing Nursing Capacity, Capability and Professional Leadership.
f. Improving the Experience and Outcome for individuals with an Intellectual Disability.

Intellectual disability nursing roles

The primary focus of nurses working in intellectual disability nursing is supporting the person with learning disability and their families in reducing health inequalities and improving access through the promotion and implementation of reasonable adjustments in primary care, community services, secondary and tertiary healthcare, education, employment, criminal justice system, the homeless, retirement, and end of life and in social care settings (Northway *et al.*, 2017; McCarron *et al.*, 2018). Intellectual disability nurses focus on effectively identifying and meeting individually determined healthcare and support needs of people with intellectual disabilities across the lifespan (McCarron *et al.*, 2018). Additionally, in the UK many intellectual disability nurses currently work as part of intellectual disability mortality reviews (Beebee and Batey, 2021).

In exploring support provided by intellectual disability nurses to people with intellectual disabilities, some of which is provided across all lifespan stages, and some at specific periods, Northway *et al.* (2017) highlight the range of interventions and supports for delivering on individualised needs and personalised outcomes facilitated in a timely manner that ensures the rights of people with learning disabilities to access healthcare. Roles undertaken by intellectual disability nurses focus on effectively identifying and meeting the health needs of people with intellectual disabilities, reducing health inequalities, and improving access through the promotion and implementation of reasonable adjustments in primary, community, secondary and tertiary healthcare, and education settings, promoting improved health outcomes (Mafuba *et al.*, 2021). In fulfilling their roles in the current demographic and policy contexts intellectual disability nurses need to be aware of the broader nursing roles (see Figure 2.3).

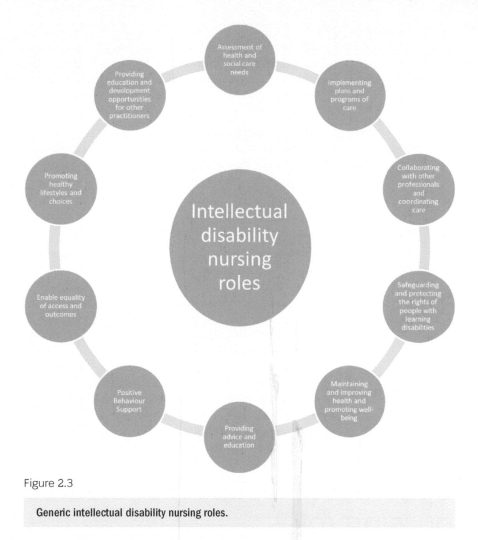

Figure 2.3

Generic intellectual disability nursing roles.

Box 2.5
Learning Activity 2.3

The role of the intellectual disability nurse in assessing the needs of people with profound and multiple disabilities

Background to care and support

Mandy is a 26-year-old lady residing at home with her mother. Mandy has a profound learning disability. Mandy's comorbid conditions include cerebral palsy, epilepsy, type-2 diabetes, and dysphagia. Mandy's support workers have recorded Mandy's weight monthly and have noted a decrease of weight over the past three months, in addition to Mandys clothes becoming too big. Mandy's seizures as reported in her care plan have increased in frequency and duration, and she has had two episodes of hypoglycemia in the fast six weeks. Mandy's care plan states that there has been no bowel motion for the past four days, with a normal pattern being every second day.

With the help of the intellectual disability nurse, Mandy has an established care plan to record the bio-psychosocial activities and help monitor Mandy's care with support workers. The care plan is written up each day, in the morning and afternoon. Identify and explore how the intellectual disability nurse applies the nursing process in Mandy's care.

Intellectual disability nurses work alongside primary, secondary, and tertiary health and social care professionals to support reasonable adjustments to the care package, nursing approach and delivery. Nurses educated in this nursing discipline are equipped with the skills to provide a consistent overview of the individual's communication needs and act as a conduit for care, as well as being a manager of care. Intellectual disability nurses have a significant role to play in developing and delivering appropriate education and training of other nurses and healthcare professionals. Intellectual disability nurses are increasingly assimilating new roles, such as health facilitator and acute health liaison roles (Mafuba *et al.*, 2021). Further key responsibilities of the role are supporting the implementation of the Mental Capacity Act 2005 and the Assisted Decision Making (Capacity) Act 2015 while integrating appropriate person-centred interactive processes (Carey and Ryan, 2019) along with associated advocacy frameworks and strategies.

Specialist intellectual disability nursing roles

Changes in UK and Irish healthcare policy and service provision embedded in health promotion, disease prevention and community integration aim to ensure the rights of people with intellectual disabilities in the United Kingdom and in the Republic of Ireland to access healthcare appropriate to their needs. Parallel with these changes has been the advancement of nurse education and training and subsequent career pathways for intellectual disability nursing roles. Intellectual disability nursing roles are increasingly focused on specialist practice and liaising with interdisciplinary and inter-agency activities in the wider community (Gates, 2011b; Mafuba *et al.*, 2021).

There is a clear difference between practising within a specialty, such as intellectual disability nursing, and holding qualification of specialist practitioner (NMC, 2022; NMBI, 2019). Determined by their qualifications and levels of expertise intellectual disability nurses now work in various clinical roles with associated differing levels of responsibility and autonomy providing support to the person with intellectual disabilities and their families. The concepts of advance practice and nurse specialist were first referred to in the American Journal of Nursing and declared within the remit of three areas: surgical, paediatric, and obstetrical nursing (DeWitt, 1900). Intellectual disability nurses educated to master's level can practice at specialist or advanced practice roles. Following periods of experiential learning, continuing professional development and post-graduate education intellectual disability nurses who gain the necessary experience and competence are suitable to engage in nursing roles with the authority to provide expert specialist services and support to people with intellectual disabilities and their families.

Terms used to describe these roles are Specialist Liaison, Clinical Nurse Specialist (CNS) and Advanced Nurse Practitioner/Nurse Practitioner (ANP/NP)/ Nurse Consultant. These are nursing roles that advance practice and McCarron *et al.* (2018) *Shaping the Future*, an example is outlined in the report envisioning a contemporary intellectual disabilities nursing practice from generalist, liaison to specialist practice levels (Figure 2.4 McCarron *et al.*, 2018).

McCarron *et al.* (2018) have acknowledged that the exemplars provided in Figure 2.5 are not exhaustive, as the role of the intellectual disability nurse will continually develop to changing needs of people with intellectual disabilities as they transition across lifespan stages, accessing different types and levels of supports at different times in their lives.

Where CNSs are expert clinicians with a focus on clinical excellence in a specialist area of practice and ANPs have a greater involvement in care activities such as diagnosis, prescription, and the treatment of conditions (Doody *et al.*, 2022), both are accountable to an advanced level and practice autonomously.

Nurse Consultants specialise in specific fields of practice, each consultant role is different. Nurse Consultants are also responsible for developing personal practice, are involved in research and evaluation, and contribute to education, training, and development. For example, many areas across the UK have developed intensive support teams as part of their community services for people with learning disabilities and learning and intellectual disability nurses (with master's level training – for example, in applied behaviour analysis/positive behaviour support) work either as consultants or team leaders (Beebee and Batey, 2021). For example, neurology departments have recruited learning disability nurses and provided training to support them to become sapphire nurses, enabling them to work as epilepsy nurse specialists in clinics that commonly see people with learning disabilities (Beebee and Batey, 2021).

In Ireland while still in its infancy stage roles are emerging such as Clinical Nurse Specialist (CNS) and Registered Advanced Nurse Practitioner (RANP). Research demonstrates the emergence of intellectual disability CNS/RANP nursing roles in areas of early intervention (infants), behaviour support (adults), and dementia (older adults), however, when matched to population need availability of these roles are limited (Carey *et al.*, 2022). Doody *et al.* (2022), identifying an absence of evidence-based literature on the roles of Advanced Nurse Practitioners in supporting people with intellectual disabilities, concluded that specialist nurses training in intellectual disabilities make meaningful contributions to the provision of care and support for families of people with intellectual disabilities, ultimately enhancing support for the person. For detailed exploration of current roles and future roles of intellectual disability nurses see Chapter 11.

Liaison roles

Research evidence demonstrates successful implementation of specialist liaison intellectual disability nursing roles supporting people with intellectual

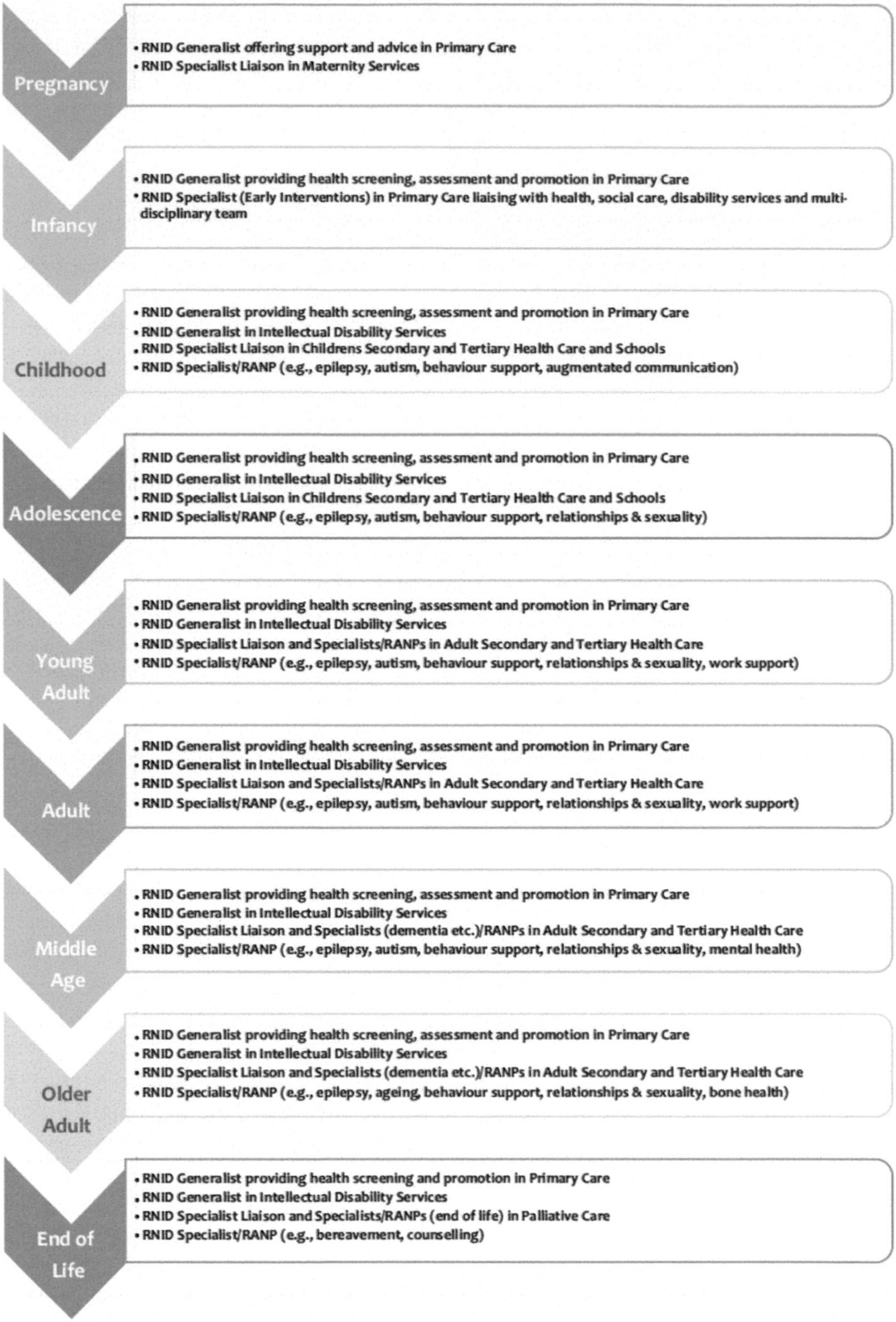

Figure 2.4   *Source:* McCarron et al., (2018)

Toward advanced practice.

disabilities access care in health screening (Marriott *et al.*, 2015); acute hospital settings (MacArthur *et al.*, 2015; Castles *et al.*, 2012) and in the criminal justice system (Shaw, 2016). In Ireland McCarron *et al.* (2018) described the pathway for specialist liaison nurse roles in maternity services, secondary and tertiary healthcare, education, and end of life (palliative care).

The development and maintenance of acute-liaison roles and strategic health facilitators who can provide leadership in designing and implementing health action plans, and in providing educational and training opportunities for generic healthcare professionals in primary and tertiary settings, is therefore important (Michael, 2008). However, the availability of intellectual disability liaison nurses remains inconsistent (Health Education England, 2020). The RCN is campaigning for every hospital in the UK to have an intellectual disability nurse on duty to advise on the best way to make reasonable adjustments (Walker, 2018). Similarly, in Ireland – recognising the unique contribution of the intellectual specialist liaison nurse roles – more work is required to ensure this service is accessible to people with intellectual disabilities across relevant services (Carey *et al.*, 2022).

For detailed discussion of current roles and liaison roles of intellectual disability nurses see Chapter 10.

Box 2.6
Learning Activity 2.4:

The specialist roles of the intellectual disability nurse in meeting the health and healthcare needs of people with profound and multiple disabilities

Refer to Mandy in Learning Activity 2.3 earlier. Having read the previous section on specialist intellectual disability nursing roles, identify those specialist roles that might be relevant in addressing Mandy's health needs.

Explore how intellectual disability nurses could develop their knowledge and skills to undertake these roles.

How would Mandy, her family, and her carers benefit from receiving support from a specialist intellectual disability nurse undertaking the roles identified?

Future intellectual disability nursing roles

Intellectual disability nurses' roles are highly valued by people with intellectual disabilities, their families, and their carers (Gates, 2011b). Intellectual disability nursing is based on the provision of safe and compassionate care, underpinned by human rights. These values and attitudes underlie the core skills learning and intellectual disability nurses and all health professionals require to deliver safe and compassionate care in the future. Current practice changes and policy developments provide opportunities for learning and intellectual disability nurses to undertake new, advanced, and extended roles in line with advances and role extensions in other fields of nursing practice. The Health Equalities Framework (Atkinson *et al.*, 2013) has detailed the determinants of health inequalities that people with intellectual disabilities experience. This provides opportunities for learning disability nurses to develop new roles focused on reducing premature death in the population of people with intellectual disabilities. The Confidential Inquiry into Premature Deaths of People with Learning Disabilities (CIPOLD) (Heslop *et al.*, 2013) has made important recommendations for reducing such premature deaths. These include, but are not limited to, the following:

i.   Clear identification of people with intellectual disabilities on the NHS/HSE record systems
ii.   A named healthcare coordinator to be allocated to people with complex or multiple health needs, or two or more long-term conditions
iii. Standardisation of Annual Health Checks and a clear pathway between Annual Health Checks and Health Action Plans
iv.   Prioritisation of advanced health and care planning.

These recommendations have clear implications for the present and future wider and specialist roles of intellectual disability nurses. These roles will become increasingly more complex and focused on health needs (see Figure 2.3).

For detailed discussion of current roles and future roles of intellectual disability nurses see Chapter 11.

Conclusion

Intellectual disability nursing has evolved over the past 100 years and there are several lessons that intellectual disability nurses of today can learn from the history of the profession to enhance their professional standing, to improve the health and healthcare outcomes of people with learning disabilities. The increasing complexity of healthcare needs of people with learning disabilities will require learning and intellectual disability nurses to possess higher levels of both skills and knowledge to meet the needs of people with learning disabilities. Although the medical model of learning and intellectual disability nursing was insufficient for meeting the holistic needs of people with learning disabilities, present and future roles of learning and intellectual disability nurses will continue to develop a repertoire of generic nursing skills and competences.

It is important for intellectual disability nurses to understand contemporary intellectual disability nursing in the light of the history of nurse education more widely. In the United Kingdom and Ireland, the past development of intellectual disability nursing and its association with mental health nursing has had a significant impact on the registration of nursing since the beginning of the twentieth century. Intellectual disability nursing remains a separate and valued registration. Historical and contemporary debates about intellectual disability nurse education have concentrated somewhat on survival of the profession. There is a need for intellectual disability nurses, and rightly so, to focus the debates on the profession's contribution to the health and healthcare outcomes of and alongside people with intellectual disabilities.

Intellectual disability nursing has survived constant re-examination and change since its inception as a specialty within the wider family of nursing. The continued survival of intellectual disability nursing will no doubt depend on intellectual disability nurses' ability to improve existing roles and to assimilate new roles in line with the needs of people with intellectual disabilities, government policy, and the evidence concerning the needs of people with learning disabilities. Intellectual disability nursing role changes are essential to ensure that such nurses can provide immediate and long-term care and support to people with learning disabilities and their families across the lifespan.

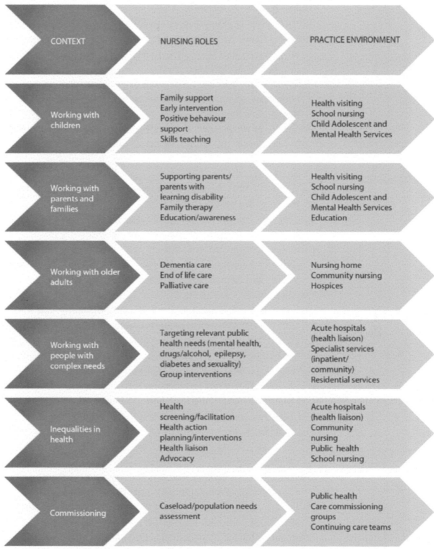

Figure 2.5

Future roles of learning disability nursing in the United Kingdom and Ireland.

References

Áras Attracta Swinford Review Group (2016) *What matters most*. Dublin: Áras Attracta Swinford Review Group.

Atkinson, D., *et al.* (2013) *The health equalities framework (HEF) – an outcomes framework based on the determinants of health inequalities*. Available at: www.ndti.org.uk/uploads/files/The_Health_Equality_Framework.pdf (Accessed 20 May 2022).

Beebee, J. and Batey, G. (2021) *Connecting for change: For the future of learning disability nursing*. Available at: www.cn.org.uk/professional-development/publications/connecting-for-change-uk-pub-009-467 (Accessed 20 April 2022).

Bollard, M. (1999) Improving primary health care for people with learning disabilities. *British Journal of Nursing*, 8(18), pp. 1216–1221.

Briggs, A. (1972) *Report of the committee on nursing*. Cmnd 5115. London: HMSO.

Bubb, S. (2014) *Winterbourne view: Time for change*. London: NHS England.

Burd, L., Burd, M., Klug, M.G., Kerbeshian, J. and Popova, S. (2019) Comorbidity and intellectual disability. In Matson, J.L. (Eds.), *Handbook of intellectual disabilities*. London: Springer.

Carey, E. and Ryan, R. (2019) Chapter 14 informed consent. In Matson, J.L. (Ed.), *Handbook of intellectual disabilities integrating theory, research and practice*. Baton Rouge, LA: Springer.

Carey, E., *et al.* (2022) The Irish perspective on placement opportunities accessed by students on undergraduate nursing (intellectual disability) programmes: A quantitative descriptive study. *British Journal of Learning Disabilities*, pp. 1–15. doi:10.1111/bld.12466.

Carr, L.T. (1995) Sexuality and people with learning disabilities. *British Journal of Nursing*, 4(19), pp. 1135–1140.

Castles, A., Bailey, C., Gates, R. and Sooben, R. (2012) Role of liaison nurses in improving communication. *Learning Disability Practice*, 15, pp. 16–19.

Clifton, M., Shaw, M. and Brown, J. (1992) *Transferability of mental handicap nursing skills from hospital to community*. York: University of York Department of Social Policy and Social Work.

Department of Health and Social Care (2019) *'Right to be heard': The government's response to the consultation on learning disability and autism training for health and care staff*. Gov.UK. Available at: https://assets.publishing.service.gov.uk/government/uploads/system/uploads/attachment_data/file/844356/autism-and-learning-disability-training-for-staff-consultation-response.pdf.

DeWitt, K. (1900) Specialties in nursing. *American Journal of Nursing*, 1(1), pp. 14–17.

DH (1995a) *Signposts to success*. London: Department of Health.

DH (1995b) *Continuing the commitment*. London: Department of Health.

DH (2007) *Good practice in learning disability nursing*. London: Department of Health.

DH, DHSSPS, Welsh Government and The Scottish Government (2012) *Strengthening the commitment: The report of the UK modernising learning disability nursing review*. Edinburgh: The Scottish Government.

Dignam, C. (2000) *Non statutory inquiry into the transfer of Mr Peter McKenna to Leas Cross Nursing Home*. Dublin: Health Service Executive.

Dingwall, R., Rafferty, A.M. and Webster, C. (1988) *An introduction to the social history of nursing*. London: Routledge.

Disability Rights Commission (2006) *Equal treatment: Closing the gap*. DRC: Stratford upon Avon.

DoH (1965) *Report of the commission of inquiry on mental handicap*. No. IRL 362.2 BRIS 632234. Department of Health. Dublin: Stationery Office.

DoHSS (1980) *Government's response to Jay Report.* Press Release 80/189. London: DoHSS.

Doody, O., Slevin, E. and Taggart, L. (2012) Intellectual disability nursing in Ireland: Identifying its development and future. *Journal of Intellectual Disabilities,* 16(1), pp. 7–16.

Doody, O., *et al.* (2022) The value and contribution of intellectual disability nurses/nurses caring for people with intellectual disability in intellectual disability settings: A scoping review. *Journal of Clinical Nursing.* doi:10.1111/jocn.16289.

Doyle, C. (2022) The importance of supportive relationships with general practitioners, hospitals and pharmacists for mothers who 'give medicines' to children with severe and profound intellectual disabilities. *Journal of Intellectual Disabilities,* 26(1), pp. 29–49.

Emerson, E., *et al.* (2011) *Health inequalities & people with learning disabilities in the UK: 2011.* Available at: www.Microsoft Word-IHaL2011healthinequalitiessocialcareguidancefinal.doc (ndti.org.uk) (Accessed 20 May 2022).

Gates, B. (2011a) The valued people project: User views of learning disability nursing. *British Journal of Nursing,* 19(22), pp. 1396–1403.

Gates, B. (2011b) *Learning disability nursing: Task and finish group: Report for the professional and advisory board for nursing and midwifery.* London: Department of Health.

Gates, B., *et al.* (2020) *Intellectual disability nursing: An oral history project.* Bingley: Emerald. ISBN: 9781839821554.

General Nursing Council (1926) *Shorthand notes of the mental nursing committee 1925–1926.* London: Public Records Office, DT6/98.

Government of Ireland (1991) *Needs and abilities: A policy for the intellectually disabled. Report of the review group on mental handicap services.* Dublin: The Stationery Office.

Health Education England (2020) *Project report: Understanding the who, where and what of learning disability liaison nurses.* London: Health Education England.

Health Service Executive (2022) *Disability services – community and social care.* Available at: www.hse.ie/eng/services/list/4/disability/ (Accessed 20 May 2022).

Herringham, W. (1926) *Letter to ministry of health 2.2.1926.* London: Public Records Office, DT48/158.

Heslop, P., *et al.* (2013) *The confidential inquiry into premature deaths of people with learning disabilities (CIPOLD).* Bristol: Norah Fry Research Centre.

Holmes, A. (1995) Self-advocacy in learning disabilities. *British Journal of Nursing,* 4(8), pp. 448–450.

Hourigan, S., Fanagan, S. and Kelly, C. (2018) *HRB statistics series 37: Annual report of the national intellectual disability database committee 2017.* Dublin: Health Research Board.

Howe Report (1969) *Report of the committee of inquiry into allegations of ill treatment of patients and other irregularities at the Ely Hospital, Cardiff.* Cmnd 3975. London: HMSO.

Jay, P. (1979) *Report on the committee of enquiry into mental handicap nursing and care.* Cmnd 7468. London: HMSO.

MacArthur, J., *et al.* (2015) Making reasonable and achievable adjustments: The contributions of learning disability liaison nurses in 'getting it right' for people with learning disabilities receiving general hospitals care. *Journal of Advanced Nursing,* 71(7), pp. 1552–1563.

Mafuba, K., *et al.* (2021) *Understanding the contribution of intellectual disability nurses: A scoping review.* London: University of West London, RCN Foundation.

Marriott, A., *et al.* (2015) Cancer screening for people with learning disabilities and the role of the screening liaison nurse. *Tizard Learning Disability Review,* 20(4), pp. 239–246.

McCarron, M., *et al.* (2018) *Shaping the future of intellectual disability nursing in Ireland.* Dublin: Health Services Executive. Available at: www.inmo.ie/tempDocs/shaping-the-future-of-intellectual-disability-nursing-in-ireland-2018.pdf (Accessed 18 October 2021).

Mella, C. (1998) *Report of the commission on nursing: A blueprint for the future.* Dublin: The Stationery Office.

Mencap (2004) *Treat me right! Better health for people with learning disabilities.* London: Mencap.

Mencap (2007) *Death by indifference.* London: Mencap.

Mencap (2012) *Death by indifference: 74 deaths and counting.* London: Mencap.

Michael, J. (2008) *Healthcare for all: Report of the independent inquiry into access to healthcare for people with learning disabilities.* London: Department of Health.

Mitchell, D. (2004) Parallel stigma? Nurses and people with learning disabilities. *British Journal of Learning Disabilities,* 28, pp. 78–81.

Moulster, G. and Turnbull, J. (2004) The purpose and practice of learning disability nursing. In Turnbull, J. (Ed.), *Learning disability nursing.* Oxford: Blackwall Science.

NAMHI (1962) *Report on day training centres for mentally handicapped children.* Dublin: National Association for the Mentally Handicapped of Ireland.

National Health Service (NHS) (2022) *Learning disability nursing.* Available at: https://learning-disability.hee.nhs.uk/careers/find-a-role-to-suit-you/learning-disability-nursing/ (Accessed 20 May 2022).

NMBI (2019) *Post registration specialist nursing and midwifery education programmes standards and requirements.* Dublin: NMBI.

Northway, R., *et al.* (2017) Supporting people across the lifespan: The role of learning disability nurses. *Learning Disability Practice,* 20(3). doi:10.7748/ldp.2017.e1841.

Nursing and Midwifery Board of Ireland (2016) *Nurse registration programmes standards and requirements* (4th edition). Dublin: Nursing and Midwifery Board of Ireland.

Nursing and Midwifery Council (2018) *Future nurse: Standards of proficiency for registered nurses.* London: NMC.

Nursing and Midwifery Council (2022) *Standards of proficiency for community spacialist practice qualifications.* London: NMC.

Office for National Statistics (2020) *Estimates of the population for the UK, England and Wales, Scotland and Northern Ireland.* London: ONS.

Parliamentary and Health Service Ombudsman and Social Services Ombudsman (2009) *Six lives: The provision of public services to people with learning disabilities.* London: TSO.

Raynes, N.V., *et al.* (1994) *The cost and quality of community residential care.* London: Fulton.

Ritchie, F. (2020) *Independent review into Thomas Oliver McGowan's LeDeR process: Phase two.* London: NHS England.

Robbins, J. (2000) *Nursing and midwifery in Ireland in the twentieth century.* Dublin: An Bord Altranais.

Shanley, E. and Guest, C. (1995) Stigmatization of people with learning disabilities in general hospitals. *British Journal of Nursing,* 4(13), pp. 759–760.

Shaw, V.L. (2016) Liaison and diversion services: Embedding the role of learning disability nurses. *Journal of Intellectual Disabilities and Offending Behaviour,* 7(2), pp. 56–65.

Sines, D.T. (1995) Empowering consumers: The caring challenge. *British Journal of Nursing,* 4(8), pp. 445–448.

Slevin, E. (1995) Student nurses' attitudes towards people with learning disabilities. *British Journal of Nursing,* 4(13), pp. 761–768.

Sweeney, J. (2010) Attitudes of Catholic religious orders towards children and adults with an intellectual disability in postcolonial Ireland. *Nursing Inquiry,* 17(2), pp. 95–110.

Sweeney, J. and Mitchell, D. (2009) A challenge to nursing: An historical review of intellectual disability nursing in the UK and Ireland. *Journal of Clinical Nursing,* 18(19), pp. 2754–2763.

Turnbull, J. (2005) *In search of the accomplished practitioner*. Unpublished PhD thesis. Reading: University of Reading.

UKCC (1997) *Registrar's letter 20/1997*. London: United Kingdom Central Council for Nursing, Midwifery and Health Visiting.

Walker, C. (2018) Specialist nurse training is essential to meet the needs of service user (Editorial). *Learning Disability Practice*. doi:10.7748/ldp.21.2.5.s1.

Further Reading

Atkinson, D., *et al.* (2013) *The health equalities framework (HEF) – an outcomes framework based on the determinants of health inequalities*. Available at: www.ndti.org.uk/uploads/files/Health_Equalities_Framework_Guide_for_Practitioners.pdf (Accessed 12 March 2020).

DH (2007) *Good practice in learning disability nursing*. London: Department of Health.

RCN (2012) *Going upstream: Nursing's contribution to public health: Prevent promote and protect*. London: Royal College of Nursing.

Scottish Government (2012) *Strengthening the commitment: The report of the UK modernising learning disability nursing review*. Edinburgh: The Scottish Government.

Wolfensberger, W. (1972) *The principle of normalization in human services*. Toronto: National Institute on Mental Retardation.

Useful Resources

BILD: www.bild.org.uk/vision-values/

Changing Our Lives: www.changingourlives.org/best-practice-2020

Contact for Families of Disabled Children: https://contact.org.uk/

Enable Scotland: www.enable.org.uk/

Foundation for People with Learning Disabilities: www.learningdisabilities.org.uk/

Inclusion Ireland: https://inclusionireland.ie/

Mencap Northern Ireland: https://northernireland.mencap.org.uk/

Mencap UK: www.mencap.org.uk/

Mencap Wales: https://wales.mencap.org.uk/

National Development Team for Inclusion: www.ndti.org.uk/projects/exploring-the-role-of-learning-disability-nurses-in-in-patient-settings

Nursing and Midwifery Board of Ireland: www.nmbi.ie/Home

Nursing and Midwifery Council UK: www.nmc.org.uk/

Royal College of Nursing: www.rcn.org.uk/clinical-topics/learning-disabilities

University of Hertfordshire: www.intellectualdisability.info/

CHAPTER 3

Carmel Doyle, Daniel Marsden, Eileen Carey and James Ridley

Intellectual disability nursing throughout the lifespan

Introduction

In this chapter, students of nursing will explore the nature of intellectual disabilities throughout the lifespan and its relationship to intellectual disability nursing. This will be contextualised within the Nursing and Midwifery Council for the United Kingdom (2018) and Nursing and Midwifery Board of Ireland (2016) standards and requirements for competence.

An intellectual disability is a lifelong condition, and it is therefore not unusual for intellectual disability nurses to work with, or offer support to, people with intellectual disabilities throughout their lifespans, quite literally from the cradle to the grave. Holistic approaches in intellectual disability nursing seek to promote interventions that adopt a whole-person-centred approach. This means providing nursing that responds to the various dimensions of being, and these typically include attention to the physical, emotional, social, economic, and spiritual needs of people.

Therefore, this chapter will focus on the knowledge and kinds of practical skills that intellectual disability nurses will need when working with people with intellectual disabilities across their lifespans. The role of the intellectual disability nurse during the childhood and adolescence of people with intellectual disabilities is explored in the context of diagnosing intellectual disability, parenting children with intellectual disabilities, transition, psychological and physical changes during adolescence, and transition into adulthood. The lifestyle and health needs of adults and older adults with intellectual disabilities, employment and retirement, personal relationships, and parenting needs of adults with intellectual disabilities will be explored. The chapter concludes by exploring end-of-life care needs, and palliative care for people with intellectual disabilities.

DOI: 10.4324/9781003296461-3

Box 3.1 This chapter will focus on the following issues:

- Childhood
    - Diagnosis of an intellectual disability
    - Parenting
    - Starting school
- Adolescence
    - Transition issue
    - Psychological and physical changes
    - The role of the intellectual disability nurse
- Adulthood
    - Maintaining healthy lifestyles and health
    - Employment
    - Personal relationships
    - Parents with intellectual disabilities
- Older adults with intellectual disabilities
    - Retirement
    - Health needs of older adults with intellectual disabilities
    - Loss
- End-of-life care
    - Breaking news
    - End-of-life decisions
    - Palliative care and people with intellectual disabilities

Box 3.2 Competences

Nursing and Midwifery Council (2018) Proficiencies

Platform 1: Being an accountable professional - 1.1, 1.9, 1.11, 1.12, 1.13, 1.14, 1.15, 1.18, 1.20

Platform 2: Promoting health and preventing ill health - 2.2, 2.4, 2.7, 2.11, 2.12

Platform 3: Assessing needs and planning care - 3.1, 3.2, 3.3, 3.4, 3.5, 3.6, 3.7 3.8, 3.9, 3.10 3.11, 3.12, 3.13, 3.14, 3.15, 3.16

Platform 4: Providing and evaluating care - 4.1, 4.7, 4.8, 4.10, 4.12, 4.13, 4.14, 4.15, **4.18**

Platform 5: Leading and managing nursing care and working in teams - 5.2

Platform 6: Improving safety and quality of care - 6.1, 6.3, 6.5, 6.6

Platform 7: Coordinating care - 7.1, 7.5

Nursing and Midwifery Board of Ireland (2016) Competences

Domain 1: Professional values and conduct of the nurse competences - 1.2

Domain 2: Nursing practice and clinical decision-making competences - 2.1, 2.2, 2.3

Childhood

Diagnosis of an intellectual disability

Pregnancy and the subsequent birth of any child leads to new circumstances that require parents and other family members to make significant changes to their lifestyles. This process of change and adaptation becomes more significant and complex if the unborn or new baby is diagnosed with or suspected of having an intellectual disability (Mencap, 2022). The diagnostic process can be challenging and defining and measuring childhood disability can be a perplexing task (Smith, 2010). Infancy to adolescence is a period marked with developmental changes and the evolving characteristics of a child can make the task of assessing function more complicated (Meggitt, 2012) with red flag signs as key indicators that prompt an assessment (Blows, Teoh and Paul, 2016). Furthermore, the multiplicity of disabilities associated with these children can make assessment and diagnosis particularly challenging. The configuration of unique levels of functioning can be so varied, a recognised assessment process is not always helpful (Nakken and Vlaskamp, 2007). Approaches to diagnosing intellectual disability include observation, developmental screening checks, noting discrepancies in the appearance of skills and the use of diagnostic assessment tools (WHO, 2012).

Emotional demands of the diagnosis of intellectual disabilities on parents must be recognised (Rivard *et al.*, 2021) primarily based on pre-, peri- or post-natal concerns (Patel *et al.*, 2020). Therefore, the communication of a diagnosis requires sensitivity. Best Practice Guidelines should be adhered to as a key support for both parents and professionals during the process (See Box 3.3).

Box 3.3 Informing Families – Best Practice Guidelines (adapted from Harnett, 2007)

- Family-centered disclosure – Provide unlimited time for face-to-face discussion of diagnosis/prognosis.
- Respect for child and family – Suitable location chosen and privacy offered.
- Sensitive and empathetic communication – Parents receive the news together from a professional and in the presence of a relative/friend that offers support. Interpreter present if required.
- Appropriate, accurate information – Written materials offered.
- Positive, realistic messages and hope – Information on how to best support child.
- Team approach and planning.
- Focused and supported implementation of best practice.

Prospective parents, and parents of a child with, or suspected of having intellectual disabilities will seek answers. This requires effective liaison, and multiagency cooperation between specialist services, primary care services, intellectual disability specialist services, and the family. During this stressful time, parents and families of children with intellectual disabilities will require coordinated and integrated support that will facilitate access to all the essential services. Integrated care has been heralded as essential to multidisciplinary mutual decision-making and organisation of care with the common goal of helping individuals to achieve positive outcomes through their healthcare experiences (HSE and RCPI, 2016). Integrated care pathways are vital for ensuring children and families are at the centre of planning for their care at home and that individual needs are responded to (Together for Short Lives, 2013). While guidelines and policies offer a map, integrated care pathways are distinct in advising on who should be doing what and how it should be undertaken with no 'one size fits all' approach to care (Pordes *et al.*, 2018). Providing an effective care pathway for children and young people with intellectual disabilities is difficult. However, distinct care pathways are important in defining and identifying services that families of children with intellectual disabilities can recognise and access easily. Defined care pathways for children with intellectual disabilities provide opportunities

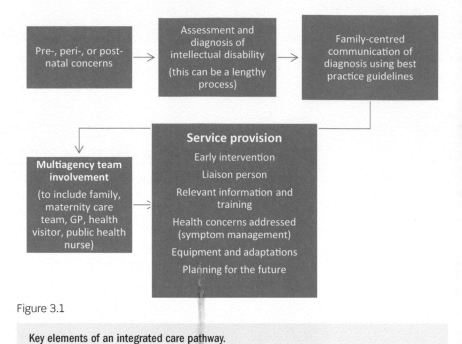

Figure 3.1

Key elements of an integrated care pathway.

for joining processes and agencies together. A variety of integrated care pathways exist for use with children with intellectual disabilities (Chambers and Kelly, 2015; Together for Short Lives, 2013; Brown *et al.*, 2019).

Figure 3.1 outlines key elements of an integrated care pathway that may be used to support families during this process of diagnosis and early intervention.

Together for Short Lives (2013) has developed an integrated care pathway as a tool for professionals who support children with complex and integrated care needs and their families throughout their care journey, from diagnosis right through to end-of-life care and bereavement support. This pathway provides a broad outline of the key events or processes that happen during the journey made by children (see Table 3.1).

Following a diagnosis or suspected diagnosis of intellectual disability, planning commences. This can be dependent upon when diagnosis is likely, whether it is prenatal, obvious at birth or whether it is a later diagnosis in the early years. The diagnosis trajectory can be disparate and very much depends on the age of the infant or child (Rivard *et al.*, 2021). Supported discharge from hospital is important with primary care services supporting this transfer. Although care coordination can be complex and challenging, a care coordinator is usually appointed for efficient management of the issues surrounding caring for children with intellectual disabilities (Ward, Glass and Ford, 2014; Currie and Szabo, 2019). This efficiency may also reduce necessity for attendance or admission to hospital on a frequent basis. The care coordinator will begin a discharge plan in collaboration with the family and will also inform relevant community health and social care services. The child's general practitioner will be involved and will be a key support. A detailed needs assessment should be undertaken, which will

Integrated Care Pathway for Children with complex and integrated care needs	
Stage one – Diagnosis or recognition	1. The prognosis – sharing significant news
	2. Transfer and liaison between hospital and community services
Stage two – Ongoing care	3. Multi-disciplinary assessment of needs
	4. A child and family care plan
Stage three – End of life:	5. An end-of-life plan
	6. Bereavement support

Table 3.1   Integrated care pathway for children

include identification of essential adaptations, equipment, and any supplies, and should be in place before discharge. Necessary training for parents and other carers should be arranged and provided prior to discharge and on an ongoing basis depending on the needs of the child and family. A multiagency support system should be put in place with early intervention as a focus also. Identifying long-term medical, healthcare, developmental, and social care needs of the child is imperative and will help in planning for short- and long-term needs.

Parenting

In general, parenting is a challenging task, and it may be more difficult if a child has an intellectual disability with more non normative requirements and challenges that extend beyond mainstream expectations creating a high level of burden (Vadivelan *et al.*, 2020). Rogers (2011) has argued that prospective parents experience pressures from internalised norms and societal expectations to produce 'perfect' children. Whilst the experience of caring can be a positive and enriching one (Whiting, 2017), it can also bring with it increased burden (Coad, Patel and Murray, 2014). When a child with an intellectual disability is expected or born, parents are likely to be traumatised and experience feelings of shock, fear, loss, disappointment, and bereavement (Ridding and Williams, 2019; Marsh, Leahy-Warren and Savage, 2018, 2020). Therefore, adequate, and timely supports, both formal and informal, are important for families of children with intellectual disabilities.

Parents often feel a burden of care, experience stress, financial problems, difficulties in accessing care, deterioration in family structures and marital problems (Nicholl and Begley, 2012; McCann, Bull and Winzenberg, 2015). The presence of an intellectual disability in a child is likely to result in other parental needs that are dependent on the degree of the child's intellectual disability and cultural background, as well as the social and economic circumstances of the family. Therefore, parents are at increased risk if necessary resources are limited or unavailable (Bourke-Taylor, Cotter and Stephan, 2014; Coad *et al.*, 2015; Woodgate *et al.*, 2015). Support needs of families are highlighted with much of the care delivery taking place at home by parents (Woodgate *et al.*, 2015; Doyle, 2020). The increasing interest in this area is due to these services wanting to be responsive to parent-identified concerns.

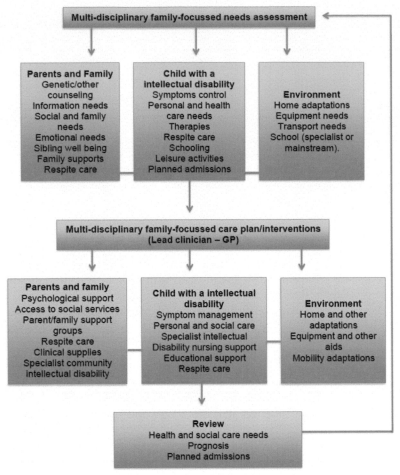

Figure 3.2

Pathways for managing children with intellectual disabilities in the community.

Family focused integrated care pathways are important because parents' and families' positive attitudes and psychological well-being are important in the intellectual, psychological, and social development of children with intellectual disabilities (Shobana and Saravanan, 2014) and are crucial in avoiding adverse impacts for both the child and family. A variety are in existence, all centred on the common goals of a thorough multi-disciplinary focused assessment with the views and preferences of the child and family clearly embedded (NICE, 2022) (see Figure 3.2). It is also important to note that the needs of a family of a child with an intellectual disability will not remain static across the lifespan but will vary with the gender, age, and level of impairment of the child.

Starting school

Support for inclusive education is a priority for the EU evident in the strategic framework for European co-operation in education and training, and the

European Disability Strategy 2010–2020 (European Commission, 2010). The need to integrate children with disabilities within mainstream education settings through the provision of individualised support was highlighted with supports in mainstream schools, special schools, and special classes. In England, 26% of children with an education, health, and care (EHC) plan which identifies educational, health and social needs and sets out the additional support to meet those needs were being educated in mainstream schools. For those children with a EHC plan, 44% of children with moderate intellectual disabilities, 12% of children with severe intellectual disabilities, and 15% of children with profound and multiple intellectual disabilities were being educated in mainstream schools (Department of Education, 2018).

For parents and carers of children with intellectual disabilities, deciding on an appropriate school may be difficult and could require professional support. In addition to the developmental limitations due to intellectual disabilities, other related conditions are likely to play a significant role in the schooling of a child with intellectual disability. Children with intellectual disabilities can sometimes have additional disabilities or conditions (multiple disabilities) such as autism spectrum disorders, medical conditions, physical and/or sensory disabilities and emotional/behavioural difficulties. Serious psychopathology affects more than 40% of children and adolescents with intellectual disability (College of Psychiatry, 2011). Furthermore, children with autism and intellectual disabilities are at increased risk of developing challenging behaviour (NICE, 2015a) and approximately 30% of children with intellectual disabilities have epilepsy impacting schooling (Robertson *et al.*, 2015).

Box 3.4
Learning Activity 3.1

Consider the needs assessment and care planning required for managing children with intellectual disabilities and complex needs (refer to Figure 3.2).

What is the role of the intellectual disability nurse who may be involved in the assessment process?

What could the positive outcomes of the involvement of intellectual disability nurses be in assessment, planning, and delivery of care for children with intellectual disabilities and complex needs?

Interventions to support children with intellectual disabilities in schools should focus on the management of additional health needs. The conditions highlighted previously may have minimal effect on some children's schooling, but these conditions may require significant support from a wide range of professionals. Individualised approaches within school environments and close collaboration among schools, parents, and healthcare professionals are in place to meet a child's needs. Intellectual disability nurses working in school nursing teams, child and adolescent mental health services, and community intellectual disability teams can provide useful interventions that could contribute to meeting the schooling needs of children with intellectual disabilities.

Adolescence

There are approximately 351,000 children aged 0–17 with an intellectual disability representing 2.5% of children in the UK (Public Health England, 2016; Office for National Statistics, 2020). Children with intellectual disabilities are likely to have poorer health and health outcomes than children without intellectual disabilities. There is a body of evidence which shows that people with intellectual disabilities have much greater health needs than those of comparable age groups who do not have intellectual disabilities, with higher incidence of osteoporosis, constipation, obesity, dementia, polypharmacy and falls risk (McCarron *et al.*, 2018). Adolescents experience many health problems but are likely to have associated mental health concerns with a diagnosable mental health condition in 36% of children compared with 8% who do not have an intellectual disability (Mental Health Foundation, 2022). This can be challenging given adolescence is a time of intense emotional and social change, having a significant negative impact on life opportunities, social inclusion, and well-being.

Adolescents with intellectual disabilities are more likely to experience poverty and social disadvantage along with higher rates of stressful life events, including physical and sexual abuse, as compared with those without intellectual disabilities (Public Health England, 2015). The presence of mental illness and experience of stressful life events result in increased levels of behaviours likely to challenge services. In addition, adolescents experience comorbid disorders, such as epilepsy, autism, and sleep disturbances which impact on their experiences during this period of their lives (Reddihough *et al.*, 2021). It is also important to recognise that some genetic conditions, such as Prader-Willi, Down, and Asperger syndromes, are associated with adolescents with intellectual disabilities. The treatment and management of health and social conditions resulting from these syndromes require careful planning. Furthermore, communication difficulties, and additional sensory disabilities such as hearing impairments, reduce adolescents' ability to interact with others or contribute meaningfully to their transition from childhood to adult services. A lack of coping strategies can make adolescence a very stressful period with adolescents experiencing low self-esteem and possibly stigmatisation. This can result in depression and anxiety, particularly in older children with intellectual disabilities as the ability gap between them and their non-disabled peers widens.

Transition issues

The transition of adolescents with intellectual disability into adulthood is challenging in that they are expected to go through psychological and social maturation just like their able counterparts. Yet, transitioning adolescents with intellectual disabilities experience lower quality of life ratings than similar-age youth (Biggs and Carter, 2016). Under-diagnosis, reduced treatment accessibility and reduced awareness of comorbid mental health disorders and intellectual disabilities among young adults can also have a negative impact on this group

(Austin *et al.*, 2018). Emerson *et al.* (2013) have reported that at the end of Key Stage 2, children with intellectual disabilities achieve significantly lower than children who do not have intellectual disabilities. For example, in 2011, only 15% of children with moderate intellectual disabilities, 3% of children with severe intellectual disabilities, and 2% of children with profound and multiple intellectual disabilities attained the expected levels in English and Mathematics versus 74% of the children who did not have intellectual disabilities. These low levels of attainment mean that adolescents with intellectual disabilities will require purposeful and planned transfer from education and other child services to adult social and healthcare services.

Survival rates of children with intellectual disabilities are now higher (Pinney, 2017) resulting in a growing need for specialised transition services to ensure that there is seamless transfer and transition from child to adult healthcare and social care services. A transition that provides uninterrupted, coordinated and developmentally appropriate care throughout the process is important (Kaufman and Pinzon, 2007). However, this can be challenging when comorbid conditions are considered (Brown *et al.*, 2021). The transition process can be fraught with poor health, difficulties accessing healthcare, using different health specialties across a variety of hospital settings (Brown *et al.*, 2021). The process of transition from child to adult health services can be particularly complex due to the different ways the two services operate. Child services are characterised by a holistic, child and family-centred approach, usually with a single coordinating pediatrician, often from Child Health Services. While child services are family-focused with parental involvement in the decision-making process, adult services are individual and condition-focused and are reliant on autonomous decision-making. Children with intellectual disabilities often remain in children's services perhaps longer than is required or appropriate with transfers sometimes abrupt and inappropriate, with some children becoming invisible by default, or voluntarily. Multidisciplinary working is essential for adolescents with intellectual disabilities going through transition from child to adult services.

For transition services for adolescents with intellectual disabilities to be effective, professionals and health and social care services need to be aware that these adolescents will be undergoing broader changes beyond their clinical needs. These adolescents, regardless of their intellectual disabilities, will desire and strive for autonomy and involvement in decision-making about their lives. It is therefore important to involve families and carers in the transition process. Effective transition services require leadership, collaboration, cross-boundary working, resources, a skilled and knowledgeable workforce, effective administration support, and clearly defined pathways. The key elements for a successful transition are identified in Figure 3.3, as suggested for a transition pathway for adolescents with intellectual disabilities (Health Education England, 2016).

There are three identified stages of transition as per Table 3.2, with each stage taking into consideration a variety of aspects that include health, education, housing, work, and social care (Together for Short Lives, 2016). Additionally, Chambers and Kelly (2015) have identified the steps in transition journeys with a detailed published report on the standards to be met.

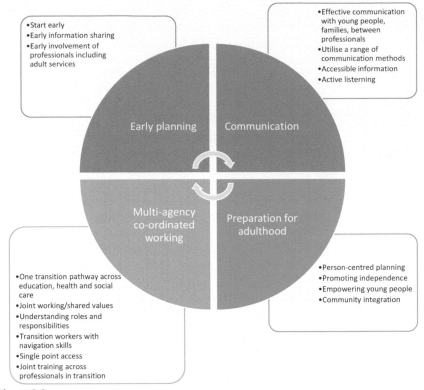

Figure 3.3

A transition pathway for adolescents with intellectual disabilities.

Stages of transition

Get ready – preparing for adulthood

Get set – moving to adult services

Go – getting the best from adult services

Table 3.2   Stages of transition

Box 3.5
Learning Activity 3.2

Consider the needs of an adolescent transitioning from child to adult health services.

What is the role of the intellectual disability nurse who may be involved in planning for the transition process?

Referring to Figure 3.3, identify the key considerations for a transition pathway that may be adopted.

The role of the intellectual disability nurse working with adolescents and families

As more people with intellectual disabilities grow into adulthood, intellectual disability nurses need to develop skills to recognise and manage disorders in adolescents with intellectual disabilities. This requires them to work in a wide range of multidisciplinary health teams. The ultimate outcome for the involvement of intellectual disability nurses with adolescents with intellectual disabilities should be supporting to achieve their full potential in terms of ability, physical, psychological, and emotional well-being. Intellectual disability nurses need to be aware that this will always require them to work in multiagency settings such as education, health, and social services. The RCN (2018) have suggested that meeting the needs of adolescents with intellectual disabilities during transition to adult services is inherent in the core skills of the registered intellectual disability nurse. A familiarity and responsibility to adopt transition pathways is important. Course curriculum requires education that encompasses information on the transition period from adolescence to adulthood and interprofessional working should be supported. This is also a key element of transition pathways.

Having a child with an intellectual disability in the family can have a major impact on individual members and the family. It is estimated that two-thirds of people living with an intellectual disability reside at home and are cared for by family members (Linehan *et al.*, 2014). It must be acknowledged that family carers are a fundamental resource in the provision of care for people with intellectual disabilities (Lafferty *et al.*, 2016). Some families will struggle with caregiving and the associated responsibilities, others will be more resilient and overcome and adapt to their situation. Nonetheless, people with intellectual disabilities experience poorer health and healthcare access. Family carers voices are important in planning person-centred care. Sardi *et al.* (2008) explored family carer opinions of intellectual disability services and established that lack of information was a core issue with the need for family carers to be consistently proactive in seeking information. This was also the case in terms of fighting for service provision across health and social care, respite care, and financial support. Recognising that the caring role would last a lifetime brought with it feelings of fear for the future. Communication challenges between interdisciplinary services and the family were also highlighted with involvement of family often tokenistic. Barr (2012) has summarised five key needs of parents of children with intellectual disability as: the need for increased certainty and control; information; acquisition of knowledge and development of skills in caring for their child; coordinated services and respite care. An awareness of all these challenges is important when working with family carers.

A requirement for professionals to work in partnership with families facilitates empowerment and supports the process of adaptation experienced by many on finding they have a child with an intellectual disability. The intellectual disability nurse is ideally positioned and plays a leading role in healthcare provision for people with intellectual disabilities and their families, supporting person-centred care approaches and health outcomes (Doody *et al.*, 2022). McCarron *et al.* (2018) highlighted the direct care provided by intellectual disability nurses to people with intellectual disabilities. Ideally, care should be delivered in a person-centred manner with positive interpersonal behaviours reflective of the relational aspect of working with the individual with intellectual disability, the family, and other professionals (Doody *et al.*, 2022). The clinical leadership role that intellectual disability nurses hold is essential in ensuring evidence-based practice is integrated in care delivery. Furthermore, intellectual disability nurses incorporate a biopsychosocial-educational model of care that in turn addresses the needs of individuals who may have complex health, social, educational, cognitive, and communication needs (Doody *et al.*, 2022). This approach allows for the physical, social, and psychological needs of the individual and their family to be addressed. Educational strategies may be adopted – for example, skills development, reinforcement, role modelling and backward/forward chaining – to educate, empower and enable the individual to reach their full potential. A person-centred approach supporting participation in decision-making, involving the individual and their family is a core element of addressing health needs, health promotion, and education. The link with family carers is likely to be the intellectual disability nurse and they tend to be in constant contact with the family, positioning them well in leading and coordinating the care team. It is also acknowledged that intellectual disability nurses are unique in their knowledge and skills related to health and well-being but also how to negotiate intricate and cross-sectoral collaborations (Wilson *et al.*, 2019). Supporting family carers requires knowledge and experience of some key considerations. See Table 3.3.

Supporting Family Carers – Points to consider

Awareness of Carers and
- Caregiving roles
- Caregiving Tasks/Responsibilities

The Family and family structure
- Adjusting and Adapting to Caregiving
- Stress
- Resilience

Coping Process
- Coping Strategies
- Coping Styles
- Coping Ability

Impact of Caring on Families and Carers
- Physical Impact
- Psychosocial Impact
- Caregiver Strain and Burden
- Depression
- Loss and Grief Associated with Caregiving
- Chronic Sorrow
- Impact on Family Roles and Relationships
- Positive Outcomes of Caregiving

Providing Support and Interventions for Families and Carers
- Assessment of Families and Caregivers' Needs
- Interventions to Support Families and Carers

Working with Families and Carers
- Relationships between Nurse and Caregivers

Table 3.3   Supporting family carers – points to consider

Underpinning the uniqueness of the role of the intellectual disability nurse in supporting family carers is the therapeutic relationship that tends to exist between the individual and the nurse which also tends to be over a protracted period due to the nature of care (Doody *et al.*, 2022). The intellectual disability nurse has an important role in the lives of people with intellectual disabilities and their families in supporting the holistic needs of the individual through care delivery across the lifespan.

Adulthood

Over the past two decades, social care services have adapted and aligned with the devolved UK governments. McMahon, Bowring and Hatton (2019) have reported that 57% of adults with intellectual disabilities live in sheltered housing compared to 2% of adults without an intellectual disability. Hatton (2017) has observed that adults with intellectual disabilities are living in a wide range of situations from residential and nursing care to supported living and tenancies, with a large proportion still living with their families.

Hatton (2017) has stated that 67% of adults with intellectual disabilities in England live in residential care with a further 4% living in nursing care. These percentages are somewhat lower in Scotland at 42%, Wales at 51% and Northern Ireland at 39%, however, the latter reports a further 43% live in nursing care. While the United Nations Convention on the Rights of Persons with Disabilities (United Nations, 2006) states that people with disabilities have the right to choose where to live with and with whom, multiple studies from western counties (Wehmeyer and Abery, 2013; Stancliffe *et al.*, 2011; McCarron *et al.*, 2011) found that much of the time these choices were not available or were afforded based on service provision rather than the wishes of the individual. A study by Kirkpatrick (2011) has demonstrated that the relocation of people with complex support needs has led to better quality of life and improved outcomes in appropriate community accommodation. Whatever the model of community residential accommodation adults with intellectual disabilities opt for, it is important to remember that their health and social support needs will need to be considered.

Maintaining healthy lifestyles and health

Unhealthy lifestyles, poor dietary habits, and physical inactivity among adults with intellectual disabilities have been widely reported (Phillips and Holland, 2011; O'Leary *et al.*, 2018a), while evidence indicates that people with intellectual disabilities are not involved or engaged in health promotion initiatives (Taggart and Cousins, 2014). Such sedentary lifestyles contribute to an increased prevalence of obesity in adults with intellectual disabilities (Gephart and Loman, 2013). Evidence from Australia (Koritsas and Iacono, 2016) indicates that 60% of adults with intellectual disabilities did not meet national physical activity standards, whilst in Sweden, Sundahl *et al.* (2016) found low levels of physical activity are common in young adults, particularly women. Cartwright *et al.* (2017) indicated three main barriers to regular physical activity for people with intellectual disabilities. Firstly, carer acceptance of physical inactivity as a norm for the people they support, secondly, restrictions and limitations implemented by carers based on their own interests and preference, and thirdly, communication issues between family and paid carers. Physical inactivity is a risk factor for hypertension, obesity, chronic health conditions, cardiovascular disease, hypercholesterolemia, type-2 diabetes, and osteoarthritis and increased cancer risk (de Rezende *et al.*, 2014; Same *et al.*, 2016), and these are significantly more prevalent in adults with intellectual disabilities. Obesity has been found to be an increasing concern in western cultures in the last decade with the systematic review evidence indicating between 17% and 43% having a Body Mass Index of 30 or above (Ranjan, Nasser and Fisher, 2018) and IDS-TILDA study in Ireland found an 13% increase in the population of people with intellectual disabilities that were obese in the decade between the first and third waves.

Poor cardiovascular fitness levels contribute to higher morbidity and mortality rates in adults with intellectual disabilities.

Box 3.6 Risks of sedentary lifestyles

- Reduced cardiovascular fitness
- Hypertension
- Obesity
- Chronic health conditions
- Cardiovascular disease
- Hypercholesterolemia
- Type-2 diabetes
- Osteoarthritis

Box 3.7 Hosking *et al.* (2017) identified 10 ambulatory care sensitive conditions for people with intellectual disabilities

1. Convulsions and epilepsy
2. Pneumonia
3. Urinary tract infection
4. Aspiration
5. Cellulitis
6. Dehydration and gastroenteritis
7. Constipation
8. COPD
9. Asthma
10. Diabetes complications

The benefits of active lifestyles across the lifespan have been well documented: Improved cardiovascular fitness (Bailey, 2006), psychological and emotional well-being (Eime *et al.*, 2013), improved motor skills (Poitras *et al.*, 2016), greater frequency of prosocial activity (Bailey, 2006) and reduced levels of obesity (Bailey, 2006), reduced risk of depression and anxiety (Hamers *et al.*, 2018), and improved mood and self-esteem (Kapsal *et al.*, 2019). Some adults with intellectual disabilities will require personal support to reduce levels of inactivity. Intellectual disability nurses can contribute to the improvement of health outcomes for adults with intellectual disabilities by engaging and supporting that adaptation of existing health promotion and public health activities that focus on dietary habits and physical activity and ultimately health, social and emotional well-being. In addition, intellectual disability nurses need to work flexibly in advocating those reasonable adjustments be made for adults with intellectual disabilities for the widely acknowledged barriers to improved lifestyles (Taggart *et al.*, 2018) to be addressed.

In addition to the impact of sedentary lifestyles, adults with intellectual disabilities are known to experience poorer health than those of comparable age groups who do not have intellectual disabilities. These include the list of 10 ambulatory care sensitive conditions outlined by Hosking *et al.* (2017) (see Box 3.3) that are often not recognised or managed effectively in primary care, higher prevalence of sensory impairments (Li *et al.*, 2015; McShea, Fulton and Hayes, 2016), mental health issues (Hughes-McCormack, 2017), aspiration and respiratory issues (University of Bristol, 2018), gastrointestinal issues such as constipation (Al Mutairi *et al.*, 2020), epilepsy (Robertson *et al.*, 2015), hypothyroidism (Hermans and Evenhuis, 2014), health inequalities and poor access to healthcare (Whittle *et al.*, 2018), unequal access to health services (Doherty *et al.*, 2020), poor uptake of public health initiatives (Heslop *et al.*, 2014), and reduced access to health screening and health promotion services (Merten *et al.*, 2015). These along with specific health inequities experienced during the Covid-19 pandemic (Public Health England, 2020a) contribute to their poorer health and well-being, and increased rates of premature and avoidable mortality compared to people with similar demographics from the wider population.

Box 3.8
Intellectual Activity 3.2

Consider the health issues presented by Hosking in Box 3.3

- How would an Intellectual Disability Nurse identify those at risk of these conditions?
- How could these risks be minimised and who would the nurse work with to manage these issues?
- How would the Intellectual disability Nurse demonstrate a person-centred approach in managing these issues?

Employment

While both England and the United States have invested significant resources to increase the numbers of people with intellectual disabilities in employment, statistics indicate employment rates remain stubbornly low (Siperstein, Heyman and Stokes, 2014; Public Health England, 2020a). There is strong evidence to indicate that paid employment is correlated with good physical and mental health (NICE, 2015b), including greater sense of autonomy, well-being, reduced anxiety, and increased social status (Modini, 2016). Employers identify a mixture of barriers to bringing people with intellectual disabilities into their workforce, including the lack of adequate jobs, in particular linked to digitisation, legal issues relating to the requirement to make adjustments, and resource issues like the perceived additional time and effort required to support someone with intellectual disabilities (Kocman, Fischer and Weber, 2018).

However, people with intellectual disabilities remain keen to be in paid employment (Rustad and Kassah, 2020), although Giri *et al.* (2022) study found that they and their carers were pessimistic about finding work, indicating the inter-dependent relationship with carers to be a significant barrier. This inter-dependance was characterised by the concerns regarding risks of being bullied, difficulties with independent travel, the perceived risks associated with work that might cause emotional strain, lack of support in the workplace, and Mencap's (2020) survey also indicated concerns regarding loss of welfare benefits.

Intellectual disability nurses may appear to have little direct involvement in the employment of people with intellectual disabilities, however, the increasing focus in participatory work and co-production activities provide for paid opportunities as experts by experience (Smith, Ooms and Marks-Maran, 2016), and recruitment interviewers (Stevens, 2017). The NHS England (2022) Intellectual Disability Employment Programme relies on advocates in all services to influence their workplace culture; in particular, Intellectual Disability Hospital Liaison nurses are well placed to influence organisational cultures in this way through the introduction of programmes like Project Search (Marsden, 2013).

Gender and sexuality

Wolfensberger's work on Normalisation (1972) heralded a new era in the care of people with intellectual disabilities that actively included personal relationships and sexuality, however, social and cultural barriers to expression of sexuality in this community have remained. Over the last decade a greater awareness of gender related issues has permeated the western media and consciousness.

Warrier *et al.* (2020) have identified elevated rates of autism and other neurodevelopmental diagnoses in transgender people – between three and six times higher than cisgender people. People with autism and intellectual disabilities who identify as transgender or non-binary report a wide range of negative experiences in healthcare and the wider community, including a social isolation (Hillier *et al.*, 2022), concerns over own safety and poor mental health (Cain and Velasco, 2021), and a lack of adequate health or care provision (Hillier *et al.*,

2022). Robinson *et al.* (2020) observes that Intellectual Disability Nurses have a unique and proactive role in supporting people with their gender and sexual expression, and the double marginalisation (Wilson *et al.*, 2018) that people with intellectual disabilities can experience.

The World Health Organisation have defined sexual health in context of pleasure and safety, and free from violence and coercion; as such the nurse's role has shifted from a biomedical position to holistic, person-centred approach (Thomas *et al.*, 2017). While human rights underpin this approach to current practice, to ignore the biopsychosocial issues associated with personal relationships within this population is also to discriminate and put people at risk. Brown *et al.* (2019) identified several themes from recent research, including the balance of risk of harm to self and others versus individual autonomy, the knowledge required for sexual relationships, the understanding and appreciation of what others may wish they would obtain from their personal relationships, facilitative support to enable self-determination including managing internal and external barriers to forming and sustaining relationships. These themes provide a vital framework for Intellectual Disability Nurse practice in proactively and reactively supporting individuals with this fundamental part of being human.

Case law A Local Authority v JB (2021) UKSC 52 presents further complexity for those needing to balance risk and autonomy. This case identified that for JB to have capacity to enter into a sexual relationship, he ought to have an appreciation of his partner's capacity to engage in sexual relations, and in this case, JB was deemed to lack capacity. This case law further defines what is necessary for someone to have capacity to consent to a sexual relationship; based on this case, a satisfactory knowledge of the risks and benefits of a sexual relationship will not suffice, as the processing ability to assess and understand if your potential partner has the pre-requisite capacity is also required. This latter activity is based on judgement and as such cannot be learnt by rote. This added complexity has far reaching implications for practice in this area, and without due consideration will lead to risk avoidance and the inevitable consequences of denying individual's rights to a personal relationship.

Supported Loving (Bates, 2019) is a network of people with intellectual disabilities, carers and care workers that believe that people with intellectual disabilities should be able to experience the same sexual freedoms as everyone else, and in doing so provides a safe space for discussion related to complex topics relating to relationships and sexuality amongst people with intellectual disabilities. As a result, good practice guidance, tools, blogs, and podcasts are available on topical areas of practice.

McCann, Marsh and Brown (2019) review of personal relationships and sexuality education with people with intellectual disabilities found some specific barriers to understanding, including abstract concepts and long sentences, which influenced comprehension and understanding. However, a reoccurring theme was the enthusiasm to participate in the programmes with improved self-esteem, positive feelings about their experiences and an improvement in the knowledge which would have a positive effect on decision-making capacity. According to Robinson *et al.* (2020) Intellectual Disability Nurses have a responsibility to understand the importance of expressing sexuality as part of Maslow's hierarchy of needs (1943) and would be wise to stay up to date on the shifting policy context and legal frameworks to empower families, care workers and ultimately individuals themselves to explore this facet of their being.

Pregnancy and parents with intellectual disabilities

Screening for intellectual disabilities

Allied to this greater awareness of gender and sexuality is an increased appreciation of the rights of people with intellectual disabilities to have a family and as such screening, pregnancy and childbirth are all issues that will be of concern to the intellectual disability nurse.

While prenatal screening for conditions which can increase the risk of disabilities has taken place for many years via amniocentesis and chorionic villus sampling, noninvasive prenatal testing (NIPT) was introduced to the UK's national Health Service in 2018. This test relies on a blood sample and therefore holds less risk to the woman and foetus, providing a probability of the baby being born with Down's, Edward's or Patau's syndromes, presenting women with a choice as to whether to continue with the pregnancy. These conditions could be considered severe medical impairments under the Abortion Act 1967 which would allow for termination at any gestation period rather than before 24 weeks that is normally accepted. While actress and advocate Sally Phillips (2016) has raised questions as to why Down's syndrome foetuses – who would have a life expectancy of 50-60 years – would be grouped here with Edwards and Patau's – who in most cases do not live beyond one year – this system for screening has remained. Ethical review (Nuffield Council of Bioethics, 2017) of this testing technology alerts to the fact that it could be applied to other conditions and disabilities, and as such greater pre-emptive consideration will be required as to whether and how these advances will be implemented. Screening and abortion laws are different around the world, and the Intellectual Disability Nurse will need to be cognizant of these issues and reflect on their personal values and how these might impact on their practice, both with women experiencing these screening processes, and in supporting Midwives and Obstetric services with ensuring services provide person-centred and evidence-based information on experience of having a child with Down's syndrome.

Parents with intellectual disabilities

Evidence indicates approximately 0.4% of parents have an intellectual disability and that this number has steadily increased since the turn of the century (Wing Man, Wade and Llewellyn, 2017; Leaviss et al., 2011), however, women with intellectual disabilities experience poorer pregnancy outcomes and are over-represented in care proceedings (Cox, Stenfert-Kroese and Evans, 2015), with between 40–60% having children taken into care (Wilson et al., 2013). Parenting capacity assessments are triggered due to concerns for the welfare of the child, with suggestion that women with intellectual disabilities often have to offer a greater level of assurance as to their abilities to undertake childcare.

Cox *et al.* (2021) have identified that resolving some of these issues required service level adjustments to the support that is provided, which included ensuring parents with intellectual disabilities are identified and effectively supported through the maternity pathway, that they were prepared for parenthood through tailoring communication and courses and supporting the progress into parenthood through collaborative and coordinated care. As a result, a Maternity toolkit named 'The Together Project' (Health Education England and University of Surrey, 2020) has been co-created and was well evaluated. Similarly, adaptations of standard support systems often appear to produce constructive and worthwhile impacts for parents with intellectual disabilities in the longer term. Glazemaker and Deboutte's (2013) project to adjust the Positive Parenting Programme for a group of 30 parents with intellectual disabilities identified that participants expressed reductions in distress and maladaptive parenting, and ultimately more settled children.

Like all aspect of daily living, the Intellectual Disability Nurse can have a key role in supporting families where parents have an intellectual disability. This can involve making information understandable, advocating, making adjustments and supporting mainstream services to make adjustments, and in working closely with other organisations and agencies. However, this area of practice is complex; nurses will want to be clear about their role, responsibilities, and accountabilities. While their primary focus will be in supporting the parent with intellectual disabilities, they will also have duty of care to the child, and these responsibilities could come into conflict. Nurses new to this area of practice will want to seek support from a more experienced colleague and seek opportunities for reflective supervisory guidance in developing knowledge and skills from the experiences.

Older adults with intellectual disabilities

Globally, increasing numbers of people with intellectual disabilities are now living into older age (Landes, Stevens and Turk, 2021; Walker and Ward, 2013; Hole, Stainton and Wilson, 2013; Doody, Markey and Doody, 2013a), however, the mean age of death in this population is still notably lower than that of their peers in the general population (Doyle 2020). O'Leary *et al.* (2018b) report that a gap of approximately 20 years exists, with greater inequality for women with intellectual disabilities than for men. And with age of death recently found to be 63 years for women and 65 years for men (Haveman, 2019), there is little evidence of closing the gap in age-standardised mortality rates or life expectancy between people with intellectual disabilities and the general population (Emerson *et al.*, 2013). People with mild intellectual disabilities are living longer, as those with mild intellectual disabilities possess the greatest independent functional capacity, and consequently live most frequently into older age (Haveman, 2019; Holland, 2000). Life expectancy remains reduced for those with moderate intellectual disability whereas those with severe and profound intellectual disability and associated complex needs live much shorter lives (Haveman, 2019; Holland, 2000). Life expectancy and mortality rates are important indicators of health status (WHO, 2015a). People with intellectual disabilities are known to die younger and from more avoidable causes amenable to change by good healthcare intervention than the general population (Heslop *et al.*, 2014; Hosking *et al.*, 2016). Adults with intellectual disabilities are known to experience 'premature aging', showing physiological, social, and cognitive signs of aging earlier than what is seen in the general population. For people with intellectual disabilities the ageing process is considered to start at a minimum of 40 years of age (McCarron *et al.*, 2011; Lin *et al.*, 2011), mainly because the frequency of illnesses suffered by people with intellectual disabilities in this age group is likened to that of adults older than 65 years without intellectual disabilities (McCarron *et al.*, 2011; Oviedo *et al.*, 2020). Adults with intellectual disabilities 'as young as 50' can experience levels of health vulnerability not normally experienced until age 80 in the wider population (Schoufour *et al.*, 2013; O'Leary *et al.*, 2018b). Interestingly, at an approximate age of 51, menopause is a highly significant natural transition in a woman's life (Bermingham, 2021). However, research is limited on menopause experience, coping mechanisms and support accessed by women growing older with intellectual disabilities (Chou, Jane Lu and Pu, 2013). An increasing lifespan for people with intellectual disabilities has consequences for an increase in numbers outliving their parents or family carers (Bibby, 2013). Many elderly parent carers now continue to be lifelong caregivers to their adult child with an intellectual disability (Perkins and Haley, 2010). Increasing numbers of sibling carers are simultaneously caring for both their ageing parents and their ageing sibling with an intellectual disability, whilst concurrently rearing a family of their own (McGarrigle, Cronin and Kenny, 2014; Brennan *et al.*, 2018). Many theorists have sought to explain what is happening internally and externally for people as they age. The following Table 3.4 presents a summary of main theories of ageing.

Biological theories of ageing centre on notions illness and decline; for example, age-related physiological consequences such as frailty, falls, depression, diseases, sensory loss, and disability are used to explain ageing (Lennartsson and Heimerson, 2012; Jaul and Barron, 2017). Shifting focus from biological theories, psychosocial theories explain ageing by introducing positive ageing concepts such as 'successful ageing', 'ageing well', 'active ageing', 'positive ageing', 'optimal ageing', and 'healthy ageing' (Rowe and Kahn, 1997). Psychosocial theory's view ageing in terms of individuals striving to maintain well-being through activity, continuity, and prioritisation (McMunn *et al.*, 2006; McCausland, McCallion and McCarron, 2021). Furthermore, psychosocial perspectives on successful ageing recognise that ageing is about adapting to change, with individuals remaining socially engaged within their safe and culturally sensitive community context (Mishra and Barratt, 2016; Thuesen *et al.*, 2021). Conversely, it is widely published that many older adults find themselves subjected to incidents of age-related discrimination and stereotyping which can ultimately affect their self-perceptions of ageing and successful ageing (Giasson *et al.*, 2017). Policies which promote and support people to age healthily and successfully are paramount drivers in societies which now accommodate increasing numbers of ageing populations. Table 3.5 presents a summary of policies related to healthy ageing.

	Psychosocial Theories	
Biological Theories	**Psychological Theories**	**Social Theories**
Wear and Tear (Wiesmann, 1882, cited in Vijg and Kennedy, 2016) Damage from everyday wear eventually exceeds the body's ability to repair itself.	**Maslow's Hierarchy of Need** (1943) A motivation theory – five categories of human needs (physiological, safety, love and belonging, esteem, self-actualisation) dictate an individual's behavior.	**Disengagement Theory** (Cummings and Henry, 1961) Older adults and society mutually withdraw from each other.
Somatic Mutation (Boveri, 1929) Genetic mutations cause cells to malfunction.	**Erikson's Eight Stages of life** (Erikson, 1950, 1982, 1997) Personality develops in a predetermined order through eight stages (infancy to adulthood).	**Activity Theory** (Havinghurst, 1961) Continue social activities of middle age or replace with others for successful ageing.
Metabolic/Caloric Restriction (McCay *et al.*, 1935) A reduction in food intake/calories delays the age-associated decline in physiological fitness and extends the life span	**Expansion of Erikson's Theory** (Peck, 1956) Additional aspects to the older adult's life. Similar to Erikson's conflicts, conflicts in middle/old age. Resolving these conflicts helps one to understand how to successfully arrive at the end of one's life.	**Person-Environment Fit** (Lawton, 1982) Interaction between individual and the environment, the individual influences his or her environment, the environment also affects the individual.
Cross-Linkage (Bjorksten, 1968) Aging results from accumulation of bonds between molecules, resulting in alteration of chemical and biological properties of the cell.	**Jung's Individualism** (Jung, 1960) Individuation is the development of consciousness – the person develops into a unique Individual. One who chooses not to be limited by collective norms.	**Age Stratification** (Riley, 1987) Age structure – Analytical framework for understanding age-related dynamic interplay between people (actors) and roles (social structures).
Free Radical (Harman, 1957) Cells are damaged by free radicals in the environment which eventually impairs their function.	**Selective Optimisation with Compensation** (Baltes and Baltes, 1990) People try to maintain a balance in their lives by looking for ways to compensate for physical/cognitive loss and be more proficient in current activities.	**Continuity Theory** (Atchley, 1989) Personality and behaviour develop over a lifetime and are key to how a person adjusts to ageing.
Endocrine/Neuroendocrine (Dilman, 1971; Dilman *et al.*, 1986) Changes in hormones that control aging lose efficiency leading to the failure of adaptive mechanisms, declining functions and death.	**Gerotranscendence** (Tornstam, 1997) Developmental theory of positive ageing – older adults develop new ways of viewing and experiencing their world.	
Immunological (Walford, 1969) The immune system is programmed to decline over time, leaving people more susceptible to diseases, ageing, and death.		

Table 3.4 Summary of main theories of ageing

Entity	Year	Policy
United Nations	1982	UN First World Assembly on Ageing
	1991	UN Principles for Older Persons
	1999	International Year of Older Persons
	2002	UN Second World Assembly on Ageing, the Madrid International Plan of Action on Ageing (MIPAA) 2002 and the MIPAA+5 and MIPAA+10 Reviews
	2015	UN Sustainable Development Goals (2015) Transforming our world: the 2030 agenda for sustainable development
	2021	Leaving no one behind
World Health Organisation	1984	The Effects of the Indoor Housing Climate on the Health of the Elderly: Report on a WHO Working Group, Graz, Austria, 20–24 September 1982
	2000	Obesity: preventing and managing the global epidemic. Report of a WHO Consultation. WHO Technical Report Series 894. Geneva: World Health Organization
	2002	Active Ageing: A Policy Framework (2002)
	2005	Strengthening active and healthy ageing World Health Assembly resolution
	2007	Demystifying the myths of ageing
	2011	European report on preventing elder maltreatment
WHO (Europe)	2012	Active Ageing Good health adds life to years
	2012	Strategy and action plan for health ageing in Europe 2012–2020
	2015	First World Report on Ageing and Health
	2017	Integrated Care for older people (ICOPE) Guidelines on community-level interventions to manage declines in intrinsic capacity
	2018	Be Healthy, Be Mobile: A handbook on how to implement mAgeing (Mobile Health for Ageing)
	2019	Integrated Care for older people (ICOPE) Guidance on person-centred assessment and pathways in primary care
	2019	Integrated care for older people (ICOPE) Implementation Framework Guidance for Systems and Services
		Global strategy and action plan on ageing and health (2016–2020)
	2020	Decade of healthy ageing: baseline report
Europe	2010	Europe 2020 – Innovation Union (2010) and the European Innovation Partnership on Active and Healthy Ageing (EIP-AHA)
	2011	European report on preventing elder maltreatment
	2011	How to promote active ageing in Europe: EU support to local and regional actors
	2012	Strategy and Action plan for healthy ageing in Europe, 2012–2020
	2016	Creating age-friendly environments in Europe. A tool for local policymakers and planners
	2017	Age-friendly environments in Europe. A handbook of domains for policy action
	2018	Age Friendly environments in Europe: Indicators, monitoring and assessments
	2012	European Year for Active Ageing and Solidarity between Generations

Table 3.5   Policies related to healthy ageing

Entity	Year	Policy
United Kingdom	2000	The Same as You? (10-year programme, Scottish Government)
	2013	The Keys to Life: Improving quality of life for people with intellectual disabilities (Scottish Government)
	2017	People with Intellectual Disabilities in Scotland: Health Needs Assessment Update Report
	2018	National Institute for Health and Care Excellence Care and support of people growing older with intellectual disabilities
Republic of Ireland	1988	The Years Ahead
	1998	Adding Years to Life and Life to Years
	2000	White Paper on Education: Intellectual for Life
	2001	Quality and Fairness
	2005	National Health Promotion Strategy
	2007	Report of the Taskforce on Active Citizenship
	2008	Report of the Interdepartmental Working Group on Long Term Care
	2010	Review of the Recommendations of Protecting our Future: Report of the Working Group on Elder Abuse
	2010	An Garda Síochána Strategy for Older People
	2010	National Clinical Programme for Older People (NCPOP)
	2012	Integrated Care Programme for Older Persons (ICPOP)
	2013	National Positive Ageing Strategy (2013)
	2015	Healthy and Positive Ageing for All Research Strategy 2015–2019
	2016	The 10 Step ICPOP Framework (ICPOP)
	2016	Supporting People's Autonomy: A Guidance Document
	2016	National Standards for Residential Care for Older People in Ireland
	2018	Positive Ageing Indicators for People with an Intellectual Disability
	2019	Housing Options for our Ageing Population Policy Statement
	2019	Focused Policy Assessment No. 8 Prevention and Early Interventions Supporting Health and Well-Being in Older Age
	2020	Ageing and Public Health (2020)

Table 3.5   (Continued)

Healthy ageing for older adults with intellectual disabilities

The World Report on Ageing and Health states that, while there is strong evidence that people today are living longer, there is little consistent evidence to support the suggestion that older people today are experiencing these added years in good health (WHO, 2015a). The Healthy Ageing framework (WHO, 2015a) defined healthy ageing as a process of developing and maintaining the functional ability that enables well-being in older age. Functional ability is having the capabilities to enable people to be and do what they value referred to as their ability to meet their basic needs, to learn, grow and make decisions, to be mobile, to build and maintain relationships, and to contribute to society (Beard *et al.*, 2016; Rudnicka *et al.*, 2020). In Ireland, 'The Intellectual Disability Supplement to the Irish Longitudinal Study on Ageing' (IDS-TILDA) study established in 2008 aimed to identify the principal influences on ageing in people with intellectual disabilities in the Republic of Ireland aged 40 years and above (McCarron *et al.*, 2011). This longitudinal study seeks to characterise and understand changes in ageing by examining healthy and successful ageing, determinants of health and longevity, and similarities or differences in ageing for those with and without intellectual disability using comparative data from the Irish Longitudinal Study on Ageing (TILDA) for the general population (McCarron *et al.*, 2011, 2014, 2020; Brennan *et al.*, 2018). The conceptual framework shown in Figure 3.4 illustrates the range of data collected by IDS-TILDA (IDS-TILDA, 2021).

And in the Republic of Ireland, the National Positive Ageing Indicators (see Figure 3.5) for people with intellectual disability (McGlinchey *et al.*, 2019) highlighted indicators relevant solely to those ageing with intellectual disability in Ireland as well as indicators applicable to the ageing population.

To understand aging well for older adults with intellectual disabilities, one needs to consider a life course approach that considers the historical, political, and social context of their lives. Heller (2004) proposes the Supports-Outcome Model of Aging Well, describing positive aging outcomes as (1) maintaining

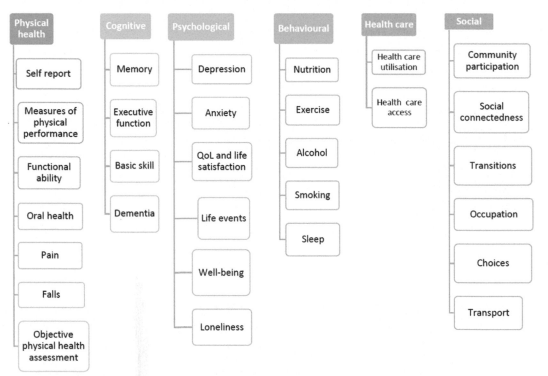

Figure 3.4   Source: IDS-TILDA (2021, p. 3)

IDS-TILDA conceptual framework.

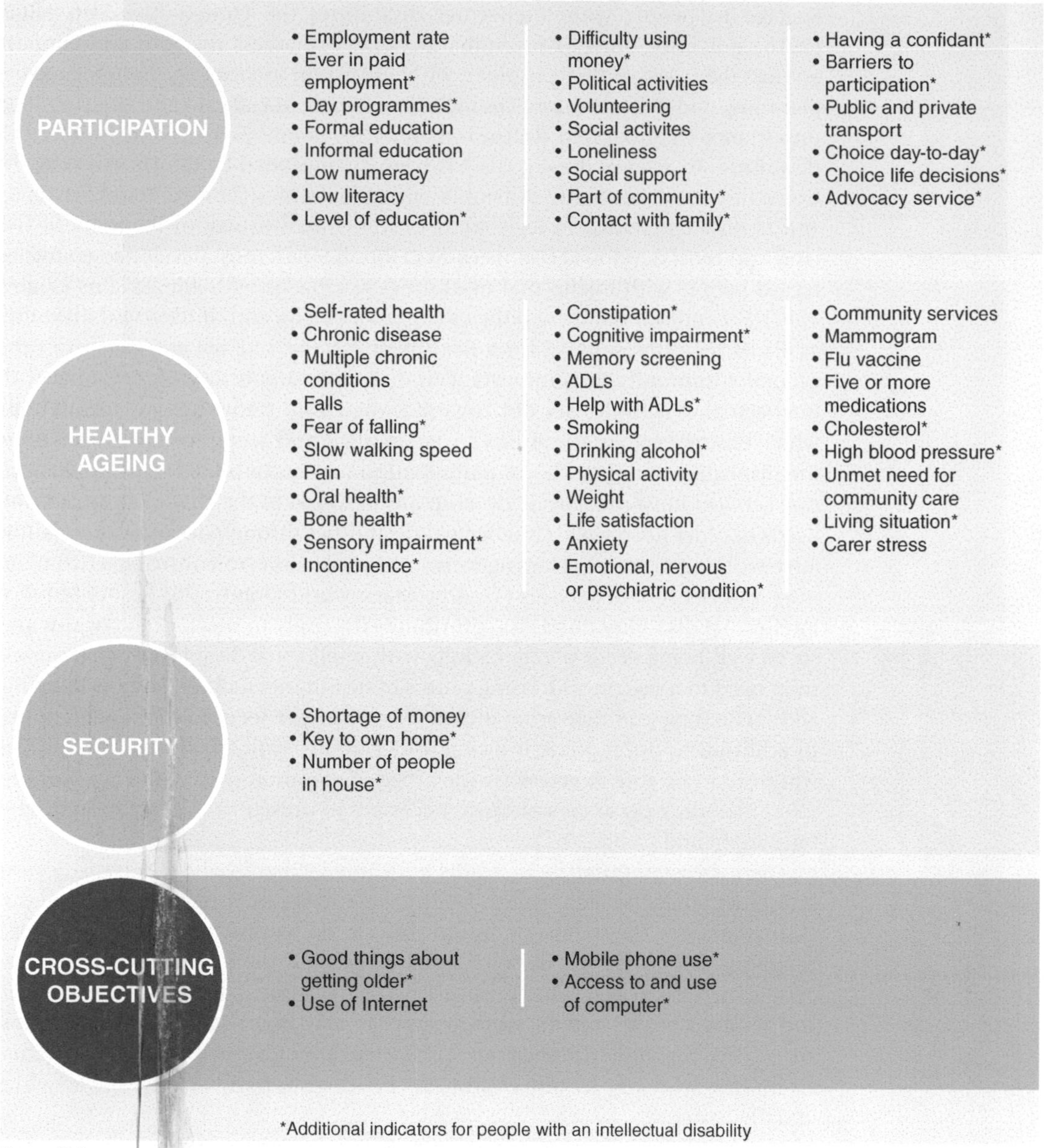

PARTICIPATION
- Employment rate
- Ever in paid employment*
- Day programmes*
- Formal education
- Informal education
- Low numeracy
- Low literacy
- Level of education*

- Difficulty using money*
- Political activities
- Volunteering
- Social activites
- Loneliness
- Social support
- Part of community*
- Contact with family*

- Having a confidant*
- Barriers to participation*
- Public and private transport
- Choice day-to-day*
- Choice life decisions*
- Advocacy service*

HEALTHY AGEING
- Self-rated health
- Chronic disease
- Multiple chronic conditions
- Falls
- Fear of falling*
- Slow walking speed
- Pain
- Oral health*
- Bone health*
- Sensory impairment*
- Incontinence*

- Constipation*
- Cognitive impairment*
- Memory screening
- ADLs
- Help with ADLs*
- Smoking
- Drinking alcohol*
- Physical activity
- Weight
- Life satisfaction
- Anxiety
- Emotional, nervous or psychiatric condition*

- Community services
- Mammogram
- Flu vaccine
- Five or more medications
- Cholesterol*
- High blood pressure*
- Unmet need for community care
- Living situation*
- Carer stress

SECURITY
- Shortage of money
- Key to own home*
- Number of people in house*

CROSS-CUTTING OBJECTIVES
- Good things about getting older*
- Use of Internet

- Mobile phone use*
- Access to and use of computer*

*Additional indicators for people with an intellectual disability

Figure 3.5

Republic of Ireland, the National Positive Ageing Indicators.

health and function and, (2) active engagement with life (Heller, 2004; Heller and Harris, 2012). These outcomes are dependent upon the interaction of a person's capabilities, their physical and emotional health and function, supports received and home, work, and community environments. Hence, aging is a dynamic process with individuals not only experiencing aging-related health changes but also changes in their supports and environments (Heller, 2019).

Specific to people with intellectual disabilities the United Kingdom NICE (2018) guideline aims to support individuals to access the care and support services they need as they get older, with a focus on identifying changing needs, planning, and delivering services including health, social care and housing. The importance of supported decision-making to enable people with intellectual disabilities to achieve these goals has been championed by the United Nations Convention on the Rights of People with Disabilities (United Nations, 2006) and is now embedded in legislation of the United Kingdom Republic of Ireland and most developed countries. Social policies in most developed countries regard people with intellectual disabilities as citizens with equal rights (Bigby, 2010). By implication, these policies suggest a person with intellectual disability avails of the same support for a healthy and active old age as a person in the general community. It is important that services supporting older adults with intellectual disabilities set out organisational care standards and regulations which ensure persons: the ability to age in place and access to care informed by the principles of rights, choice participation and autonomy. Health and social care services must proactively develop and respond to the changing profile and needs of older people with intellectual disabilities through developing collaborative working practices across agencies and professions to ensure effective planning and delivery of services (Doody, Markey and Doody, 2013a, 2013b). For intellectual disability nurses to contribute effectively to meeting the health and social well-being needs of older adults with intellectual disabilities, such nurses' roles need to focus on addressing causes of health inequalities, such as housing, and facilitating and delivering inclusive service-user focused care and support. In addition to appropriate housing, older adults with intellectual disabilities will need to be able to access a wide range of community care and support services, including personal assistance necessary to prevent social isolation (Shaw, Cartwright and Craig, 2011).

The increasing numbers of adults with intellectual disabilities transitioning into older adults is significant to health and social care roles of intellectual disability nurses in the context of radical shifts in policy and practice in the United Kingdom and in the Republic of Ireland. As with the general population, as people increase in age, issues regarding work, retirement, loss and bereavement, and reduced health and social care support may occur (Glaesser and Perkins, 2013). This presents challenges and difficulties for older people with intellectual disabilities who may require continuing lifelong support with routine activities of daily living.

Retirement

Older people with intellectual disabilities remain mostly invisible in mainstream retirement research and policy (Heller, 2019). The employment rates of people with intellectual disabilities are recorded as low (approximately 6% in the UK in 2015) (Bigby, 2021). Of those employed working in supported employment schemes tends to be the norm (McDermott and Edwards, 2012). A substantial decrease in rates of employment have been noted for people with intellectual disabilities due to the onset of age-related mobility impairments such as increased difficulties with travel or undertaking work tasks (Stancliffe *et al.*, 2019). For many people with intellectual disabilities retirement is more likely to be a sudden, unplanned, and involuntary event (Engeland, Kittelsaa and Langballe, 2018; Stancliffe *et al.*, 2019). In countries such as Ireland, the United States and Australia, adults with intellectual disabilities continue to rely heavily on day centres for engagement in regular activities and social connections (Stancliffe, Kramme, and Nye-Lengerman, 2018). In Scotland, while people must retire from day services at the age of 65, there are suggestions for continued informal day service access for these retirees (Engeland, Kittelsaa and Langballe, 2018). Studies from Ireland and the UK also suggest that day centres are the most common type of service used by older people with intellectual disabilities (McConkey *et al.*, 2018). The significance of day centres in terms of social connections for older people is reinforced by data from a representative sample of older people with intellectual disabilities in Ireland. More than two in five older people had no friends outside their own home, and although most had some contact with family, they did not participate with them in social activities, and relied on support staff for engagement in social activities (McCausland *et al.*, 2016). Early research on the retirement transition has largely focused on financial conditions and physical health and less on psychological aspects, but this trend has changed in recent years as more interest in psychological factors has been noted (Shultz and Wang, 2011). In the United Kingdom and in the Republic of Ireland the promotion of rights, choice, inclusion, and independence have been essential values of health and social care service provision for people with intellectual disabilities for a considerable time. There is very limited support for older people with intellectual disabilities working in these supported employment schemes to make intentional and informed decisions about their retirement. It is important that transition planning from sheltered or other forms of supported employment or day service types take account of the health and social care needs of older adults with intellectual disabilities. Systems to enable successful transition to retirement for older adults with intellectual disabilities will need to focus on the individuals' perspectives of retirement and individual support to enable people in making informed choices about their retirement. Reforms of disability service systems such as individualised funding schemes have the potential to enable support to be adapted to individual need and allow flexibility in possibilities for individuals to participate in a range of programmes, activities, groups, and voluntary roles (Bigby, 2021). Intellectual disability nurses working with older adults with intellectual disabilities have a significant role in promoting and facilitating active ageing. In addition, nurses at all levels of health and social care can play a useful role in informing policies and strategies that need to be implemented to ensure that appropriate services are delivered to older adults with intellectual disabilities.

Health and social well-being needs of older adults with intellectual disabilities

As people age, they are more likely to experience health conditions such as visual and hearing impairments, osteoarthritis, back and neck pain, chronic obstructive pulmonary disease, diabetes, depression, and dementia (WHO, 2018).

Many older adults experience multimorbidity, defined as two or more chronic conditions in the same individual (van den Akker, Buntinx and Knottnerus, 1996). Older adults are more likely to present with complex health states which are commonly regarded as 'geriatric syndromes', including frailty, urinary incontinence, falls, delirium, and pressure ulcers (WHO, 2018). Depression and anxiety are two of the most common mental disorders affecting older people, with 7 and 3.8% of the world's older population being affected, respectively (WHO, 2015a). As previously mentioned, the reality of greater life longevity now exists for people with intellectual disabilities. And emerging research is now beginning to detail similarities and differences in patterns of ageing for people with intellectual disabilities when compared to their peers in the general population. Apart from 'premature ageing' older adults with intellectual disabilities also experience high rates of health risk factors such as obesity (Ryan et al., 2021), physical inactivity (van Schijndel-Speet et al., 2017), sedentary lifestyles (Carmeli, 2015), loneliness and poor emotional health (Wormald et al., 2019). Older adults with intellectual disabilities are more frequently affected by certain chronic health conditions such as respiratory disease (Axmon, Höglund and Ahlström, 2017), cardiovascular disease (De Winter et al., 2016), epilepsy (Monaghan et al., 2021), gastrointestinal tract anomalies such as constipation (Morad et al., 2007), dementia (Arvio), kidney disease (De Winter et al., 2014), osteoarticular disorders such as osteoporosis (Fritz, Edwards and Jacob, 2021), and thyroid disorders (Hermans et al., 2013), some of which they have endured throughout their life. Furthermore, people with intellectual disabilities are more prone to accidents and associated injuries than their peers in the general population. Depression and anxiety are considered common disorders in individuals with intellectual disabilities, and they frequently occur together (Hsieh, Scott and Murthy, 2020). McCarron et al. (2013) report multi-morbidity rates as high as 63% in their study sample. The leading cause of death for adults with intellectual disability is frequently reported as respiratory disease, followed closely by, or superseded by, heart disease, then followed in varying order by neoplasms, external causes of death and diseases of the nervous system (Glover et al., 2017; Heslop et al., 2014; O'Leary et al., 2018a; Oppewal et al., 2018). Landes, Stevens and Turk (2021) found that, regardless of the severity of the disability, adults with intellectual disabilities had substantially higher risk of death from pneumonitis, influenza/pneumonia and choking, whereas those with mild/moderate intellectual disabilities a higher risk of death from diabetes mellitus. In a life course perspective, there are also cumulative effects of health inequalities that compound over time. Inequities in determinants of social well-being for people with intellectual disabilities are reported as: access to appropriate housing and poor neighbourhood cohesion (Beard et al., 2009) and poverty (Commission on Social Determinants of Health, 2008). Healthy aging is about creating the environments and opportunities that enable people to be and do what they value throughout their lives (WHO, 2019b). Adults with intellectual disabilities as a group with generally low incomes and who experience discrimination often feel socially excluded and are less likely to engage in community activities (Emerson et al., 2011). Moreover, adults with intellectual disabilities often lack health knowledge (i.e., health literacy) about what contributes to healthy lifestyles (Kuijken et al., 2016).

For many people with intellectual disabilities such health inequalities begin early in their lives, and their cumulative effect and adverse health outcomes inevitably impact most heavily as they get older (McCausland, McCallion and McCarron, 2021). This is particularly common with underdiagnosed or inadequately managed preventable health conditions (Haverman *et al.*, 2011), which in many cases lead to premature deaths. To characterise health complexity, some who study the aging process in adults with intellectual disabilities have turned to measures of frailty (Schoufour *et al.*, 2013; McKenzie *et al.*, 2017).

As the population of older adults with intellectual disabilities increases, intellectual disability nurses need to play a significant role in understanding frailty in the context of caring for older adults with intellectual disabilities and in early screening, assessment, and diagnosis of preventable conditions, along with symptomatic treatment of manageable long-term conditions. Intellectual disability nurses need to ensure older adults with intellectual disability receive appropriate and timely access to services and promote health and social well-being of older adults with intellectual disabilities (Dixon-Ibarra, Lee and Dugala, 2013; Krinsky-McHale and Silverman, 2013). Collection, analysis and dissemination of good quality data on health conditions experienced by people with an intellectual disability is essential to influence, shape and resource future planning, policies, services, and supports to meet the health needs of people with intellectual disabilities (McCarron *et al.*, 2018).

Loss

Loss can be an incredibly painful, complex, and confusing mix of experiences for someone with intellectual disabilities (Read, 2014; Young, 2017). Types of loss are attributed to loss of a significant loved or valued person; loss of a part of self – including several physical, social, and role-related losses; loss of external objects and loss as encountered by human beings as they mature from infancy to old age (Peretz, 1970). As adults with intellectual disabilities age, they are more likely to experience a greater number of losses. Feelings of loss represent an emotional response to separation from subjectively important persons or things (Yang and Lee, 2012). The longer a person with intellectual disability lives, the more likely they are to experience the loss of significant people or the death of someone important (Blackman, 2002, 2013, 2016). As many individuals with intellectual disabilities are now beginning to outlive their parents (Clute, 2010, 2017), approximately 54% of people with intellectual disability experience the death of their parents (Rodríguez *et al.*, 2018). People with intellectual disabilities are more likely to experience peer deaths (Emerson *et al.*, 2012a). Secondary losses refer to the additional losses experienced following bereavement. These can be substantial (loss of the family home) or more subtle (loss of family rituals). Secondary losses can be momentous for the individual but are often unrecognised by others, which can compound the original grief (Blackman, 2008). When experiencing bereavement, people with intellectual disabilities are particularly vulnerable because they are usually dependent upon others to facilitate their bereavement needs (Read and Elliott, 2003) and provide them with factually correct information (McEvoy *et al.*, 2017; Thorp *et al.*, 2017). It has been suggested that the presence of intellectual disability is a strong predictor of mental health problems following the loss of a loved one (Bonell-Pascual *et al.*, 1999; Rodríguez *et al.*, 2018; Emerson *et al.*, 2012b; Thorp *et al.*, 2017). Literature suggests that spirituality and religion can provide meaning and purpose to life, support people with intellectual disabilities during stressful life events, and comfort at times such as when a bereavement occurs (Stancliffe *et al.*, 2015; Wiese *et al.*, 2015).

Historically, people with intellectual disabilities have been excluded from end-of-life services. Many people with intellectual disabilities are not informed of the deaths of friends or family and may be excluded from associated rituals (McRitchie *et al.*, 2014). Similarly, people with intellectual disabilities have often been excluded from discussions around their own mortality, terminal diagnosis, and terminal care (Tuffrey-Wijne, 2013). Possible reasons for excluding people with intellectual disabilities have been identified as: the person having difficulty understanding or not fully appreciating the timescale of the illness; fear of the person becoming upset and or being harmed psychologically; avoiding potential burden on the individual; caregiver difficulty or discomfort in managing their own emotions; lack of caregiver knowledge, skill, training or resources – not knowing what to say; organisational constraints, confidentiality issues and absent/unclear disability service policies (Lord, Field and Smith, 2017; Ryan *et al.*, 2010; Tuffrey-Wijne, 2013; Wiese *et al.*, 2013, 2015). While some people with intellectual disabilities have limited understanding of death (McEvoy *et al.*, 2017; Stancliffe *et al.*, 2015), not having opportunities to learn about end of life perpetuates misunderstandings that may contribute to complicated grief (Dodd *et al.*, 2008).

Involving people with intellectual disabilities when death is predictable has been highlighted as beneficial (Ryan *et al.*, 2010). Involvement in bereavement rituals can be positive for people with intellectual disabilities (Hall, 2014) including viewing the body, attending funerals, visiting the grave and reminiscing about the deceased (McEvoy *et al.*, 2017; McRitchie *et al.*, 2014), helping the person accept the reality of loss (Gilrane-McGarry and Taggart, 2007), expressing their grief and recalling positive memories of the deceased (Gray and Abendroth, 2016) offering a sense of finality, and facilitating opportunity for continuing bonds with the deceased (Morgan and McEvoy, 2014). Staff in intellectual disability services should be well placed to recognise and support issues of bereavement (Dodd *et al.*, 2008; Wiese *et al.*, 2013) and people with intellectual disabilities' own mortality (Wiese *et al.*, 2013). Most staff working in intellectual disability services will be confronted with people with intellectual disabilities who need support around death, dying and bereavement (Tuffrey-Wijne and Watchman, 2015) and support provided must be adapted to the individual person's cognitive understanding, communication style and need (Tuffrey-Wijne, 2013). It is, however, important to recognise that people with intellectual disabilities will go through the grieving process like any other person who has suffered the loss of a close relation. It could be argued that perhaps because of cognitive limitations, older adults' ability to cope with loss would require more support. McEvoy *et al.* (2017) and Tuffrey-Wijne (2013), emphasise that the level of involvement should be responsive to individuals' preferences, as some people may prefer not to participate in some respects. Intellectual disability nurses need to understand the spiritual and religious needs of individuals and engage strategies to support the person, their families, peers, and carers to cope in times of anticipated loss, loss, or bereavement. Like any other older adult, older adults with intellectual disabilities have a fundamental human right to be supported to know about death and dying (Wiese *et al.*, 2013). Older adults with intellectual disabilities will need to be prepared physically, emotionally and psychologically to adjust to the age-related losses and stressors that may result in alterations to their thinking, experiences and actions (Kessel *et al.*, 2002).

Coping with and minimising the impact of aging and loss that may lead to emotional and psychological problems for older adults with intellectual disabilities will require:

- End-of-life education from appropriately trained professionals
- Grief counseling
- Bereavement services
- Responsive end-of-life care services.

BOX 3.9
CASE STUDY 3.1

John Jacobs is a 53-year-old man with a Down syndrome and a moderate intellectual disability. His parents, who have been his sole carers for most of his life, are both now well into their 80s and require health and social care support now, so they visit less often. His sister Anne, to whom he was close, died a year ago from cancer. A year ago, John moved from living at home into a group residential home, with three other males who are older than him and supported by experienced carers who provide assistance with his self-care and daily activities. Since he was 25 years old John has worked in a local sheltered employment scheme and makes a small contribution into his pension.

John and his support worker Thomas attend his scheduled three-monthly meeting with his community intellectual disability nurse, Luke who has known John for over 11 years. Thomas reports that he is concerned by recent changes in John's behaviour. Over the last two months John has become disinterested in going to work

and when at work has been struggling to cope with expectations, tending to become stressed and agitated, which has not previously been normal behaviour for John. John's employer is concerned that he can no longer cope with the job. Thomas also reports that John is less engaged in activities at home and is now failing to complete tasks which he has previously enjoyed and been good at. He no longer takes part in bingo nights and is requesting to spend more time in his room. John is having accidents, with incontinence and faecal soiling needing prompting with self-care, which is also not normal for him. Luke is acutely aware that there have been numerous recent changes in John's life. John is finding the loss of personal and social skills difficult to cope with and staff are concerned that he is getting depressed. They are also concerned that the level of his health needs requires him to be in a nursing home rather than a residential home. Luke draws on available information in nursing care plans and subjective opinions from others. Using the nursing process he coordinates the development of a revised plan of care and makes appropriate referrals. What is your opinion of what is going on with John, and how you help Luke and John?

Box 3.10
Student Activity 3.3

a. Given what you have learned so far in this chapter, discuss your understanding of ageing as applicable to John's situation.

b. Explore the role of intellectual disability nurses in meeting John's health and social well-being needs. You need to consider this in the wider context of the complex health, health and social well-being needs of older adults with intellectual disabilities.

c. Given John's age, consider the intellectual disability nursing roles in supporting John if it is recommended that he transition services (e.g., if it is recommended that John go to a nursing home), challenges the key worker will have to address if John is assessed as needing to be cared for in a nursing home rather than a residential home.

d. Given what you have learned so far in this chapter, explore the role an intellectual disability nurse will play in meeting John's health and social care needs. You need to consider this in the wider context of the complex health and healthcare needs of older adults with intellectual disabilities.

e. Identify and describe the roles of the health and social care professionals who may need to be involved in this case.

Intellectual disability nurses must be vigilant for the increasing frailty likely to be experienced by many older adults with intellectual disabilities and work to ensure health promotion and disease prevention while enabling the person to live in their communities and access appropriate and timely healthcare ensuring health and well-being. Intellectual disability nurses engage the nursing process when caring for adults growing older with intellectual disabilities, advocate and make referrals when required, communicate and coordinate care liaising between person, family, multidisciplinary team, specialists, and other agencies as required ensuring access to appropriate healthcare. Intellectual disability nurses have important roles in providing training and support for care staff working directly with older adults with intellectual disabilities. Intellectual disability nurses will need to develop adequate coordination skills to ensure that older adults with intellectual disabilities experiencing the various effects of ageing are appropriately supported.

The *People with Intellectual Disabilities in Scotland: 2017 Health Needs Assessment Update Report* (Truesdale and Brown, 2017) presents a broad overview of the evidence of health needs of adults with intellectual disabilities as presented in Box 3.4

Box 3.11 Health needs of adults with intellectual disabilities

1. Accidents
2. Bone Health
3. Cardiovascular Disease

4. Communication
5. Diabetes
6. Epilepsy
7. Gastrointestinal Disorders
8. Hematological Disorders
9. Infections
10. Mobility, Balance, Coordination, and Foot Care
11. Nutrition
12. Obesity & Metabolic Disorders
13. Oral and Dental health
14. Physical Activity
15. Respiratory Disorders
16. Sensory Impairments
17. Visual/Hearing Impairments
18. Sleep Disorders
19. Sexuality & Sexual Health
20. Mental Ill-Health
21. Behaviour Challenges
22. Dementia
23. Forensic Care & People Who Offend
24. Life Events & Trauma
25. Pharmacotherapy
26. Psychological Intervention
27. Health Checks
28. Healthy Lifestyles, Health Improvement & Health Promotion

End-of-life and people with intellectual disabilities

When compared to their peers in the wider population people with intellectual disabilities tend to have higher morbidity rates, experience greater healthcare disparities, premature deaths, and are more likely to die unexpectedly and to die from conditions that are treatable (Doyle *et al.*, 2021; Heslop *et al.*, 2014; Williamson *et al.*, 2017). Many children with intellectual disabilities are born with a life-limiting condition (LLC) and many young people with intellectual disabilities, who have a life-limiting condition, are now frequently surviving due to advances in healthcare (National End of Life Care Programme, 2011). Life-limiting conditions have been defined by International Children's Palliative Care Network as conditions for which there is no cure and death is inevitable, either in childhood or early adulthood and where some life-limiting illnesses progress quickly, and others may cause a slow deterioration over many years

(ICPCN, 2020). The burden of life-limiting conditions increases with age, with one in three adults suffering from multiple chronic conditions (MCC) (Marengoni *et al.*, 2011), and from a UK perspective, the proportion of people living with four or more diseases is predicted to almost double between 2015 and 2035 (Kingston *et al.*, 2018). When compared to the general population the impact of life-limiting conditions can be higher for people with intellectual disabilities and especially those with multiple and complex needs who are more likely to experience higher rates of hospitalisation and readmissions (Schalock *et al.*, 2007; Balogh *et al.*, 2018; Lunsky *et al.*, 2019). Increases in hospitalisations and death from conditions that are treatable have been reported to be caused by discrimination, poor access to or acquisition of primary care and a lack of care coordination (Glover *et al.*, 2017; Hosking *et al.*, 2016).

As people with intellectual disabilities, especially those with life-limiting conditions approach end of life, intellectual disability nurses must provide support by anticipating and addressing their needs, coordinating support, communicating appropriately, respecting their autonomy to make informed choices about their life and when necessary, advocating on their behalf, especially at end of life. Specifically, intellectual disability nurses provide comfort care by doing basic nursing care, for example bathing, hair/mouth care, and emotional support, whilst upholding the person's dignity. Additionally, at the end of life a primary focus for intellectual disability nurses is the management of pain and symptoms, and provision of psychosocial and spiritual care.

The World Health Organisation advocates for countries to establish integrated care systems which ensure individuals across the lifespan living with long-term conditions and end-of-life care requirements are adequately supported in their communities. In Ireland the '*Integrated Model of Care for the Prevention and Management of Chronic Disease*' is at the heart of the '*National Framework for the Integrated Prevention and Management of Chronic Disease*' and demonstrates how 'end-to-end' care can be provided within the Irish health services (HSE, 2020). In the UK '*Ambitions for Palliative and End of Life Care: A national framework for local action 2021–2026 framework*' (NHS, 2021), complimented with '*Delivering high quality end of life care for people who have an intellectual disability*' (Palliative Care for People with Disabilities (2017) set out aims for quality end-of-life care and provide information on resources and tips for commissioners, service providers and health and social care staff who care for people with intellectual disabilities at the end-of-life. People with intellectual disabilities with life-limiting illnesses are as entitled to receive good end-of-life care in places of their choice as any other terminally ill individual (Reddall, 2010). Person-centeredness is a vital component of healthcare quality, particularly near the end of life when care is provided to people with intellectual disabilities and their families who have widely varying treatment goals and preferences. However, inadequacies of the current approaches to end-of-life and palliative care for people with intellectual disabilities have been noted (Ryan *et al.*, 2010). The 'Confidential Inquiry into Premature Deaths of People with Intellectual Disabilities' (Heslop *et al.*, 2013) found that people with intellectual disabilities receive poor end-of-life care when compared with their nondisabled counterparts and has recommended good practice in the end-of-life care of people with intellectual disabilities (Marriot, Marriott and Heslop, 2013). End-of-life or palliative care is often complex: in terms of morbidity, presenting symptoms, interventions to be applied, and of the type and number of service providers involved (Meyer, 2019). It is important to acknowledge that providing end-of-life care for people with intellectual disabilities can be complex and challenging for both the professionals and relatives involved (Read, 1998). Many healthcare professionals not educated in the field of intellectual disabilities often struggle to communicate with a dying person with intellectual disabilities, or their family members, due to cultural prejudices, the individual's complex clinical conditions, and a lack of knowledge and skills regarding how to hold such a conversation (Sue, Mazzotta and Grier, 2019). In addition, it has been observed that healthcare professionals caring for terminally ill people with intellectual disabilities are generally unaware of the meaning of end-of-life care in practice or how they can support people with intellectual disabilities to access palliative care support (Reddall, 2010; Reilly, Raymond and O'Donnell, 2020).

Intellectual disability nurses have professional responsibilities to ensure quality end-of-life and palliative care to people with intellectual disabilities and their families, grounded in the essence of nursing practice and supported by the Nursing and Midwifery Council in the UK and the Nursing and Midwifery Board of Ireland's code of ethics. Intellectual disability nurses are crucial to the provision of comprehensive person-centred care supporting their needs and personal wishes, inclusive of timely and appropriate assessment and treatment of physical, emotional, spiritual health and well-being. Intellectual disability nurses must be vigilant in the recognition of changes in the health status of the individual, identifying when to necessitate the introduction of palliative care. Intellectual disability nurses have a pivotal role in coordinating multidisciplinary care approaches for people with intellectual disabilities and palliative care needs. Crucial to the role is the timely referral of the individual to specialist palliative care support accessed via intellectual or intellectual disability palliative care specialist nurses and other palliative care specialists to ensure quality of life for the person. When a person dies intellectual disability nurses ensure the person's body is treated with utmost dignity respectful of individual and family cultural and spiritual preferences and provides bereavement support to family members.

Intellectual disability nurses and other healthcare professionals caring for terminally ill or potentially terminally ill people with intellectual disabilities will find 'the dying trajectory' useful (Brown *et al.*, 2005) (see Figure 3.6). 'The dying trajectory' is important in that it provides a framework for assessing the possibility of terminal illness where there is significant alteration of a person with an intellectual disability's health status. Considering evidence from a study by Ng and Li (2003) showing that 50% of the professionals who had cared for terminally ill people with profound intellectual disabilities were unable to identify signs and symptoms of end of life, this framework is an indispensable tool for professionals, such as intellectual disability nurses, working in a variety of settings. The use of this framework is likely to prevent the delay in the diagnosis of terminal illness that may impact the provision of appropriate palliative care in the right environment. Healthcare professionals who work with people with intellectual disabilities who require end-of-life care have advocated the availability of appropriate frameworks and guidelines (Morton-Nance

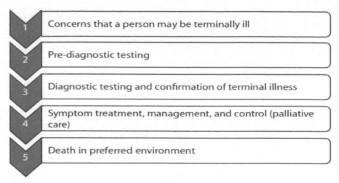

Figure 3.6   *Source:* Adapted from Brown *et al.*, (2010)

The dying trajectory.

and Schafer, 2012). Successful provision of end-of-life and palliative care for people with intellectual disabilities will require person-centred modifications of current approaches. The Confidential Inquiry into Premature Deaths of People with Intellectual Disabilities (Heslop *et al.*, 2013) highlighted the need to address inequalities experienced by people with intellectual disabilities with life-limiting conditions through improved joint working and coordination, reasonable adjustments, advance planning, shared decision-making, and proactive assessments (Marriott, Marriott and Heslop, 2013).

Breaking the news

While life expectancy remains stubbornly low compared to people with similar health condition in the rest of the population (University of Bristol, 2018), practice debates and discussion pertaining to the sharing of bad news with people with intellectual disabilities about diagnoses and prognoses remain. Truth telling initiatives and activities (Tuffrey-Wijne and Watchman, 2015) are generally accepted to be enabling individuals' autonomy toward end of life, however, evidence indicates that non-disclosure is still prevalent in practice. According to Lord *et al.* (2017) staff will often avoid conversations relating to death due to a lack of confidence and experience in managing this topic.

Brownrigg's (2018) review of the literature highlights the ethical considerations associated with this area of practice, indicating that different stakeholder groups would disclose a greater or lesser amount of information depending on the individual's perceived ability to understand. However, when considering outcomes, patients, families, and carers often spoke of more positively regarding circumstances where they had greater choice and control of aspects of care. According to Tuffrey-Wijne and Watchman (2015) communicating news of a terminal diagnosis to an individual with intellectual disabilities sensitively but with clarity, can be complex. Their model for this important element of practice guides intellectual disabilities nurses in being able to undertake the activity, to model this for others and to teach, train and support carers and families with doing the same. Chunking the information in elements relating to the individual's background knowledge of illness and death, memories, and life experiences, and linking this to their understanding of what is happening to them now including their diagnosis, and how this might impact on their life in the future. These elements of the conversation need to be prioritised, and planned out, with a requirement to ensure that clarifying questions are employed to check retention and comprehension. Within this model, sufficient forethought will be required to ensure the communication is adapted for the individual's understanding and involve the relevant family members and carers to ensure the clarity of and consistency of understanding.

Similarly, friends and peers, sometimes fellow residents, will be aware of the individual's deterioration in health and consideration will need to be given to the sharing of this information. Wherever possible the individual and/or a member of the family should be consulted as to the wishes of the individual. In a residential care service, carers and nurses will need to be prepared for potential conflicts of interest as to the amount of information they might be able to share with concerned friends. The welfare of those around the individual will also need to be considered, and nurses may have a role in supporting the bereavement process of people with learning disabilities, families and carers. There are some excellent contemporary resources available for nurses to undertake this work directly or teaching and training families and care teams in exploring their own grief and enabling others to do the same.

End-of-life decisions

The United Nations Convention on the Rights of People with Disabilities (2006) enshrines the capacity of people with intellectual disabilities for social, physical, emotional, and intellectual development. In doing so, concepts of autonomy and independence have become central structures in supporting people with intellectual disabilities make informed decisions (Carey and Ryan, 2019). Infusing values of self-determination and choice can be challenging when people experience complex communication needs, impaired social interaction, and limited experience of choice in addition to difficulty making informed choices for themselves (Bigby *et al.*, 2004) and even more so at the end of life. Supported decision-making frameworks have been developed to involve people with intellectual disabilities in meaningful ways enabling them to provide informed consent (Bach and Kerzner, 2010; Flynn and Arstein-Kerslake, 2014; Carey and Ryan, 2019). To uphold the right of self-determination for people with intellectual disabilities, especially for those at the end-of-life, intellectual disability must be equipped with skills to support the person make decisions. It is vitally important for these nurses to understand and apply the principles of the United Nations Convention on the Rights of People with Disabilities (United Nations, 2006) in line with national legislation, e.g., Mental Capacity Act 2005 in the United Kingdom. In Ireland the Assisted Decision Making (Capacity) Act 2015 requires legally recognised decision-makers to support a person to maximise their decision-making powers and places a legal requirement on service providers to enable a person to decide through the provision of a range of supports and information tailored to individual need (McCarron *et al.*, 2018).

Having a central role in supporting people with intellectual disabilities and their families make decisions about end of life, intellectual disability nurses are ideally placed to provide education, commence discussions, and engage people with intellectual disabilities to plan and prepare for end-of-life decisions. This process ensures foundations for and development of Advance Care Plans, long before these decisions are required to be made. Planning and preparing for end-of-life decisions encompass identifying the personal preferences and priorities of a person with an intellectual disability in relation to possibilities of terminal diagnosis and associated treatment goals, circles of support, living arrangements, place of death, and funeral arrangements along with other individual aspirations so as to be prepared should the person undergo diagnostic testing and receive confirmation of a terminal illness. Advance Care Planning (ACP) has been found to have had positive outcomes for people with intellectual disabilities, in terms of discussing matters at people's own pace, getting support to make their own choices, having the process adapted to who they are, and continually working to shape life choices of their choosing (McKenzie *et al.*, 2017). Once such plans have been initiated and are in place, they can be updated in the event of the person undergoing diagnostic testing and receiving confirmation of a terminal illness.

All healthcare professionals involved in end-of-life decisions need to have knowledge and experience of the healthcare needs and preferences of the person with intellectual disabilities. Noorlandt *et al.* (2021) propose that when medical decisions are required for people with intellectual disabilities in the palliative phase, Shared Decision-Making (SDM) has been identified as the preferred practice. Shared decision-making is a process in which healthcare professionals communicate and collaborate effectively with the person, family and care providers, to discuss care and treatment options and enable a person to reach a decision about their care (National Institute for Health and Care Excellence (NICE) (2021a, 2021b). This process of shared decision-making is important because it provides an inclusive framework, which ensures that the person with an intellectual disability, his or her family, and his or her carers are central to the end-of-life and palliative care interventions (see Figure 3.7).

Knowledgeable about the preferences of people with intellectual disabilities, their families, and their carers, working multidisciplinary, interdisciplinary, and transdisciplinary platforms, intellectual disability nurses are ideally placed to advocate with and for people with intellectual disabilities in end-of-life care decisions. Noorlandt *et al.* (2021) provide an aid for shared decision-making with people with intellectual disabilities in the palliative phase.

Palliative care and people with intellectual disabilities

The World Health Organisation (WHO) defines palliative care as an approach that improves the quality of life of persons and their families facing the problems associated with life threatening illness, through the prevention and relief of suffering by means of early identification and impeccable assessment and treatment of pain and other problems, physical, psychosocial and spiritual

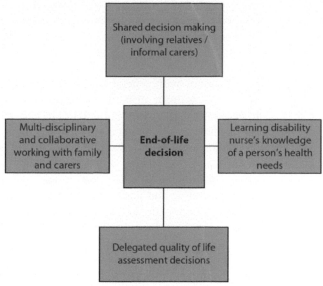

Figure 3.7 *Source:* Adapted from Wagemans *et al.* (2013)

Factors affecting end-of-life decisions for people with intellectual disabilities.

(Rudnicka *et al.*, 2020). Palliative care is applicable early in the course of ill-ness, in conjunction with other therapies that are intended to prolong life, such as chemotherapy or radiation therapy, and it includes investigations needed to better understand and manage distressing clinical complications, and uses a team approach to address the needs of persons and their families (WHO, 2020). In Ireland, the National Clinical Programme for Palliative Care (NCPPC) have developed a Palliative Care Model of Care for the organisation of care for people with life-limiting or life-threatening conditions (National Clinical Programme for Palliative Care, 2018). The model of care recommends palliative care services should be structured in three levels of increasing specialisation. Palliative care provided at Level 1: in any setting by all healthcare practitioners as part of their role and using a palliative care approach; at Level 2: in any setting using a pallia-tive care approach by healthcare professionals who have additional knowledge of palliative care principles and use this as part of their role; at Level 3 Specialist palliative care provided by healthcare professionals who work solely in pallia-tive care, and who have extensive knowledge and skills in this area (Ryan *et al.*, 2010). In the UK existing guidance to improve palliative and end-of-life care for people with intellectual disabilities is mostly based on Guidance from the National Institute for Health and Care Excellence (NICE) (NICE, 2018, 2022).

Intellectual disability nurses use problem solving frameworks, such as the nursing process to ensure a systematic process is enlisted to prioritise need and ensure quality care. Palliative care involves the management and control of symptoms such as pain. Although not all people who are terminally ill will experience pain, it is a common feature in end-of-life care. For people with intellectual disabilities and particularly those using a variety of communication methods, it may be complex and challenging for those who are not familiar with the person to assess pain. Relatives and carers may be able to assist with pain assessment. Where pain is assessed or suspected, intellectual disability nurses caring for people with intellectual disabilities receiving end-of-life care need to collaborate with general practitioners and other palliative care specialists to ensure that appropriate pain relief is provided. Intellectual disability nurses need to be aware of alternative approaches to pain relief, such as physiotherapy, massage, reflexology, or other complementary therapies that can facilitate relaxation.

Other complications associated with end of life include loss of appetite, dehydration, and constipation. Intellectual disability nurses need to maintain nutritional and fluid intake and output records, ensure that the diets of such individuals are high in fiber and liaise with relevant dietitian. Medication can also contribute to loss of appetite and lead to increasing occurrence of constipation. Where constipation is an issue, intellectual disability nurses need to liaise with general practitioners to ensure that appropriate laxatives are prescribed and administered. Intellectual disability nurses need to monitor excretion and ensure continence care, rotations of postural positioning and maintenance of skin integrity. Where dysphagia becomes an issue, intellectual disability nurses providing end-of-life care to people with intellectual disabilities need to undertake appropriate screening and timely referral for comprehensive assessment to relevant multidisciplinary team members when required. Intellectual disability nurses must be vigilant of and respond to psychological changes presenting, for example, fear, anxiety, and agitation. It is important also to note that use of opioid analgesics will result in chemical imbalance of the brain, and this can cause confusion or hallucinations. This may result in restlessness, verbal aggression, or physical aggression. This can be particularly difficult to assess where such behaviours already existed prior to terminal illness. Intellectual disability nurses must accommodate spiritual needs for individuals who, for example, are lacking hope, accepting impending death and needing to say goodbye to loved ones. As end-of-life approaches, it is likely that a person will become tired and drowsy and will spend more time sleeping. Breathing is likely to become irregular and noisy because of increased mucus in the lungs. Blood circulation will reduce, resulting in cyanosis. Intellectual disability nurses who provide end-of-life care will require wide ranging knowledge, and nursing skills to facilitate appropriate end-of-life and palliative care.

Conclusion

There are several lessons that intellectual disability nurses of today and tomorrow can learn from a cradle-to-the-grave approach to nursing those with intellectual disabilities, to improve the health and healthcare outcomes for people with intellectual disabilities. The increasing complexity of the health and healthcare needs of people with intellectual disability and the increasing complexity of health and social care provision will require intellectual disability nurses to possess higher levels of knowledge about the changing, complex needs of people with intellectual disabilities. In meeting the holistic needs of people with intellectual disabilities across the lifespan, present and future roles of intellectual disability nurses will require a wide range of nursing skills and competences across the lifespan of people with intellectual disabilities.

It is important for intellectual disability nurses to understand contemporary intellectual disability nursing in the context of the normal lifespan of people with intellectual disabilities. Intellectual disability nurses need to be aware that the diagnosis of an intellectual disability in a child has a significant and often long-term impact on the family and wider society. Intellectual disability nurses will require the knowledge, skills, competence, and sensitivity to support parents as they respond to and face significant challenges. Effectively supporting adolescents with intellectual disabilities is complex and challenging. Intellectual disability nurses will need to work in partnership and collaborate with other agencies and professionals to improve access to appropriate services, to improve the health and healthcare outcomes of this vulnerable group. The lifestyles, health and healthcare needs of people with intellectual disabilities are often complex and challenging. This is more so today than ever before because of an increased life expectancy for people with intellectual disabilities. To meet the changing needs of this population, intellectual disability nurses will need to develop and continue to develop new ways of working with people with intellectual disabilities, their families and their carers, and other professionals across a wide range of agencies and organisations. People with intellectual disabilities are now living longer with complex and often long-term conditions in a wide range of community-based residential facilities. Intellectual disability nurses working in these settings and other NHS community-based services will need to develop their knowledge and skills to enhance the care experience of people with intellectual disabilities, especially in end-of-life care. While this may be a new and complex area for many intellectual disability nurses, efforts can be focused on building relationships with people with intellectual disabilities, their families and carers, and other professionals and palliative care organisations to enhance end-of-life care experiences for people with intellectual disabilities.

References

Al Mutairi, H., *et al.* (2020) Laxative use among older adults with intellectual disability: A cross-sectional observational study. *International Journal of Clinical Pharmacy*, 42, pp. 89–99.

Atchley, R.C. (1989) A continuity theory of normal aging. *The Gerontologist*, 29(2), pp. 183–190.

Austin, K.L., *et al.* (2018) Depression and anxiety symptoms during the transition to early adulthood for people with intellectual disabilities. *Journal of Intellectual Disability Research*, 62(5), pp. 407– 421.

Axmon, A., Höglund, P. and Ahlström, G. (2017) Chronic respiratory disorders and their treatment among older people with intellectual disability and/or autism spectrum disorder in comparison with the general population. *Healthcare*, 5(3), p. 40. Doi:10.3390/healthcare5030040.

Bach, M. and Kerzner, L. (2010) *A new paradigm for protecting autonomy and the right to legal capacity.* Available at: www.lco-cdo.org/disabilities/bach-kerzner.pdf (Accessed 2 August 2022).

Bailey, R. (2006) Physical education and sport in schools: A review of benefits and outcomes. *Journal of School Health*, 76(8), pp. 397–401.

Balogh, R., *et al.* (2018) All-cause, 30-day readmissions among persons with intellectual and developmental disabilities and mental illness. *Psychiatric Services*, 69(3), pp. 353–357.

Baltes, P.B. and Baltes, M.M. (1990) Psychological perspectives on successful aging: The model of selective optimization with compensation. In Baltes, P.B. and Baltes, M.M. (Eds.), *Successful aging: Perspectives from the behavioral sciences*. Cambridge: Cambridge University Press.

Barr, O. (2012) Supporting the families of learning-disabled children. *Independent Nurse*, 4. Available at: www.independentnurse.co.uk/professional-article/supporting-the-families-of-learning-disabled-children/64218 (Accessed 22 July 2022).

Bates, C. (2019) Supported loving – developing a national network to support positive intimate relationships for people with intellectual disabilities. *Tizard Intellectual Disability Review*, 24(1), pp. 13–19.

Beard, J.R., *et al.* (2009) Neighborhood characteristics and change in depressive symptoms among older residents of New York City. *American Journal of Public Health*, 99(7), pp. 1308–1314. Doi:10.2105/AJPH.2007.125104.

Beard, J.R., *et al.* (2016) The World report on ageing and health: A policy framework for healthy ageing. *The Lancet*, 387, pp. 10033, 2145–2154. Doi:10.1016/S0140-6736(15)00516-4.

Bermingham, B. (2021) *Midlife women rock: A menopause story for a new generation*. Cork: Oral Kelly Publishing.

Bibby, R. (2013) 'I hope he goes first': Exploring determinants of engagement in future planning for adults with a learning disability living with ageing parents. What are the issues? *British Journal of Learning Disabilities*, 41(2), pp. 94–105.

Bigby, C. (2010) Beset by obstacles: A review of Australian policy development to support ageing in place for people with intellectual disability. *Journal of Intellectual and Developmental Disability*, 33(1), pp. 76–86.

Bigby, C. (2021) Retirement for people with intellectual disability, policy, pitfalls, and promising practices. In Putnam, M. and Bigby, C. (Eds.), *Handbook on ageing with disability* (1st edition). London: Routledge, Chapter 21. Doi:10.4324/9780429465352.

Bigby, C., *et al.* (2004) Retirement or just a change of pace? An Australian national survey of disability day services used by older people with disabilities. *Journal of Intellectual & Developmental Disability*, 29(3), pp. 239–254.

Biggs, E.E. and Carter, E.W. (2016) Quality of life for transition-age youth with autism or intellectual disability. *Journal of Autism and Developmental Disorders*, 46(1), pp. 190–204.

Bjorksten, J. (1968) The cross-linkage theory of aging. *Journal of the American Geriatrics Society*, 16(4), pp. 408–427.

Blackman, N. (2002) Grief and intellectual disability: A systemic approach. *Journal of Gerontological Social Work*, 38(1–2), pp. 253–263.

Blackman, N. (2008) The development of an assessment tool for the bereavement needs of people with learning disabilities. *British Journal of Learning Disabilities*, 36(3), pp. 165–170.

Blackman, N. (2013) *The use of psychotherapy in supporting people with intellectual disabilities who have experienced bereavement*. Unpublished PhD thesis. Hatfield: University of Hertfordshire.

Blackman, N. (2016) Supporting people with learning disabilities through a bereavement. *Tizard Learning Disability Review*, 21(4), pp. 199–202.

Blows, E.S., Teoh, L. and Paul, S.P. (2016) Recognition and management of learning disabilities in early childhood by community practitioners. *Community Practitioner*, 89(5), pp. 32–35.

Bonell-Pascual, E., *et al.* (1999) Bereavement and grief in adults with learning disabilities: A follow-up study. *British Journal of Psychiatry*, 175(4) pp. 348–350.

Bourke-Taylor, H., Cotter, C. and Stephan, R. (2014) Young children with cerebral palsy: Families self-reported equipment needs and out of pocket expenditure. *Child Care Health Development*, 40, pp. 454–462.

Boveri, T. (1929) *The origin of malignant tumors*. Baltimore, MD: Williams and Wilkins.

Brennan, D., *et al.* (2018) What's going to happen when we're gone? Family caregiving capacity for older people with an intellectual disability in Ireland. *Journal of Applied Research ins Intellectual Disabilities*, 31(2), pp. 226–235.

Brown, M., *et al.* (2005) The internal struggle between the wish to die and the wish to live: A risk factor for suicide. *The American Journal of Psychiatry*, 162(10), pp. 1977–1979.

Brown., M., *et al.* (2010) Equality and access to general healthcare for people with learning disabilities: Reality or rhetoric? *Journal of Research in Nursing*, 15(4), pp. 351–361.

Brown, M., *et al.* (2019) Transitions from child to adult health care for young people with intellectual disabilities: A systematic review. *Journal of Advanced Nursing*, 75(11), pp. 2418–2434. https://doi.org/10.1111/jan.13985.

Brown, M., *et al.* (2021) *Transition from child to adult health services for people with complex learning disabilities*. Belfast: Queens University.

Brownrigg, S. (2018) Breaking bad news to people with intellectual disabilities: A literature review. *British Journal of Learning Disabilities*, 46(4), pp. 225–232.

Cain, L.K. and Velasco, J.C. (2021) Stranded at the intersection of gender, sexuality, and autism: Gray's story. *Disability & Society*, 36(3), pp. 358–375.

Carey, E. and Ryan, R. (2019) Informed consent. In Matson, J.L. (Ed.), *Handbook of intellectual disabilities integrating theory, research and practice*. New York, NJ: Springer, pp. 221–247.

Carmeli, E., *et al.* (2015) Oxidative stress and nitric oxide in sedentary older adults with intellectual and developmental disabilities. In *Pathophysiology of respiration*. New York: Springer, pp. 21–27.

Cartwright, L., *et al.* (2017) Barriers to increasing the physical activity of people with intellectual disabilities. *British Journal of Learning Disabilities*, 45(1), pp. 47–55.

Case law A Local Authority v JB (2021) UKSC 52. Available at: https://www.supremecourt.uk/cases/docs/uksc-2020-0133-judgment.pdf (Accessed 24 November 2022).

Chambers, L. and Kelly, K. (2015) *Stepping up: A guide to developing a good transition to adulthood for young people with life-limiting and life-threatening conditions*. Bristol: Together for Short Lives.

Chou, Y.C., Jane Lu, Z.Y. and Pu, C.Y. (2013) Menopause experiences and attitudes in women with intellectual disability and in their family carers. *Journal of Intellectual and Developmental Disability*, 38(2), pp. 114–123.

Clute, M.A. (2010) Bereavement interventions with adults with intellectual disabilities: What works? *OMEGA – Journal of Death and Dying*, 61(2), pp. 163–177.

Clute, M.A. (2017) Living disconnected: Building a grounded theory view of bereavement for adults with intellectual disabilities. *OMEGA-Journal of Death and Dying*, 76(1), pp. 15–34.

Coad, J., Patel, R. and Murray, S. (2014) Disclosing terminal diagnosis to children and their families: Palliative professionals' communication barriers. *Death Studies*, 38(1–5), pp. 302–307.

Coad, J., *et al.* (2015) Exploring the perceived met and unmet need of life-limited children, young people and families. *Journal of Pediatric Nursing*, 30(1), pp. 45–53.

College of Psychiatry of Ireland (2011) *Mental health provision for children with a learning disability, a position paper*. Dublin: College of Psychiatry of Ireland.

Commission on Social Determinants of Health (2008) *Closing the gap in a generation: Health equity through action on the social determinants of health*. Geneva: World Health Organization.

Cox, A., *et al.* (2021) Supporting the delivery of good maternity care for parents with intellectual disabilities. *Midwifery*, 102, p. 103073. Doi:10.1016/j.midw.2021.103073.

Cox, R., Stenfert-Kroese, B. and Evans, R. (2015) Solicitors' experiences of representing parents with intellectual disabilities in care proceedings: Attitudes, influence and legal processes. *Disability & Society*, 30(2), pp. 84–298.

Cumming, E. and Henry, W. (1961) *Growing old: The process of disengagement*. New York: Basic Books.

Currie, G. and Szabo, J. (2019) It is like a jungle gym, and everything is under construction": The parent's perspective of caring for a child with a rare disease. *Child: Care, Health and Development*, 45(1), pp. 96–103.

Department for Education (2018) *Special educational needs in England: January 2018*. London: Department for Education.

De Rezende, L.F.M., *et al.* (2014) Sedentary behavior and health outcomes among older adults: A systematic review. *BMC Public Health*, 14(1), p. 333.

De Winter, C.F., *et al.* (2014) Cardiovascular risk factors (diabetes, hypertension, hypercholesterolemia and metabolic syndrome) in older people with intellectual disability: Results of the HA-ID study. *Research in Developmental Disabilities*, 33(6), pp. 1722–1731.

De Winter, C.F., *et al.* (2016) A 3-year follow-up study on cardiovascular disease and mortality in older people with intellectual disabilities. *Research in Developmental Disabilities*, 53, pp. 115–126.

Dilman, V.M. (1971) Age-associated elevation of hypothalamic, threshold to feedback control, and its role in development, ageing, and disease. *The Lancet*, 1(7711), pp. 1211–1219.

Dilman, V.M., Revskoy, S.Y. and Golubev, A.G. (1986) Neuroendocrine-ontogenetic mechanism of aging: Toward an integrated theory of aging. *International Review of Neurobiology*, 28, pp. 89–156.

Dixon-Ibarra, A., Lee, M. and Dugala, A. (2013) Physical activity and sedentary behavior in older adults with intellectual disabilities: A comparative study. *Adapted Physical Activity Quarterly*, 30(1), pp. 1–19.

Dodd, P., *et al.* (2008) A study of complicated grief symptoms in people with intellectual disabilities. *Journal of Intellectual Disability Research*, 52(5), pp. 415–425.

Doherty, A.J., *et al.* (2020) Barriers and facilitators to primary health care for people with intellectual disabilities and/or autism: An integrative review. *BJGP Open*, 4(3). Doi:10.3399/bjgpopen20X101030.

Doody, C.M., Markey, K. and Doody, O. (2013a) Future need of ageing people with an intellectual disability in the Republic of Ireland: Lessons learned from the literature. *British Journal of Learning Disabilities*, 41(1), pp. 13–21.

Doody, C.M., Markey, K. and Doody, O. (2013b) The experiences of registered intellectual disability nurses caring for the older person with intellectual disability. *Journal of Clinical Nursing*, 22(7–8), pp. 1112–1123.

Doody, O., *et al.* (2022) The value and contribution of intellectual disability nurses/ nurses caring for people with intellectual disability in intellectual disability settings: A scoping review. *Journal of Clinical Nursing*, pp. 1– 48. Doi:10.1111/ jocn.16289.

Doyle, A., *et al.* (2021) People with intellectual disability in Ireland are still dying young. *Journal of Applied Research in Intellectual Disabilities*, 34(4), pp. 1057–1065.

Doyle, C. (2020) The importance of supportive relationships with general practitioners, hospitals and pharmacists for mothers who 'give medicines' to children with severe and profound intellectual disabilities. *Journal of Intellectual Disabilities*, 26(1), pp. 29–49.

Eime, R.M., *et al.* (2013) A systematic review of the psychological and social benefits of participation in sport for children and adolescents: Informing development of a conceptual model of health through sport. *International Journal of Behavioural Nutrition and Physical Activity*, 10(98). Doi:10.1186/1479-5868-10-98.

Emerson, E., *et al.* (2011) The health of disabled people and the social determinants of health. *Public Health*, 125(3), pp. 145–147.

Emerson, E., *et al.* (2012a) *Health inequalities & people with learning disabilities in the UK: 2012*. Learning Disabilities Observatory. Available at: http://com plexneeds.org.uk/modules/Module-4.1-Workingwith-other-professionals/All/ downloads/m13p020c/emerson_baines_health_inequalities.pdf (Accessed 28 July 2022).

Emerson, E., *et al.* (2012b) *People with learning disabilities in England 2011*. Lancaster: Learning Disabilities Observatory, University of Lancaster.

Emerson, E., *et al.* (2013) *People with learning disabilities in England 2012*. Lancaster: Learning Disabilities Observatory, University of Lancaster.

Engeland, J., Kittelsaa, A.M. and Langballe, E.M. (2018) How do people with intellectual disabilities in Norway experience the transition to retirement and life as retirees? *Scandinavian Journal of Disability Research*, 20(1), pp. 72–81.

Erikson, E.H. (1950) *Childhood and society*. New York: W.W. Norton.

Erikson, E.H. (1982) *The life cycle completed*. New York: W.W. Norton.

Erikson, J.M. (1997) *The lifecycle completed – extended version with chapters on the ninth stage of development*. New York: W.W. Norton.

European Commission (2010) *European disability strategy 2010–2020: A renewed commitment to a barrier-free Europe*. Brussels: European Commission.

Flynn, E. and Arstein-Kerslake, A. (2014) Legislating personhood: Realising the right to support in exercising legal capacity. *International Journal of Law in Context*, 10(1), pp. 81–104.

Fritz, R., Edwards, L. and Jacob, R. (2021) Osteoporosis in adult patients with intellectual and developmental disabilities: Special considerations for diagnosis, prevention, and management. *Southern Medical Journal*, 114(4), pp. 246–251.

Gephart, E.F. and Loman, D.G. (2013) Use of prevention and prevention plus weight management guidelines for youth with developmental disabilities living in group homes. *Journal of Pediatric Health Care*, 27(2), pp. 98–108.

Giasson, H. L., *et al.* (2017) Age group differences in perceived age discrimination: Associations with self-perceptions of aging. *The Gerontologist*, 57(Suppl 2), S160–S168.

Gilrane-McGarry, U. and Taggart, L. (2007) An exploration of the support received by people with intellectual disabilities who have been bereaved. *Journal of Research in Nursing*, 12(2), pp. 129–144.

Giri, A., *et al.* (2022) Lived experience and the social model of disability: Conflicted and interdependent ambitions for employment of people with a learning disability and their family carers. *British Journal of Learning Disabilities*, 50(1), pp. 98–106.

Glaesser, R.S. and Perkins, E.A. (2013) Self-injurious behavior in older adults with intellectual disabilities. *Social Work*, 58(3), pp. 213–221.

Glazemakers, I. and Deboutte, D. (2013) Modifying the 'positive parenting program' for parents with intellectual disabilities. *Journal of Intellectual Disability Research*, 57(7), pp. 616–626.

Glover, G., *et al.* (2017) Mortality in people with intellectual disabilities in England. *Journal of Intellectual Disability Research*, 61(1), pp. 62–74.

Gray, J.A. and Abendroth, M. (2016) Perspectives of US direct care workers on the grief process of persons with intellectual and developmental disabilities: Implications for practice. *Journal of Applied Research in Intellectual Disabilities*, 29(5), pp. 468–480.

Hall, C. (2014) Bereavement theory: Recent developments in our understanding of grief and bereavement. *Bereavement Care*, 33(1), pp. 7–12.

Hamers, P.C.M., Festen, D.A.M. and Hermans, H. (2018) Non-pharmacological interventions for adults with intellectual disabilities and depression: A systematic review. *Journal of Intellectual Disability Research*, 62(8), pp. 684–700.

Harman, D. (1957) Prolongation of the normal life span by radiation protection chemicals. *Journal of Gerontology*, 12(3), pp. 257–263.

Harnett, A. (2007) *Informing families of their child's disability national best practice guidelines consultation and research report.* Dublin: National Federation of Voluntary Bodies Providing Services to People with Intellectual Disability.

Hatton, C. (2017) Living arrangements of adults with intellectual disabilities across the UK. *Tizard Intellectual Disability Review*, 22(1), pp. 43–50.

Haveman, M. (2019) Ageing and physical health. In Prasher, V.P. and Janick, P. (Eds.), *Physical health of adults with intellectual and developmental disabilities.* Geneva: Springer Nature, pp. 305–334.

Haverman, M., *et al.* (2011) Ageing and health status in adults with intellectual disabilities: Results of the European POMONA II study. *Journal of Intellectual and Developmental Disability*, 36(1), pp. 49–60.

Havighurst, R.J. (1961) Successful aging. *The Gerontologist*, 1(1), pp. 8–13.

Health Education England (2016) *Learning disabilities transition pathway competency framework.* London: NHS.

Health Education England and University of Surrey (2020) *The together project.* Available at: https://www.surrey.ac.uk/together-project (Accessed 24 November 2022).

Health Service Executive (HSE) (2020) *National framework for the integrated prevention and management of chronic disease in Ireland 2020–2025 integrated care programme for the prevention and management of chronic disease.* Available at: www.hse.ie/eng/about/who/cspd/icp/chronic-disease/documents/national-framework-integrated-care.pdf (Accessed 2 August 2022).

Health Service Executive and Royal College of Physicians (2016) *Pediatric model of care.* Dublin: Health Service Executive and Royal College of Physicians.

Heller, T. (2004) Aging with developmental disabilities: Emerging models for promoting health, independence, and quality of life. In Kemp, B.J. and Mosqueda, L. (Eds.), *Aging with a disability: What a clinician needs to know.* Baltimore, MD: Johns Hopkins University Press, pp. 213–233.

Heller, T. (2019) Bridging aging and intellectual/developmental disabilities in research, policy, and practice. *Journal of Policy and Practice in Intellectual Disabilities*, 16(1), pp. 53–57.

Heller, T. and Harris, S.P. (2012) *Disability through the life course.* London: Sage.

Hermans, H., Beekman, A.T. and Evenhuis, H.M. (2013) Prevalence of depression and anxiety in older users of formal Dutch intellectual disability services. *Journal of Affective Disorders*, 144(1–2), pp. 94–100.

Hermans, H. and Evenhuis, H.M. (2014) Multimorbidity in older adults with intellectual disabilities. *Research in Developmental Disabilities*, 35(4), pp. 776–783.

Heslop, P., et al. (2013) *Confidential inquiry into premature deaths of people with learning disabilities (CIPOLD)*. Bristol: University of Bristol.

Heslop, P., et al. (2014) The confidential inquiry into premature deaths of people with intellectual disabilities in the UK: A population-based study. *The Lancet*, 383, pp. 889–895.

Hillier, A., et al. (2022) Overview of a life skills coaching program for adults on the autism spectrum: Coaches' perspectives. *Psychological Reports*, 125(2), pp. 937–963.

Hole, R.D., Stainton, T. and Wilson, L. (2013) Ageing adults with intellectual disabilities: Self-advocates' and family members' perspectives about the future. *Australian Social Work*, 66(4), pp. 571–589.

Holland, A.J. (2000) Ageing and learning disability. *British Journal of Psychiatry*, 174, pp. 26–31.

Hosking, F.J., et al. (2016) Mortality among adults with intellectual disability in England: Comparisons with the general population. *American Journal of Public Health*, 106(8), pp. 1483–1490.

Hosking, F.J., et al. (2017) Preventable emergency hospital admissions among adults with intellectual disability in England. *The Annals of Family Medicine*, 15(5), pp. 462–470.

Hsieh, K., Scott, H.M. and Murthy, S. (2020) Associated risk factors for depression and anxiety in adults with intellectual and developmental disabilities: Five-year follow up. *American Journal on Intellectual and Developmental Disabilities*, 125(1), pp. 49–63.

Hughes-McCormack, L., et al. (2017) Prevalence of mental health conditions and relationship with general health in a whole-country population of people with intellectual disabilities compared with the general population. *BJPsych Open*, 3(5), pp. 243–248.

ICPCN (2020) *Basic symptom control in paediatric palliative care*. Available at: https://www.icpcn.org/clinical-care-resources/ (Accessed 27 November 2022).

Intellectual Disability Supplement to the Irish Longitudinal Study on Ageing'(IDS-TILDA) (2021) *User information guide*. Dublin: Centre for Ageing and Intellectual Disability (TCAID), Trinity College Dublin, The University of Dublin.

Jaul, E. and Barron, J. (2017) Age-related diseases and clinical and public health implications for the 85 years old and over population. *Frontiers in Public Health*, 5, p. 335.

Jung, C.G. (1960) On the nature of the psyche. In Read, H., Fordham, M. and Adler, G. (Eds.) and Hull, R.F.C. (Trans.), *The collected works of C.G. Jung* (Vol. 8). New York: Pantheon Books, pp. 159–234.

Kapsal, N.J., et al. (2019) Effects of physical activity on the physical and psychosocial health of youth with intellectual disabilities: A systematic review and meta-analysis. *Journal of Physical Activity and Health*, 16(12), pp. 1187–1195.

Kaufman, M. and Pinzon, J. (2007) Transition to adult care for youth with special health care needs. *Paediatrics & Child Health*, 12(9), pp. 785–788.

Kessel, S., et al. (2002) Use of group counseling to support aging-related losses in older adults with intellectual disabilities. *Journal of Gerontological Social Work*, 38(1–2), pp. 241–251.

Kingston, A., et al. (2018) Projections of multi-morbidity in the older population in England to 2035: Estimates from the population ageing and care simulation (PACSim) model. *Ageing*, 47, pp. 374–380.

Kirkpatrick, K. (2011) A home of my own - progress on enabling people with learning disabilities to have choice and control over where and with whom they live. *Tizard Intellectual Disability Review*, 16(2), pp. 7–13.

Kocman, A., Fischer, L. and Weber, G. (2018) The employers' perspective on barriers and facilitators to employment of people with intellectual disability: A differential mixed-method approach. *Journal of Applied Research in Intellectual Disabilities*, 31(1), pp. 120–131.

Koritsas, S. and Iacono, T. (2016) Weight, nutrition, food choice and physical activity in adults with intellectual disability. *Journal of Intellectual Disability Research*, 2(60), pp. 355–364.

Krinsky-McHale, S.J. and Silverman, W. (2013) Dementia and mild cognitive impairment in adults with intellectual disability: Issues of diagnosis. *Developmental Disabilities Research Review*, 18(1), pp. 31–42.

Kuijken, N. M. *et al.* (2016). Healthy living according to adults with intellectual disabilities: towards tailoring health promotion initiatives. *Journal of Intellectual Disability Research*, 60(3), pp.228–241. https://doi.org/10.1111/jir.12243

Lafferty, A., *et al.* (2016) *Family carers' experiences of caring for a person with intellectual disability*. Dublin: University College Dublin.

Landes, S.D., Stevens, J.D. and Turk, M.A. (2021) Cause of death in adults with intellectual disability in the United States. *Journal of Intellectual Disability Research*, 65(1), pp. 47–59.

Lawton, M.P. (1982) Competence, environmental press, and the adaptation of older people. In Lawton, M.P., Windley, P.G. and Byens, T.O. (Eds.), *Aging and the environment: Theoretical approaches*. New York: Springer.

Leaviss, J., *et al.* (2011) *Inclusive support for parents with a learning disability*. London: Mencap.

Lennartsson, C. and Heimerson, I. (2012) Elderly people's health: Health in Sweden: The national public health report. *Scandinavian Journal of Public Health*, 40(9), pp. 95–120.

Li, J.C.H., *et al.* (2015) The challenges of providing eye care for adults with intellectual disabilities. *Clinical & Experimental Optometry*, 98(5), pp. 420–429.

Lin, J.D., *et al.* (2011) Early onset ageing and service preparation in people with intellectual disabilities: Institutional managers' perspective. *Research in Developmental Disabilities*, 32(1), pp. 188–193.

Linehan, C., *et al.* (2014) *Mapping the national disability policy landscape*. Dublin: School of Social Work and Social Policy, Trinity College.

Lord, A.J., Field, S. and Smith, I.C. (2017) The experiences of staff who support people with intellectual disability on issues about death, dying and bereavement: A metasynthesis. *Journal of Applied Research in Intellectual Disabilities*, 30(6), pp. 1007–1021.

Lord, A.J., *et al.* (2017) The experiences of staff who support people with intellectual disability on issues about death, dying and bereavement: A metasynthesis. *Journal of Applied Research in Intellectual Disabilities*, 30(6), pp. 1007–1021.

Lunsky, Y., *et al.* (2019) High health care costs among adults with intellectual and developmental disabilities: A population-based study. *Journal of Intellectual Disability Research*, 63(2), pp. 124–137.

Marengoni, A., *et al.* (2011) Aging with multimorbidity: A systematic review of the literature. *Ageing Research Reviews*, 10(4), pp. 430–439.

Marriott, A., Marriott, J. and Heslop, P. (2013) Good practice in helping people cope with terminal illnesses. *Learning Disability Practice*, 16(6), pp. 22–25.

Marsden, D. (2013) *How East Kent is making the NHS workforce more inclusive*. Available at: www.hsj.co.uk/topics/technology-and-innovation/how-east-kent-is-making-the-nhs-workforce-more-inclusive/5061285.article (Accessed 2 August 2022).

Marsh, L., Brown, M. and McCann, E. (2020) The views and experiences of fathers regarding their young child's intellectual and developmental disability diagnosis: Findings from a qualitative study. *Journal of Clinical Nursing*, 29(17–18), pp. 3373–3381.

Marsh, L., Leahy-Warren, P. and Savage, E. (2018) "Something was wrong": A narrative inquiry of becoming a father of a child with an intellectual disability in Ireland. *British Journal of Learning Disabilities*, 46(4), pp. 216–224.

Maslow, A.H. (1943) A theory of human motivation. *Psychological Review*, 50(4), pp. 370–396.

McCann, D., Bull, R. and Winzenberg, T. (2015) Sleep deprivation in parents caring for children with complex needs at home: A mixed methods systematic review. *Journal of Family Nursing*, 21(1), pp. 86–118.

McCann, E., Marsh, L. and Brown, M. (2019) People with intellectual disabilities, relationship and sex education programmes: A systematic review. *Health Education Journal*, 78(8), pp. 885–900.

McCarron, M., *et al.* (2011) *Growing older with an intellectual disability in Ireland 2011: First results from the intellectual disability supplement to the Irish longitudinal study on ageing.* Dublin: School of Nursing and Midwifery, Trinity College Dublin.

McCarron, M., *et al.* (2013) Patterns of multimorbidity in an older population of persons with an intellectual disability: Results from the intellectual disability supplement to the Irish longitudinal study on aging (IDS-TILDA). *Research in Developmental Disabilities*, 34(1), pp. 521–527.

McCarron, M., *et al.* (2014) Epidemiology of epilepsy in older adults with an intellectual disability in Ireland: Associations and service implications. *American Journal on Intellectual and Developmental Disabilities*, 119(3), pp. 253–260.

McCarron, M., *et al.* (2018) *Shaping the future of intellectual disability nursing in Ireland.* Dublin: Health Services Executive.

McCarron, M., *et al.* (2020) *The impact of COVID-19 on people ageing with an intellectual disability in Ireland.* Dublin. Available at: www.tcd.ie/tcaid/assets/pdf/wave4idstildareport.pdf (Accessed 20 July 2022).

McCausland, D., McCallion, P. and McCarron, M. (2021) Health and wellness among persons ageing with intellectual disability. In Putnam, M. and Bigby, C. (Eds.), *Handbook on ageing with disability* (1st edition). London: Routledge, Chapter 20.

McCausland, D., *et al.* (2016) Social connections for older people with intellectual disability in Ireland: Results from wave one of IDS-TILDA. *Journal of Applied Research in Intellectual Disabilities*, 29(1), pp. 71–82.

McCay, C.M., Crowell, M.F. and Maynard, L.A. (1935) The effect of retarded growth upon the length of life span and upon the ultimate body size. *Journal of Nutrition*, 10, pp. 63–79.

McConkey, R., *et al.* (2018) Changes in the provision of day services in Ireland to adult persons with intellectual disability. *Journal of Policy and Practice in Intellectual Disabilities*, 16(3). DOI: 10.1111/jppi.12261.

McDermott, S. and Edwards, R. (2012) Enabling self-determination for older workers with intellectual disabilities in supported employment in Australia. *Journal of Applied Research in Intellectual Disabilities*, 25(5), pp. 423–432.

McEvoy, J., Treacy, B. and Quigley, J. (2017) A matter of life and death: Knowledge about the body and concept of death in adults with intellectual disabilities. *Journal of Intellectual Disability Research*, 61(1), pp. 89–98.

McGarrigle, C.A., Cronin, H. and Kenny, R.A. (2014) The impact of being the intermediate caring generation and intergenerational transfers on self-reported health of women in Ireland. *International Journal of Public Health*, 59(2), pp. 301–308.

McGlinchey, E., *et al.* (2019) *Positive ageing indicators for people with an intellectual disability 2018.* Dublin: Trinity Centre for Ageing and Intellectual Disability.

McKenzie, K., Ouellette-Kuntz, H. and Martin, L. (2017) Applying a general measure of frailty to assess the aging related needs of adults with intellectual and developmental disabilities. *Journal of Policy and Practice in Intellectual Disabilities*, 14(2), pp. 124–128.

McMahon, M., Bowring, D.L. and Hatton, C. (2019) Not such an ordinary life: A comparison of employment, marital status and housing profiles of adults with and without intellectual disabilities. *Tizard Intellectual Disability Review*, 24(4), pp. 213–221.

McMunn, A., *et al.* (2006) Social determinants of health in older age. *Social Determinants of Health*, 2, pp. 267–298.

McRitchie, R., *et al.* (2014) How adults with an intellectual disability experience bereavement and grief: A qualitative exploration. *Death Studies*, 38(1–5), pp. 179–185.

McShea, L., Fulton, J. and Hayes, C. (2016) Paid support workers for adults with intellectual disabilities; their current knowledge of hearing loss and future training needs. *Journal of Applied Research in Intellectual Disabilities*, 29(5), pp. 422–432.

Meggitt, C. (2012) *Child development: An illustrated guide* (3rd edition). China: Heinemann Press.

Mencap (2020) *Employment vision statement.* Available at: www.mencap.org.uk/about-us/what-we-think/employment-what-we-think (Accessed 2 August 2022).

Mencap (2022) *Getting a diagnosis after your child is born.* London: Mencap.

Mental Health Foundation (2022) *Learning disabilities statistics.* Available at: https://www.mentalhealth.org.uk/explore-mental-health/mental-health-statistics/learning-disabilities-statistics (Accessed 24 November 2022).

Merten, J.W., *et al.* (2015) Barriers to cancer screening for people with disabilities: A literature review. *Disability and Health Journal*, 8(1), pp. 9–16.

Meyer, I. (2019) The complexity of caring for the dying – an empirical approach to understanding palliative care as integrated care in the German healthcare system. *International Journal of Integrated Care*, 19(S1), pp. 1–8.

Mishra, V. and Barratt, J. (2016) *Reablement and older people: Final report from Copenhagen summit.* Available at: www.ifa-copenhagen-summit.com/wp-content/uploads/2016/04/CopenhagenSummit-Final-Report.pdf (Accessed 28 July 2022).

Modini, M., *et al.* (2016) The mental health benefits of employment: Results of a systematic meta-review. *Australasian Psychiatry*, 24(4), pp. 331–336.

Monaghan, R. *et al.* (2021) The relationship between antiepileptic drug load and challenging behaviors in older adults with intellectual disability and epilepsy. Epilepsy & Behaviour, 122. https://doi.org/10.1016/j.yebeh.2021.108191

Morad, M., *et al.* (2007) Prevalence and risk factors of constipation in adults with intellectual disability in residential care centers in Israel. *Research in Developmental Disabilities*, 28(6), pp. 580–586.

Morgan, N. and McEvoy, J. (2014) Exploring the bereavement experiences of older women with intellectual disabilities in long-term residential care: A staff perspective. *Omega-Journal of Death and Dying*, 69(2), pp. 117–135.

Morton-Nance, S. and Schafer, T. (2012) End of life care for people with a learning disability. *Nursing Standard*, 27(1), pp. 40–47. https://doi.org/10.7748/ns2012.09.27.1.40.c9270

Nakken, H. and Vlaskamp, C. (2007) A need for a taxonomy for profound intellectual and multiple disabilities. *Journal of Policy and Practice in Intellectual Disabilities*, 4(2), pp. 83–87.

National Clinical Programme for Palliative Care (2018) *Adult palliative care services, model of care for Ireland.* Available at: https://www.hse.ie/eng/about/who/cspd/ncps/palliative-care/ (Accessed 27 November 2022).

National End of Life Care Programme (2011) *The route to success in end-of-life care – achieving quality for people with learning disabilities*. Leicester: National End of Life Care Programme.

National Health Service (2021) *National palliative and end of life care partnership. Ambitions for palliative and end of life care: A national framework for local action 2021–2026*. Aavailable at: www.england.nhs.uk/wp-content/uploads/2022/02/ambitions-for-palliative-and-of-life-care-2nd-edition.pdf (Accessed 29 July 2022).

National Institute for Health and Care Excellence (2018) *Care and support for people growing older with learning disabilities*. Available at: www.nice.org.uk/guidance/ng96/ (Accessed 28 July 2022).

National Institute for Health and Care Excellence (2021a) *Shared decision making*. Available at: nice.org.uk/about/what-we-do/our-programmes/nice-guidance/nice-guidelines/shared-decision-making (Accessed 29 July 2022).

National Institute for Health and Care Excellence (2021b) *Managing symptoms for an adult in the last days of life*. Available at: pathways.nice.org.uk/pathways/end-of-life-care-for-people-with-lifelimiting-conditions#path=view%3A/pathways/end-of-life-care-for-people-with-life-limitingconditions/managing-symptoms-for-an-adult-in-the-last-days-of-life.xml&content=view-index (Accessed 29 July 2022).

Ng, J. and Li, S. (2003) A survey exploring the educational needs of care practitioners in learning disability (LD) settings in relation to death, dying and people with learning disabilities. *European Journal of Cancer Care*, 12, pp. 12–19.

NHS England (2022) *NHS England learning disability employment programme*. Available at: www.england.nhs.uk/about/equality/equality-hub/ld-emp-prog/ (Accessed 2 August 2022).

NICE (2015a) *Workplace health: Management practices (NG13)*. Available at: www.nice.org.uk/guidance/ng13# (Accessed 2 August 2022).

NICE (2015b) *Challenging behaviour and learning disabilities: Prevention and interventions for people with learning disabilities whose behaviour challenges*. London: NICE.

NICE (2022) *Disabled children and young people up to 25 with severe complex needs: Integrated service delivery and organisation across health, social care and education (NG213)*. London: NICE.

Nicholl, H. and Begley, C. (2012) Explicating caregiving by mothers of children with complex needs in Ireland: A phenomenological study. *Journal of Pediatric Nursing*, 27(6), pp. 642–651.

Noorlandt, H.W. *et al.* (2021) Consensus on a conversation aid for shared decision making with people with intellectual disabilities in the palliative phase. *Journal of Applied Research in Intellectual Disabilities*, 34(6), pp. 1538–1548.

Nuffield Council on Bioethics (2017) *Non-invasive prenatal testing: Ethical issues*. Available at: www.nuffieldbioethics.org/assets/pdfs/NIPT-ethical-issues-full-report.pdf (Accessed 2 August 2022).

Nursing and Midwifery Board of Ireland (2016) *Nurse registration programmes standards and requirements* (4th edition). Dublin: Nursing and Midwifery Board of Ireland.

Nursing and Midwifery Council (2018) *Future nurse: Standards of proficiency for registered nurses*. London: NMC.

Office for National Statistics (2020) *Estimates of the population for the UK, England and Wales, Scotland and Northern Ireland*. London: Office for National Statistics.

O'Leary, L., Cooper, S.A. and Hughes-McCormack, L. (2018a) Early death and causes of death of people with intellectual disabilities: A systematic review. *Journal of Applied Research in Intellectual Disabilities*, 31(3), pp. 325–342.

O'Leary, L., Taggart, L. and Cousins, W. (2018b) Healthy lifestyle behaviours for people with intellectual disabilities: An exploration of organizational barriers and enablers. *Journal of Applied Research Intellectual Disabilities*, 31(Suppl. 1), pp. 122–135.

Oppewal, A., *et al.* (2018) Causes of mortality in older people with intellectual disability: Results from the HA-ID study. *American Journal on Intellectual and Developmental Disabilities*, 123(1), pp. 61–71.

Oviedo, G.R., *et al.* (2020) Intellectual disability, exercise and aging: The IDEA study: Study protocol for a randomized controlled trial. *BMC Public Health*, 20(1), pp. 1–16.

Palliative Care for People with Disabilities (PCPLD) (2017) Delivering high quality end of life care for people who have a learning disability: Resources and tips for commissioners, service providers and health and social care staff. Developed by NHS England in association with the PCPLD Network. Available at: www.england.nhs.uk/publication/delivering-high-quality-end-of-life-care-for-people-who-have-a-learning-disability/ (Accessed 2 August 2022).

Patel, D.R., *et al.* (2020) A clinical primer on intellectual disability. *Translational Pediatrics*, 9(Suppl 1), pp. S23–S35.

Peck, R. (1956) Psychological developments in the second half of life. In Anderson, J.E. (Ed.), *Psychological aspects of aging*. Washington, DC: American Psychological Association, pp. 42–53.

Peretz, D. (1970) Development, object-relationships, and loss. In Schoenberg, B., Carr, A., Peretz, D. and Kutscher, A. (Eds.), *Loss and grief: Psychological management in medical practice*. New York: Columbia University Press, pp. 3–19.

Perkins, E.A. and Haley, W.E. (2010) Compound caregiving: When lifelong caregivers undertake additional caregiving roles. *Rehabilitation Psychology*, 55(4), pp. 409–417.

Phillips, A.C. and Holland, A.J. (2011) Assessment of objectively measured physical activity levels in individuals with intellectual disabilities with and without down's syndrome. *PloS One*, 6(12), e84031. Doi:10.1371/journal.pone.0028618.

Phillips, S. (2016) *A world without down's syndrome*. Available at: https://login.intellectualonscreen.ac.uk/wayfless.php?entityID=https%3A%2F%2Fidp.canterbury.ac.uk%2Fshibboleth&target=https%3A%2F%2Fintellectualonscreen.ac.uk%2Fondemand%2Findex.php%2Fprog%2F0DA04B5A%3Fbcast%3D122944894 (Accessed 2 August 2022).

Pinney, A. (2017) *Understanding the needs of disabled children with complex needs or life-limiting conditions*. London: Council for Disabled Children and True Colours Trust.

Poitras, J.V., *et al.* (2016) Systematic review of the relationships between objectively measured physical activity and health indicators in school-aged children and youth. *Applied Physiology, Nutrition and Metabolism*, 41(6 Suppl 3), pp. S197–S239.

Pordes, E., *et al.* (2018) Models of care delivery for children with medical complexity. *Pediatrics*, 141(Suppl 3), pp. S212–S223.

Public Health England (2015) *The determinants of health inequities experienced by children with learning disabilities*. London: Public Health England.

Public Health England (2016) *People with learning disabilities in England 2015*. London: Public Health England.

Public Health England (2020a) *Deaths of people identified as having intellectual disabilities with COVID-19 in England in the spring of 2020*. Available at: https://assets.publishing.service.gov.uk/government/uploads/system/uploads/attachment_data/file/933612/COVID-19__intellectual_disabilities_mortality_report.pdf (Accessed 29 July 2022).

Public Health England (2020b) *People with intellectual disabilities in England.* Available at: www.gov.uk/government/publications/people-with-intellectual-disabilities-in-england/chapter-2-employment (Accessed 29 July 2022).

Ranjan, S., Nasser, J.A. and Fisher, K. (2018) Prevalence and potential factors associated with overweight and obesity status in adults with intellectual developmental disorders. *Journal of Applied Research in Intellectual Disabilities,* 31(Suppl 1), pp. 29–38.

RCN (2018) *The registered nurse – learning disability skills, knowledge and expertise across the lifespan.* London: Royal College of Nursing.

Read, S. (1998) Learning disabilities: The palliative care needs of people with learning disabilities. *International Journal of Palliative Nursing,* 4(5), pp. 246–251.

Read, S. (2014) *Supporting people with intellectual disabilities experiencing loss and bereavement: Theory and compassionate practice.* London: Jessica Kingsley.

Read, S. and Elliott, D. (2003) Death and learning disability: A vulnerability perspective. *The Journal of Adult Protection,* 5(1), pp. 5–14.

Reddall, C. (2010) A palliative care resource for professional carers of people with learning disabilities. *Journal of Cancer Care,* 19(4), pp. 469–475.

Reddihough, D., *et al.* (2021) Comorbidities and quality of life in children with intellectual disability. *Child Care Health Development,* 47(5), pp. 654–666.

Reilly, D.E., Raymond, K. and O'Donnell, C. (2020) "It was emotional" – a group for people with learning disabilities to talk about end of life. *British Journal of Learning Disabilities,* 48(3), pp. 199–205.

Ridding, A. and Williams, J. (2019) Being a dad to a child with down's syndrome: Overcoming the challenges to adjustment. *Journal of Applied Research in Intellectual Disabilities,* 32(3), pp. 678– 690.

Riley, M.W. (1987) On the significance of age in sociology. *American Sociological Review,* 52(1), pp. 1–14.

Rivard, M., *et al.* (2021) The diagnostic trajectory in autism and intellectual disability in Quebec: Pathways and parents' perspective. *BMC Pediatrics,* 21, p. 393.

Robertson, J., *et al.* (2015) Prevalence of epilepsy among people with intellectual disabilities: A systematic review. *Seizure,* 29, pp. 46–62.

Robinson, Z.M., *et al.* (2020) Supporting people with intellectual disabilities who identify as LGBT to express their sexual and gender identities. *Learning Disability Practice.* Doi:10.7748/ldp.2020.e2094.

Rodríguez, M.Á., *et al.* (2018) Evaluating the characteristics of the grieving process in people with intellectual disability. *Journal of Applied Research in Intellectual Disabilities,* 31(6), pp. 999–1007.

Rogers, C. (2011) Disabling a family? Emotional dilemmas experienced in becoming a parent of a child with learning disabilities. *British Journal of Special Education,* 34(3), pp. 136–143.

Rowe, J. and Kahn, R. (1997) Successful aging. *The Gerontologist,* 27(4), pp. 433–440.

Rudnicka, E., *et al.* (2020) The world health organization (WHO) approach to healthy ageing. *Maturitas,* 139, pp. 6–11.

Rustad, M. and Kassah, K.A. (2020) Intellectual disability and work inclusion: On the experiences, aspirations and empowerment of sheltered employment workers in Norway. *Disability & Society,* 37(3), pp. 496–521.

Ryan, J., *et al.* (2021) Overweight/obesity and chronic health conditions in older people with intellectual disability in Ireland. *Journal of Intellectual Disability Research,* 65(12), pp. 1097–1109.

Ryan, K., *et al.* (2010) An exploration of the experience, confidence and attitudes of staff to the provision of palliative care to people with intellectual disabilities. *Palliative Medicine,* 24(6), pp. 566–572.

Same, R.V., *et al.* (2016) Relationship between sedentary behavior and cardiovascular risk. *Current Cardiology Reports*, 18(1), p. 6. Doi:10.1007/s11886-015-0678-5.

Sardi, I., *et al.* (2008) Family carers' opinions on learning disability services. *Nursing Times*, 104(11), pp. 30–31.

Schalock, R.L., *et al.* (2007) Intellectual disability: Definition, classification, and systems of supports. AAIDD. The renaming of mental retardation: Understanding the change to the term intellectual disability. *Journal of Intellectual and Developmental Disabilities*, 45(2), pp. 116–124.

Schoufour, J.D., *et al.* (2013) Multimorbidity and polypharmacy are independently associated with mortality in older people with intellectual disabilities: A 5-year follow-up from the HA-ID study. *American Journal on Intellectual and Developmental Disabilities*, 123(1), pp. 72–82.

Shaw, K., Cartwright, C. and Craig, J. (2011) The housing and support needs of people with an intellectual disability into older age. *Journal of Intellectual Disability Research*, 55(9), pp. 895–903.

Shobana, M. and Saravanan, C. (2014) Comparative study on attitudes and psychological problems of mothers towards their children with developmental disability. *East Asian Archives of Psychiatry*, 24(1), pp. 16–22.

Shultz, K.S. and Wang, M. (2011) Psychological perspectives on the changing nature of retirement. *American Psychologist*, 66(3), p. 170.

Siperstein, G.N., Heyman, M. and Stokes, J.E. (2014) Pathways to employment: A national survey of adults with intellectual disabilities. *Journal of Vocational Rehabilitation*, 41, pp. 165–178.

Smith, P., Ooms, A. and Marks-Maran, D. (2016) Active involvement of intellectual disabilities service users in the development and delivery of a teaching session to pre-registration nurses: Students' perspectives. *Nurse Education in Practice*, 16(1), pp. 111–118.

Smith, R.A. (2010) The history of childhood disabilities. *Journal of Disability and Oral Health*, 11(2), pp. 77–88.

Stancliffe, R.J., Kramme, J.E. and Nye-Lengerman, K. (2018) Exploring retirement for individuals with intellectual and developmental disabilities: An analysis of national core indicators data. *Intellectual and Developmental Disabilities*, 56(4), pp. 217–233.

Stancliffe, R.J., *et al.* (2011) Choice of living arrangements. *Journal of Intellectual Disability Research*, 55(8), pp. 746–762.

Stancliffe, R.J., *et al.* (2015) Transition to retirement and participation in inclusive community groups using active mentoring: An outcomes evaluation with a matched comparison group. *Journal of Intellectual Disability Research*, 59(8), pp. 703–718.

Stancliffe, R.J., *et al.* (2019) Aging, community-based employment, mobility impairment, and retirement: National core indicators – adult consumer survey data. *Research and Practice for Persons with Severe Disabilities*, 44(4), pp. 251–266.

Stevens, K., *et al.* (2017) Experiences of service users involved in recruitment for nursing courses: A phenomenological research study. *Nurse Education Today*, 58, pp. 59–64.

Sue, K., Mazzotta, P. and Grier, E. (2019) Palliative care for patients with communication and cognitive difficulties. *Canadian Family Physician Canadian Family Physician*, 65(1), pp. S19–S24.

Sundahl, L., *et al.* (2016) Physical activity levels among adolescents and young adult women and men with or without intellectual disability. *Journal of Applied Research in Intellectual Disabilities*, 29(1), pp. 93–98.

Taggart, L. and Cousins, W. (2014) *Health promotion for people with intellectual and developmental disabilities*. Berkshire, UK: McGraw-Hill Education.

Taggart, L., *et al.* (2018) Health promotion and wellness initiatives targeting chronic disease prevention and management for adults with intellectual and developmental disabilities: Recent advancements in type 2 diabetes. *Current Developmental Disorders Reports*, 5(3), pp. 132–142.

Thomas, R., *et al.* (2017) Ensuring an inclusive global health agenda for transgender people. *Bulletin of the World Health Organization*, 95(2), pp. 154–156.

Thorp, N., Stedmon, J. and Lloyd, H. (2017) 'I carry her in my heart': An exploration of the experience of bereavement for people with learning disability. *British Journal of Learning Disabilities*, 46(1), pp. 45–53.

Thuesen, J., *et al.* (2021) Reablement in need of theories of ageing: Would theories of successful ageing do? *Ageing & Society*, pp. 1–13. Doi:10.1017/S0144686X21001203.

Together for Short Lives (2013) *A core care pathway for children with life-limiting and life-threatening conditions* (3rd edition). Bristol: Together for Short Lives.

Together for Short Lives (2016) *Moving to adult services: What to expect. A guide for young people with life-threatening conditions making the transition to adult services.* Bristol: Together for Short Lives.

Tornstam., L. (1997) Gerotranscendence: The contemplative dimension of ageing. *Journal of Aging Studies*, 11(2), pp. 143–145.

Truesdale, M. and Brown, M. (2017) *People with learning disabilities in Scotland: 2017 health needs assessment update report.* Glasgow: NHS Health.

Tuffrey-Wijne, I. (2013) *How to break bad news: To people with learning disabilities.* London: Jessica Kingsley.

Tuffrey-Wijne, I. and Watchman, K. (2015) Breaking bad news to people with intellectual disabilities and dementia. *Learning Disability Practice*, 18(7), pp. 16–23.

United Nations (2006) *Convention on the rights of persons with disabilities (CRPD).* Available at: www.un.org/development/desa/disabilities/convention-on-the-rights-of-persons-with-disabilities.html#menu-header-menu (Accessed 22 July 2022).

University of Bristol (2018) *Intellectual disability mortality review (LeDeR) programme: Learning into action bulletin.* Available at: www.bristol.ac.uk/media-library/sites/sps/leder/WORKINGAspirpneumJulynewsletterfinal2.pdf (Accessed 22 July 2022).

Vadivelan, K., *et al.* (2020) Burden of caregivers of children with cerebral palsy: An intersectional analysis of gender, poverty, stigma, and public policy. *BMC Public Health*, 20, p. 645. Doi:10.1186/s12889-020-08808-0.

Van den Akker, M., Buntinx, F. and Knottnerus, J.A. (1996) Comorbidity or multimorbidity. *European Journal of General Practice*, 2(2), pp. 65–70.

Van Schijndel-Speet, M., *et al.* (2017) A structured physical activity and fitness programme for older adults with intellectual disabilities: Results of a cluster-randomised clinical trial. *Journal of Intellectual Disability Research*, 61(1), pp. 16–29.

Vijg, J. and Kennedy, B.K. (2016) The essence of aging. *Gerontology*, 62(4), pp. 381–385. Doi:10.1159/000439348.

Wagemans, A., *et al.* (2013) The factors affecting end-of-life decision-making by physicians of patients with intellectual disabilities in the Netherlands: A qualitative study. *Journal of Intellectual Disability Research*, 57(4), pp. 380–389.

Walford, R.L. (1969) The immunologic theory of aging. *Immunological Reviews*, 2(1), p. 171.

Walker, C. and Ward, C. (2013) Growing older together: Ageing and people with learning disabilities and their family carers. *Tizard Learning Disability Review*, 18(3), pp. 112–119.

Ward, C., Glass, N. and Ford, R. (2014) Care in the home for seriously ill children with complex needs: A narrative literature review. *Journal of Child Health Care*, 19(4), pp. 1–8.

Warrier, V., *et al.* (2020) Elevated rates of autism, other neurodevelopmental and psychiatric diagnoses, and autistic traits in transgender and gender-diverse individuals. *Nature Communications*, 11, p. 3959. Doi:10.1038/s41467-020-17794-1.

Wehmeyer, M.L. and Abery, B.H. (2013) Self-determination and choice. *Intellectual and Developmental Disabilities*, 51(5), pp. 399–411.

Whiting, M. (2017) Caring for children '24–7' – the experience of well child nurses and the families of whom they are providing care and support. *Journal of Child Health Care*, 23(1), pp. 35–44.

Whittle, E., *et al.* (2018) Barriers and enablers to accessing mental health services for people with intellectual disability: A scoping review. *Journal of Mental Health Research in Intellectual Disabilities*, 11(1), pp. 69–102.

Wiese, M., *et al.* (2013) 'If and when?' – The beliefs and experiences of community living staff in supporting older people with intellectual disability to know about dying. *Journal of Intellectual Disability Research*, 57(10), pp. 980–992.

Wiese, M., *et al.* (2015) Intellectual about dying, death, and end-of-life planning: Current issues informing future actions. *Journal of Intellectual and Developmental Disability*, 40(2), pp. 230–235.

Williamson, H.J., *et al.* (2017) Health care access for adults with intellectual and developmental disabilities: A scoping review. *OTJR: Occupation, Participation and Health*, 37, pp. 227–236.

Wilson, N.J., *et al.* (2018) A narrative review of the literature about people with intellectual disability who identify as lesbian, gay, bisexual, transgender, intersex or questioning. *Journal of Intellectual Disabilities*, 22(2), pp. 171–196.

Wilson, N.J., *et al.* (2019) Nurses working in intellectual disability-specific settings talk about the uniqueness of their role: A qualitative study. *Journal of Advanced Nursing*, 75(4), pp. 812–822.

Wilson, S., *et al.* (2013) A systematic review of interventions to promote social support and parenting skills in parents with an intellectual disability. *Child: Care, Health and Development*, 40(1), pp. 7–19.

Wing Man, N., Wade, C. and Llewellyn, G. (2017) Prevalence of parents with intellectual disability in Australia. *Journal of Intellectual & Developmental Disability*, 42(2), pp. 173–179.

Wolfensberger, W.P. (1972) *The principle of normalization in human services*. Toronto: National Institute on Mental Retardation.

Woodgate, R.L., *et al.* (2015) Intense parenting: A qualitative study detailing the experiences of parenting children with complex care needs. *BMC Pediatrics*, 15(197), pp. 1–15.

World Health Organisation (2012) *Early childhood development and disability: A discussion paper*. Geneva: World Health Organisation.

World Health Organization (2015a) *World report on aging and health*. Geneva: World Health Organisation.

World Health Organisation (2015b) *Sexual health*. Geneva: World Health Organisation.

World Health Organization (2018) *Handbook for national quality policy and strategy: A practical approach for developing policy and strategy to improve quality of care*. Geneva: World Health Organisation.

World Health Organization (2019b) *Integrated care for older people (ICOPE) implementation network – guidance for systems and services*. Geneva: World Health Organization.

Wormald, A.D., McCallion, P. and McCarron, M. (2019) The antecedents of loneliness in older people with an intellectual disability. Research in Developmental Disabilities, 85, pp.116–130.

Yang, Y.Y. and Lee, F.P. (2012) Concept analysis of feelings of loss among elderly nursing home residents. *Hu Li Za Zhi*, 59(4), pp. 99–104.

Young, H. (2017) Overcoming barriers to grief: Supporting bereaved people with profound intellectual and multiple disabilities. *International Journal of Developmental Disabilities*, 63(3), pp. 131–137.

Further Reading

Emerson, E., *et al.* (2013) *People with learning disabilities in England 2012.* Lancaster: Learning Disabilities Observatory, University of Lancaster.
Heslop, P., *et al.* (2013) *Confidential inquiry into premature deaths of people with learning disabilities (CIPOLD).* Bristol: University of Bristol.

Useful Resources

AIIHPC (All Ireland Institute of Hospice and Palliative Care): https://aiihpc.org/
BILD (British Institute of Learning Disabilities): www.bild.org.uk/
Breaking Bad News http: www.breakingbadnews.org/ and Irene Tuffrey-Wijne
Foundation for People with Learning Disabilities: www.intellectualdisabilities.org.uk/
IDS-TILDA (Intellectual Disability Supplement to the Irish Longitudinal Study on Ageing) Trinity Centre for Ageing and Intellectual Disability (TCAID): www.idstilda.tcd.ie/
Improving Health and Lives – Learning Disability Observatory: https://improvinghealthandlives.org.uk/
Inclusion Ireland: https://inclusionireland.ie/
NHS Choices – End-of-life care: www.nhs.uk/planners/end-of-life-care/pages/end-of-life-care.aspx
NHS Choices – Learning disability: www.nhs.uk/Livewell/Childrenwithaintellectualdisability/Pages/Childrenwithalearningdisabilityhome.aspx
NHS Easy Read Resources: www.cwp.nhs.uk/resources/easy-read-leaflets/
NHS Specialist Services for Children with Learning Disabilities: https://cchp.nhs.uk/cchp/explore-cchp/specialist-service-children-learning-disabilities
NICE (National Institute for Health Care and Excellence: www.nice.org.uk/
Palliative Care of People with Learning Disabilities Network: www.pcpld.org
Professor of Intellectual Disability and Palliative Care: www.tuffrey-wijne.com/?page_id=90
Scottish Learning Disabilities Observatory: www.sldo.ac.uk/

CHAPTER 4

Lynette Harper, Kirsty Henry, Lisa Oluyinka and Louise Cogher

Role of the intellectual disability nurse in promoting health and well-being

Introduction

In this chapter, students of nursing will explore the role of the intellectual disability nurse in promoting the health and well-being of people with intellectual disabilities. This will be contextualised within the Nursing and Midwifery Council (NMC) for the United Kingdom (2018) and Nursing and Midwifery Board of Ireland (NMBI) (2016) standards and requirements for competence.

This chapter incorporates key concepts and policies in public health and includes the key policy drivers that are refocusing nursing interventions to be centrally concerned with prevention. The role of intellectual disability nurses in helping people with intellectual disabilities plan for good health and well-being will be explored. We also explore intellectual disability nurses' public health roles, and the importance of health promotion in care planning, health facilitation, and health action planning will be addressed, as well as newer roles such as health liaison nursing in primary care and acute settings. These roles are explored in the context of well-known health issues, such as cardiovascular fitness, obesity, epilepsy, mental ill health, sexuality, diet, and smoking. Many of these conditions require intellectual disability nurses to develop careful and imaginative ways of constructing nursing interventions to improve or maintain the health status of people with intellectual disabilities.

DOI: 10.4324/9781003296461-4

Box 4.1 This chapter will focus on the following issues:

- Key concepts and policies
  - What is public health?
- Health promotion
  - Why health promotion?
  - Characteristics of successful health promotion
- Health facilitation
  - Why health facilitation?
  - Essential skills for health facilitation
- Health action planning
  - Why health action planning?
- Health liaison
  - Why health liaison?
- Public health policies
  - England
  - Scotland
  - Northern Ireland
  - Wales
  - UK frameworks
- Intellectual disability public health nursing practice
- Current public health roles of intellectual disability nurses
  - Facilitating access to healthcare
  - Health screening and health surveillance
  - Health promotion and health education
  - Health protection and health prevention
- Factors that influence intellectual disability nurses' public health practice
  - Public health role clarity
  - Demographic intelligence
  - Interprofessional and interagency collaboration
  - Leadership
  - Resources
  - Politics

Box 4.2 Competences

Nursing and Midwifery Council (2018) Proficiencies

Platform 1: Being an accountable professional – 1.9, 1.14

Platform 2: Promoting health and preventing ill-health – 2.1, 2.2, 2.3, 2.4, 2.5, 2.6, 2.7, 2.10, 2.11, 2.12

Platform 3: Assessing needs and planning care – 3.6, 3.15

Platform 5: Leading and managing nursing care and working in teams – 5.12

Platform 7: Coordinating care – 7.1, 7.2, 7.3, 7.4

Nursing and Midwifery Board of Ireland (2016) Competences

Domain 2: Nursing practice and clinical decision-making competences – 2.1, 2.2, 2.3, 2.5

Domain 3: Knowledge and cognitive competences – 3.1

Key concepts and policies

What is public health?

The Acheson Report has described public health as

> the science and art of preventing disease, prolonging life and promoting health through organised efforts of society.

(Acheson, 1988, p. 27)

This definition has been accepted by public health policy, the World Health Organisation (2012) and the professional standards body for public health specialists and practitioners in the UK and Ireland (Faculty of Public Health, 2019; Institute of Public Health, 2020). However, the concept of public health is contentious (Dawson and Verweij, 2007), as there is no globally agreed definition of what 'public health' means (Baggott, 2011; Kaiser and Mackenbach, 2008). The lack of an agreed dialogical definition is not surprising, given that the meaning of 'health' itself is a subject of endless debate (Blaxter, 2004). An all-encompassing definition of public health (Baggott, 2011) is problematic, and a source of significant confusion (Griffiths and Hunter, 1999). Recent efforts have been made to develop conceptual models of public health to clarify the concept. The most notable model was developed by Griffiths, Jewell, and Donelly (2005). The framework has three interrelated domains of 'health prevention', 'health, improvement', and 'health service delivery and quality'.

Winslow's observations remain pertinent in the literature; he advocated that health is interconnected with social life, the environment in which populations live, grow and age and furthermore, that the education of individuals within identified populations is key.

According to Winslow.

Box 4.3 Ten essential public health operations (EPHOs)

1. Surveillance of population health and well-being
2. Monitoring and response to health hazards and emergencies
3. Health protection including environmental, occupational, food safety and others
4. Health promotion including action to address social determinants and health inequity
5. Disease prevention, including early detection of illness
6. Assuring governance for health and well-being
7. Assuring a sufficient and competent public health workforce
8. Assuring sustainable organisational structures and financing
9. Advocacy, communication, and social mobilisation for health
10. Advancing public health research to inform policy and practice

(Taken from World Health Organisation (2022). Available at: www. euro.who.int/en/health-topics/Health-systems/public-health-ser vices/policy/the-10-essential-public-health-operations (Accessed 9 August 2022).)

Public health is the science and the art of preventing disease, prolonging life and promoting physical health and efficiency through rioritiz community efforts for the sanitation of the environment, the control of community infections, the education of the individual in principles of personal hygiene, the organisation of medical and nursing service for the early diagnosis and preventative treatment of disease, and the development of social machinery which will ensure to every individual in the community a standard of living adequate for the maintenance of health.

(Winslow, 1920, p. 23)

This approach to public health highlights the importance of public health roles, including those of intellectual disability nurses in meeting the public health needs of people with intellectual disabilities. Intellectual disability nurses play a key role in public health through improving the health literacy of people with intellectual disabilities through provision of resources in accessible formats relating to health needs, healthy lifestyles, and health and social policy. Furthermore, intellectual disability nurses advocate for and with people with intellectual disabilities and enable equality of service provision.

The FPH organises public health practice into three domains (health improvement, health protection, and improving services) (Faculty of Public Health, 2020). These domains are like Griffiths *et al.*'s model (Griffiths, Jewell and Donelly, 2005). In addition to the three domains, the FPH identifies nine key areas of public health practice, and these are given in Figure 4.1.

On the other hand, the World Health Organisation (2022) provides details of essential public health operations (EPHOs). The WHO top 10 EPHOs have emphasised the importance of social determinants to health, environment, and social needs of populations.

Health promotion

Health promotion is a process of enabling people to have control over the determinants of their health to improve their health and well-being (WHO, 1986). As

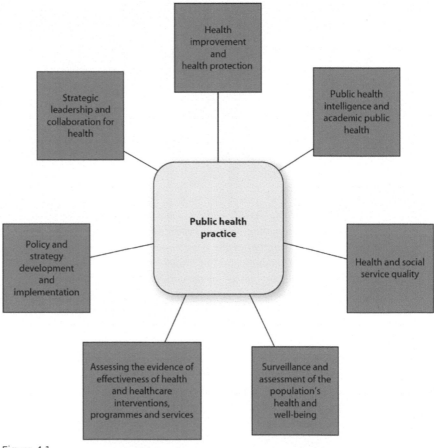

Figure 4.1

Key areas of public health practice.

a concept and set of practical strategies, it remains an essential guide in addressing the major health challenges that people with intellectual disabilities face, including communicable and non-communicable diseases, and issues related to their human development and health. Health promotion is a process directed toward enabling people with learning disabilities to act. Health promotion is therefore not something that is done on or to people with intellectual disabilities; it is done by, with, and for people with intellectual disabilities either as individuals or as groups. The purpose of health promotion is to strengthen the skills and capabilities of individuals with intellectual disabilities to act and the capacity of groups or communities to act collectively to exert control over the determinants of their health and achieve positive change. The health promotion role of intellectual disability nurses is concerned with making healthier choices easier choices for people with intellectual disabilities. Health promotion involves the overlapping activities of health education, health protection, and prevention.

Why health promotion?

Broadly, health promotion focuses on prolonging healthy life, reducing inequalities in health, and reducing pressure on health services. People with intellectual disabilities have increased comorbidity, communication difficulties, a high prevalence of serious conditions such as epilepsy, and specific patterns of health needs associated with the etiology of their disability. Unfortunately, this combination of need is mirrored by a consistent picture of poor health promotion uptake, inadequate care for serious morbidity, unrecognised health needs, and poor access to healthcare.

There is a great disparity between the health of people with intellectual disabilities and that of the general population (McMahon and Hatton, 2021; Heslop *et al.*, 2013; Public Health England, 2018; Michael, 2008). These studies or reviews suggest that examination of any community-based population of people with intellectual disabilities consistently uncovers serious health problems such as:

- Untreated, yet treatable, medical conditions
- Delayed diagnosis of health conditions
- Multi-morbidity and complex care and treatment plans involving polypharmacy.
- A lack of uptake of health promotion to reduce the likelihood of developing health conditions.

This shows a need for education and training to raise awareness of specific health issues related to people with intellectual disabilities for both staff working in healthcare services, carers, and for people with intellectual disabilities. For people with intellectual disabilities, health promotion is important because there is a disparity between the health and healthcare needs of this group of people compared to that of the general population (Hott and Flores, 2021; DH, 2001). It is important to recognise that these disparities in health and health outcomes are avoidable and could be improved with appropriate early interventions (Heslop *et al.*, 2013; Glover *et al.*, 2017). For people with intellectual disabilities, these disparities result from poor access to health services, limited options in lifestyle, and poor living standards (Whitehead, 1992).

Health promotion is important for people with intellectual disabilities because international studies have shown poor uptake of public health initiatives by people with intellectual disabilities (McConkey, Taggart and Kane, 2015; Turner, Giraud-Saunders and Marriott, 2013). Doherty et al.'s (2020) systematic review reported that people with intellectual disabilities face barriers to primary healthcare which reduces access to health screening and health promotion services. Barriers included a lack of knowledge and awareness of people with intellectual disabilities, poor communication, and lack of knowledge on how to increase people with intellectual disabilities' involvement in decision-making. Lennox, Beange, and Edwards (2000) and Iacano et al. (2014) have noted the need for effective health advocacy for people with intellectual disabilities from relevant health professionals. In the last decade acting as advocates and promoting inclusion, equity, and fairness to improve health outcomes have remained common themes in the discourse of intellectual disability nurses (Cope and Shaw, 2019). Healthcare outcomes are dependent on safe, effective, and holistic care and therefore, the role of intellectual disability nurses in promoting the health of people with intellectual disabilities is important. However, there remains a lack of agreement on how to conceptualise health promotion for people with intellectual disabilities and how to gain optimum health and well-being outcomes through adapting generic health promotion initiatives for people with intellectual disabilities (Roll, 2018).

A significant proportion of people with intellectual disabilities and their carers will need professional support to be able to access public health and other healthcare services. Doody, Lyons, and Ryan (2019) have pointed to a lack of evidence that shows the involvement of people with intellectual disabilities in engaging in care planning within health services. This suggests that people with intellectual disabilities can be passive participants in their health and healthcare, despite evidence that involvement in decision-making enables people with intellectual disabilities to feel empowered and supports understanding of their diagnosis and treatment (Doherty et al., 2020) and thus concordance with nursing care plans (Chapman, 2018).

In the United Kingdom the introduction of the Quality Outcomes Framework (QOF) in 2004, and the later introduction of Directed Enhanced Services (DES) in England (Scottish Enhanced Services Programme [SESP] in Scotland), placed the responsibility of preventive health service provision for people with intellectual disability on general practitioners. The QOF and DES has incentivised primary care providers to maintain registers of people with intellectual disabilities and complete personalised annual health checks (Chauhan et al., 2012).

Intellectual disability nurses have an important role in developing and implementing health promotion strategies that meet the health needs of people with intellectual disabilities (Table 4.1). Recent studies have demonstrated that preventive interventions such as health screenings are effective in identifying the health needs of people with intellectual disabilities to reduce preventable hospital admissions and identify gaps in health services (Robertson et al., 2011, 2014; Carey et al., 2017; Emerson and Glover, 2010; Emerson, Copeland and Glover, 2011). However, Taggart et al.'s (2018) cost analysis of annual health

Approach	Objective	Activity	Examples
Education	To provide information and create well-informed people. To empower choice and foster personal growth through provision of knowledge. To prevent disease by persuading people to adopt lifestyles that promote freedom from disease. To raise awareness of the need for health policy, to stimulate people to tackle the social, environmental, and political influences on health.	Information giving regarding cause of illnesses and effect of lifestyles. Develop knowledge and skills for people to be able to make healthier choices. Educate people to change attitudes and behaviour and adopt healthier lifestyles.	Persuasive education. Provision of education (one to one, groups, peers, media).
Protection	To influence individuals' choices. To modify individuals' risks. To modify the environment.	Political and social action.	Public health policy development. Changes to the environment.
Prevention	*Primary prevention* – Seeks to prevent onset of disease. *Secondary prevention* – Aims to halt the progression of disease. *Tertiary prevention* – Rehabilitation to minimise risk.	Diagnosis and treatment.	Screening. Diagnostic tests. Medical or surgical intervention.

Table 4.1   Approaches to health promotion

checks in an aging population of people with intellectual disabilities found that identifying health conditions did not improve health related quality of life or mortality if effective treatment options are not accessible. Therefore, access to interventions and follow-up care is equally important to intellectual disability nurses as identification of health needs. Furthermore, promoting healthy lifestyle choices from an early age can reduce the risk of developing diseases in later life. These public health and health promotion initiatives should be targeted towards people with intellectual disabilities, be proactive, work at multiple levels of the system develop through collaboration with individuals with intellectual disabilities, and involve the wider professional team.

Characteristics of successful health promotion

Effectively promoting the health and well-being of people with intellectual disabilities requires:

- Knowledge and competence of the health promotion among a workforce that includes intellectual disability nurses and others
- Knowledge-based public health and health promotion practice
- Evidence-based public health and health promotion practice
- Integrated and seamless local and national health promotion policies
- Integrated and collaborative health-promoting services
- Active participation by people with intellectual disabilities

- Healthy local and national public policy
- Structures and systems that are effective in putting healthy public policy into practice
- Strengthening and empowering local community actions and strategies
- Reorientation of health services from treatment to prevention
- Strengthening structures and processes in all sectors, to create supportive environments that promote the health and well-being of people with intellectual disabilities
- Funding and availability of resources specifically targeted at meeting the public health needs and promoting the health and well-being of people with intellectual disabilities.

Health facilitation

Health facilitation involves both case work to help people access mainstream services and service improvement within mainstream services to help parts of the NHS to develop the necessary skills for other healthcare professionals (National Learning Disability Professional Senate, 2015). The impetus for both is to help ensure that good healthcare is delivered in primary and secondary care (DH, 2002). Health facilitation needs to occur on several levels, e.g., individual, operational, and strategic. Ultimately, health facilitation is about ensuring healthier lives and better health for people with intellectual disabilities (DH, 2002). Health facilitation is important because good healthcare needs to be delivered by ordinary services, as well as specialist intellectual disability services. Health facilitation includes working directly with people with intellectual disabilities and their carers to

- Undertake holistic health needs assessments
- Trace individual problems to their source and seek their resolution
- Develop the ability of people with intellectual disabilities to recognise and address their own health needs.

Health facilitation also includes working with a wide range of health services to help them plan better to meet people with intellectual disabilities' health needs (DH, 2002). The most common public health role of community nurses working in facilitation and liaison roles is to advocate and support implementation of public health policies and better access to resources, to enable people with intellectual disabilities to gain full access to the healthcare they need in both primary and secondary NHS services (Mafuba and Gates, 2013).

Why health facilitation?

People with intellectual disabilities experience unequal access to health services and delays to diagnosis of treatable conditions (Heslop et al., 2013; Mencap,

2004, 2007, 2020; DH, 2007a, 2007b). In the United Kingdom, access to public health is primarily through the primary healthcare system. Current literature shows that a significant proportion of health inequalities in people with
intellectual disabilities are linked to poor quality healthcare provision (DH,
2013; Michael, 2008; Mencap, 2012; Parliamentary Health Ombudsman and
Social Services Ombudsman, 2009). This rather suggests that these inequalities
are preventable. UK government policy has focused on improving people with
intellectual disabilities' access to generic and preventive health services for some
considerable time (DH, 1992, 1995, 2001, 2009a; NHS Executive, 1998; Ruddick, 2005). However, the continuing disparities in health in people with intellectual disabilities suggest that policies alone are not enough.

Barriers to accessing services contribute to health inequalities for people with
intellectual disabilities. A significant number of barriers that contribute to failure in meeting the healthcare needs of people with intellectual disabilities have
been identified (Doherty *et al.*, 2020; Tuffrey-Wijne *et al.*, 2014). Identification
of people with intellectual disabilities and flagging the need to consider reasonable adjustments has been consistently identified as a common barrier (Public
Health England, 2016; Tuffrey-Wijne *et al.*, 2014). Furthermore, lack of training
of how to make reasonable adjustments and the lack of knowledge of what support is available from professionals with specialist knowledge of working with
people with intellectual disabilities has been highlighted (Doherty *et al.*, 2020).
Effective health facilitation is therefore important in ensuring that people with
learning disabilities can access appropriate healthcare.

Essential skills for health facilitation

Appropriate subject knowledge: Successful health facilitation requires relevant
background knowledge regarding the health and social care needs of people
with intellectual disabilities.

Clinical skills: To function effectively as a health facilitator, intellectual disability nurses will have to be competent in complex and comprehensive health
needs assessments and risk assessments to be able to assist with screening or
assessment and clinical procedures, in a wide range of clinical settings in which
they practice.

Health and social care needs: Knowledge of health and social care needs of
people with intellectual disabilities is indispensable for intellectual disability
nurses to be able to provide advice and share their knowledge and expertise with
other health and social care professionals.

Determinants of health: The impact of the wider determinants of health
and their impact on people with intellectual disabilities was discussed earlier.
Knowledge of wider determinants of health and barriers to services experienced
by people with intellectual disabilities is important for intellectual disability
nurses to be able to develop systems and protocols that are essential to meeting
the health and social care needs of people with intellectual disabilities.

Communication and collaborative working: Health facilitation involves a wide
range of stakeholders. Intellectual disability nurses will require effective communication and negotiation skills in dealing with other professionals, agencies,
carers, and people with intellectual disabilities. Nurses need to advocate and

actively encourage people with intellectual disabilities and the family or carers to be productively involved in decision-making and planning for healthcare needs. Communication skills are also vital in developing partnership working arrangements with other agencies and professionals. In addition, to fulfill their roles as health facilitators, intellectual disability nurses need to be familiar with health services in the areas in which they practice, to facilitate access to appropriate services. Appropriate experience of how health services operate is also important for learning disability nurses to fulfill this role.

Health action planning

Health action plans provide details of the actions essential to maintaining and improving the health of people with intellectual disabilities and any support that may be required for the implementation of the plans. Health action planning links people with intellectual disabilities to a wide range of health services and support mechanisms necessary for attaining better health. For health action plans to work, reasonable adjustments may need to be made and it is therefore essential that health action plans are produced in partnership with the person concerned. Co-creation ensures that people, together with their carers, understand their health and how they can maintain and improve it, as well as ensuring that healthcare services are able to respond to the person's health needs. In addition, health action plans are important for influencing wider healthcare services to inform changes that are important in developing systems and structures that positively impact the health and healthcare of people with learning disabilities.

Points to note:

- Health action plans are simply plans about what people can do to be fit and healthy.
- Health action plans list any help and support that might be needed to achieve and maintain good health.
- Health action plans may be reactive or proactive, or both reactive and proactive. They aim to
  - Ensure that individual health needs, including those needs specifically relating to syndromes, are properly addressed for people with intellectual disabilities.
  - Address the wider determinants of health.
  - Remove the barriers to good health for people with intellectual disabilities.
  - Support the mainstream health agenda and the drive to reduce health inequalities.

Why health action planning?

People with intellectual disabilities are known to have much greater health needs than those of comparable age groups who do not have intellectual

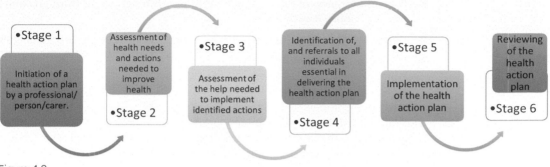

Figure 4.2

Stages in health action planning.

disabilities (Emerson and McGrother, 2010; Heslop *et al.*, 2013; McMahon and Hatton, 2021). These include higher rates of mental health problems (Buckles *et al.*, 2013; Hughes-McCormack *et al.*, 2017); sensory impairments (Kiani and Miller, 2010); epilepsy (Robertson *et al.*, 2015); and obesity and weight-related disorders (Hsieh, Rimmer and Heller, 2014; Ryan *et al.*, 2021). People with intellectual disabilities are more likely to die from preventable causes (Mencap, 2007; DH, 2007a, 2007b; Heslop *et al.*, 2013; McCarron *et al.*, 2015; McMahon and Hatton, 2021). Studies have shown that the health problems that people with intellectual disabilities experience are commonly and widely undiagnosed, misdiagnosed, and untreated (Ramsey *et al.*, 2022). Although the life expectancy of people with learning disabilities has increased with that of the general population, overall life expectancy remains lower, and mortality rates remain significantly higher than those of the general population (McCarron *et al.*, 2015). It is therefore important in the context of public health that intellectual disability nurses understand the risk factors associated with intellectual disabilities to prevent premature deaths. If used appropriately, health action planning could improve the health and healthcare outcomes for people with learning disabilities (see Figure 4.2).

Health Liaison

The key focus of health liaison is the facilitation of access to mainstream healthcare services. The role of the liaison nurse is varied, and might include:

■ Supporting the assessment of mental capacity to consent to treatment.
■ Supporting professionals and organisations to make reasonable adjustments to overcome environmental and system barriers.
■ Assistance with diagnosis and treatment.
■ Directly supporting and/or advocating for patients with intellectual disabilities who are receiving assessments or treatment for health conditions.

■ Raising awareness of intellectual disability within staff teams through education and policy development.

■ Providing advice and support with augmentative communication strategies.

■ Providing advice on discharge planning or the need for continuing care.

In their role health liaison intellectual disability nurses liaise with other services and professionals such as the medical team who will be treating the person with intellectual disabilities, care managers, and primary care services. To effectively undertake the health liaison role, liaison nurses need to have a visible and accessible base (Brown *et al.*, 2011). In addition, there is a need for collaboration between intellectual disability specialist services, primary care, and acute services (Tuffrey-Wijne *et al.*, 2013)

Why health liaison?

Health liaison is important for learning disability and intellectual disability nursing because people with intellectual disabilities have greater health needs than the general population (McMahon and Hatton, 2021), yet experience poorer access to healthcare (Brown *et al.*, 2011; Tuffrey-Wijne *et al.*, 2013). Studies have shown that people with learning disabilities are considered a low priority by healthcare professionals (Tromans *et al.*, 2020; Ramsey *et al.*, 2022), and that barriers to accessing health for people with intellectual disabilities are often compounded by communication challenges (Norah Fry Research Centre, 2021). Healthcare professionals often have limited augmentative communication skills, which further limits their ability to diagnose and treat people with

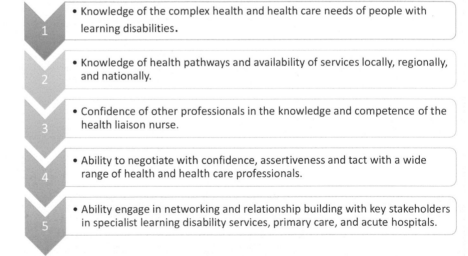

Figure 4.3

Skills for health liaison.

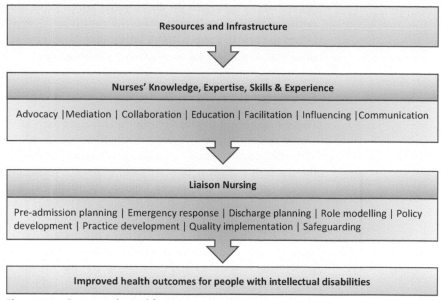

Figure 4.4   *Source:* Adapted from Brown *et al.* (2011)

Conceptual model of learning disability liaison nursing service.

intellectual disabilities effectively (Hemm, Dagnan and Meyer, 2015; Gregson, Randle-Phillips and Hillman, 2022). Intellectual disability nurses have important roles in facilitating communication between people with intellectual disabilities and health services, and in overcoming the barriers that they may face in accessing services.

To effectively liaise with other professionals and agencies, learning disability and intellectual disability nurses require specialist health liaison skills (see Figure 4.3). Brown *et al.* (2011) have suggested a conceptual model of learning disability and intellectual disability liaison nursing (see Figure 4.4).

Public health policies

Each of the four countries of the United Kingdom has different public health policies, and this divergence has been increasing (Greer, 2009).

England

In England, prioritising the health of people with an intellectual disability has been developing since Valuing People (DH, 2001) *Tackling Health Inequalities* (DH, 2007a), *Healthy Lives, Healthy People* (DH, 2010), CIPOLD (Heslop *et al.*, 2013). And the LeDeR reviews. The NHS long term plan (2019) sets out a vision for the twenty-first century, identifying the tackling of health inequalities for people with intellectual disabilities as a key priority, alongside offering a commitment to improved integration of health and social care. These measures affirm the role of the intellectual disability liaison nurse to connect services for people and facilitate access to generic health services.

Scotland

There has been a distinct public health approach in Scotland for a considerable time; *Scotland's Health: A Challenge to Us All* (Scottish Office, 1992) identified coronary heart disease and cancer as key public health targets. Since then, a series of other policies have emerged, including *Our National Health: A Plan for Action, a Plan for Change* (Scottish Executive, 2000a), *Improving Health in Scotland* (Scottish Executive, 2003), *Better Health, Better Care: Action Plan* (Scottish Government, 2007), and *Equally Well* (Scottish Government, 2008). Like in England, none of these policies specifically addressed the public health needs of people with intellectual disabilities, but they applied to the whole population. In 2021, the Scottish government consolidated its plans to transform intellectual disability services to address inequalities in health: Learning/Intellectual Disability and Autism Transformation Plan (Scottish Government, 2021).

BOX 4.4
CASE STUDY 4.1

Ash is 30 years old and has a moderate intellectual disability and Prader-Willi syndrome. Ash lives at home with his parents and attends a supported employment project for four days each week. He has limited social contacts and therefore relies on his immediate family for social support. Ash is severely overweight and has type two diabetes. He also has epilepsy, which is managed by medication. Ash has not been receiving any support from the local community team for people with intellectual disabilities.

Ash has a long history of weight-management challenges associated with his Prader-Willi syndrome. Prader-Willi syndrome is a genetic condition where there can be associated obsessions including behaviours relating to food and an unsatisfied appetite. The syndrome is complex, and there are a range of characteristics present that include episodes of mental ill health and behaviour that can be challenging to manage (see Chapter 1).

Ash has been admitted to an assessment and treatment service following a series of increasingly challenging conflicts at home. His parents describe an 'unmanageable obsession with food' that has led to several 'incidents' in supermarkets and cafes where Ash has 'lashed out' at members of the public that have tried to confront him stealing food. They explain that they try to restrict his diet because of his diabetes, however, this is making him resentful and aggressive.

Box 4.5
Student Activity 4.1

You are a student nurse on placement in the Assessment and Treatment service. Your practice supervisor asks you to undertake a physical health assessment with Ash.

Describe how you would use health promotion to support Ash to managing his weight-related health issues.

Using a recognised model, construct a health action plan for Ash to manage his diabetes. Explore how you would use health facilitation to meet Ash's health and social care needs.

Discuss the role(s) of other professionals in the assessment process.

Explore the role of health liaison nursing while Ash is in an acute assessment and treatment unit.

Identify relevant NMC/An Bord Altranais competencies that are applicable in this scenario.

Northern Ireland

Northern Ireland has adopted a much more focused and sustained public health policy approach (Wilde, 2007; NI Executive, 2008). Since the 1990s, key policy documents have emerged, including *Health and Wellbeing: Towards the New Millennium* (DHSSNI, 1996), *Well in 2000* (DHSSNI, 1997), *Investing for Health* (DHSSPSNI, 2002), and *A Healthier Future* (DHSSPS, 2004).

In 2002 the DHSSPS initiated *The Bamford Review of Mental Health and Learning Disability* (Department of Health, 2007) which called for a wide range of improvements to mental health and intellectual disability services, policy and legislation setting out a 10–15-year plan. This vision established a series of action plans over the next decade led by the Public Health Agency which have strengthened this position for people with intellectual disabilities in Northern Ireland. These have been incorporated into the *Making Life Better Charter – A Whole System Strategic Framework For Public Health 2013–2023* (DHSSPSNI, 2014).

Wales

Wales was the first UK country to develop a comprehensive and inclusive public health strategy (Welsh Office NHS Directorate, 1989, 1992) that was quite distinct (Greer, 2009; Coyle, 2007). The identified priority areas were cancer, maternal and child health, emotional health, respiratory illness, cardiovascular diseases, intellectual disabilities, mental distress and illness, injuries, healthy environments, and physical disabilities. Since then, a series of other public health policy initiatives emerged and include *Better Health, Better Wales* (Welsh

Office, 1998), *Improving Health in Wales* (NAfW, 2001), *Wellbeing in Wales* (Welsh Assembly Government, 2002), *Wales – A Better Country* (Welsh Assembly Government, 2003), and *Designed for Life* (Welsh Assembly Government, 2005). Commitment to reduce health inequalities experienced by people with intellectual disabilities in Wales was renewed in the Improving Lives project (Welsh Government, 2018) and outlined in the *Learning Disability Strategy Action Plan 2022–2026* (Welsh Government, 2022).

Other developments

The UK-wide general practitioner contract specifies three distinct groups of services: essential services (compulsory – consultations), additional services (optional – immunisation and screening), and enhanced services (optional – specialised services). There were originally 10 indicators on the *Quality Outcomes Framework* (QOF), and this has been repeatedly revised, and has included intellectual disabilities since 2006. In 2008, additional payment for the provision of *Clinical Directed Enhanced Services* (NHS England, 2022) for people with intellectual disabilities was introduced. This was intended to improve access to generic public health services by people with intellectual disabilities at the primary healthcare level.

Valuing People: A New Strategy for Learning Disability for the 21st Century (DH, 2001) highlighted the need to improve the health of people with intellectual disabilities in England and Wales (*The Same as You* in Scotland) (Scottish Executive, 2000b). The complexity of the healthcare needs of people with intellectual disabilities is acknowledged, and the inadequacies of existing models of healthcare provision for people with intellectual disabilities in generic healthcare settings highlighted. In Scotland, the *Health Needs Assessment Report: People with Learning Disabilities in Scotland* (NHS Health Scotland, 2004) highlighted the needs of people with intellectual disabilities and provided guidance to healthcare professionals about how these could be met.

Since *Valuing People* was published in 2001 (DH, 2001), there have been other notable developments which have affected the implementation of public health policy for people with intellectual disabilities. Although these are not discussed at this point in any detail, they are worth noting for students and practitioners to widen their understanding of the practice environment. These notable developments include the *Treat Me Right* report (Mencap, 2004), which highlighted the health needs of people with learning disabilities and suggested how access to services could be improved. *Equal Treatment: Closing the Gap* (DRC, 2006) revealed an inadequate response from the NHS and the English and Welsh governments to the major physical health inequalities experienced by people with mental health needs and people with intellectual disabilities. *Death by Indifference* (Mencap, 2007) alleged institutional discrimination within the NHS, which resulted in people with learning disabilities receiving ineffective healthcare. The report presented the stories of six people who the authors believe died unnecessarily because of healthcare professionals' lack of understanding of the complexity of the healthcare needs of people with intellectual disabilities. *Healthcare for All* (Michael, 2008) highlighted the high levels of unmet health needs of people with intellectual disabilities, poor access to services, and ineffectiveness of the treatment they received. *Six Lives* (Parliamentary and Health Service Ombuds-man and Social Services Ombudsman, 2009) was the government's response to *Death by Indifference* (Mencap, 2007). *Death by Indifference: 74 Deaths and Counting* (Mencap, 2012) has reported further avoidable deaths of people with intellectual disabilities. *Confidential Inquiry into Premature Deaths of People with Learning Disabilities (CIPOLD)* concluded that the effectiveness and quality of healthcare provided to people with intellectual disabilities was inadequate and recommended proactive interventions to address these deficiencies (Helsop *et al.*, 2013). These reports triggered the Annual *Learning Disability Mortality Review* which requires the reporting of deaths of people with intellectual disabilities (and this now includes people with Autism) for review (LeDeR) (NHS, 2021).

Learning disability public health nursing practice

Brief history of public health roles of learning disability nurses

Jukes (1994) has traced to the 1960s the origins of the intellectual disability nurse's involvement with public health for people with intellectual disabilities. Several attempts have been made to identify and clarify the contribution of intellectual disability nurses to health promotion (Elliot-Cannon, 1981). The Griffiths Report (Griffiths, 1988), and the NHS and Community Care Act (DH, 1990) emphasised the *'health'* contribution of intellectual disability nursing. The Department of Health has clearly emphasised the public health role of the intellectual disability nurse in England (DH, 2001, <u>2007c</u>). However, defining the public health role of intellectual disability nurses has been difficult (Mobbs *et al.*, 2002). As a result, the public health role of intellectual disability nurses has evolved differently across the United Kingdom (Mobbs *et al.*, 2002). Primary care and social care services have a conflicting understanding of the role and contribution of intellectual disability nurses to the delivery of public health services to people with learning disabilities (McGarry and Arthur, 2001). There is very little research into the learning disability nurse's role, practice, and contribution to public health services for people with intellectual disabilities (Boarder, 2002). Research on the role of intellectual disability nurses has concentrated on their broader professional roles such as advocacy (Gates, 1994; Jukes, 1994; Mobbs *et al.*, 2002; Llewellyn and Northway, 2007), and generic community nursing roles (Holloway, 2004; Boarder, 2002; Powell, Murray and McKenzie, 2004).

Intellectual disability nurses have a key public health role in several key areas, including contributing to public health policy development, planning public health policy implementation, and taking a lead role in the implementation and delivery of public health policy for people with intellectual disabilities (Mafuba and Gates, 2013).

Current public health roles of learning disability nurses

Studies have noted increasing involvement of intellectual disability nurses with public health in England (Boarder, 2002; Mobbs *et al.*, 2002; Barr, 2006; Barr *et al.*, 1999). McConkey, Moore and Marshall (2002) and have reported the increasing involvement of community intellectual disability nurses with health promotion and health screening of people with intellectual disabilities in Northern Ireland. In Ireland, intellectual disability nurses are identified as having the knowledge and skills to support people with intellectual disabilities to achieve optimum health outcomes in a public health role (McCarron *et al.*, 2018). The public health roles of intellectual disability nurses are changing because of policy initiatives such as health facilitation and health action planning (Scottish Executive, 2000b; DH, 2001; DHSSPS, 2004). Intellectual disability nursing students and practitioners need to be aware that the influences on how they undertake their public health roles are likely to be complex and may not necessarily be consistent with the descriptions provided here.

A study by Mafuba and Gates (2013) has demonstrated that intellectual disability nurses are involved with healthcare delivery, health education, health prevention and protection, facilitating access to health, health promotion, and health surveillance in meeting the public health needs of people with learning disabilities.

Facilitating access to healthcare

Facilitating access to healthcare is the most common public health role of intellectual disability nurses (Marshall and Moore, 2003; Barr *et al.*, 1999; Abbott, 2007; Mafuba and Gates, 2013). The public health roles of intellectual disability nurses are becoming more facilitatory as a result of recent policy initiatives (Scottish Executive, 2000b; DH, 2001; DHSSPS, 2004). For detailed discussion on the facilitatory roles of intellectual disability nurses, refer to Chapter 10.

Health screening and health surveillance

Health screening is an important role for intellectual disability nurses in improving the health and healthcare of people with intellectual disabilities. First, the number of health problems among people with intellectual disabilities has been estimated to be 2.5 times greater than among people without intellectual disabilities, and mortality rates are higher than those of the wider population. People with intellectual disabilities are disproportionately affected by respiratory disease, epilepsy, dysphagia, constipation, mental health problems, communication difficulties, visual impairments, dental problems, coronary heart disease, diabetes, and obesity. Mortality from these conditions is preventable, and intellectual disability nurses play an important role in assessing these needs. Causes for higher mortality rates are diverse and complex but include co-morbid conditions, reduced access and barriers to services, and poor diagnosis and poor treatment by health professionals. People with intellectual disabilities experience poor access to mainstream public health and health promotion services, such as health screening and health protection services and immunisation programmes. The involvement of intellectual disability nurses with health screening and health surveillance across the United Kingdom and Northern Ireland is varied. One explanation could be that health screening is part of the general practitioner contract, and intellectual disability nurses' involvement in this area is only through collaboration with general practitioners who might not see these activities as a priority. Another explanation could be that UK health has been target-driven in the recent past (Bevan, 2006), resulting in people with intellectual disabilities being part of the national statistics. The incorporation of the Improving Health and Lives Learning Disabilities Observatory into Public Health England in 2013 has continued to highlight the importance of detailed health screening and health surveillance for people with intellectual disabilities. Similarly in Northern Ireland, public health services for people with intellectual disabilities have been the remit of the Public Health Agency since 2009.

Health promotion and health education

Health promotion involves enabling people with intellectual disabilities to increase control over their health to improve their experience of health and healthcare. In undertaking health promotion, intellectual disability nurses work with people with intellectual disabilities and their carers to deal with:

- Factors that influence health, such as lifestyle and healthcare-seeking behaviours.
- Broader determinants of health, which are outside the control of people with intellectual disabilities, such as their living environment, employment, and the provision and availability of and accessibility of health services.

In this role intellectual disability nurses work with individuals with intellectual disabilities and their families/carers to provide knowledge, values, and skills that are essential for them to take positive and preventive health actions.

In undertaking health education intellectual disability nurses focus on influencing the attitudes to determinants of health and healthcare of individuals with intellectual disabilities and their carers. The focus of health education is to use the health experiences of people with intellectual disabilities and their communities to increase health literacy necessary for health improvement.

Health protection and health prevention

Health protection involves important responsive activities of public health practice that affect whole populations, such as infectious diseases, food, hygiene, water, environmental health, medicines control, and a wide range of other activities. The aim of these activities is to minimise the risk of adverse impact to health of environmental determinants of health.

Health prevention involves immunisation, health screening, and other public health activities that focus on the prevention and early detection of intellectual disability, disease, and illness. Health prevention programmes are implemented in communities and primary and acute healthcare settings. For people with intellectual disabilities, health prevention may include annual health checks and screening tests. Health prevention activities can occur at six levels:

- *Primary prevention*: Focuses on activities that prevent cases of illness or disease in a population and diminish as far as possible the risk of undesirable health outcomes occurring. Intellectual disability nurses could support people with learning disabilities to have annual seasonal flu vaccinations, for example.
- *Secondary prevention*: Focuses on activities that detect pre-symptomatic illness and where pre-symptomatic early intervention can be taken. In intellectual disability public health nursing practice, secondary and selective activities may involve working with individuals and groups at risk of developing specific health problems, for example, providing screening services for early onset of dementia for people with Down syndrome.
- *Tertiary prevention*: Focuses on maximising optimal healthy lifestyles for individuals or groups who have or are experiencing illness or disease that are at risk of becoming chronic without support and intervention. In intellectual disability nursing practice this could be supporting an individual with diabetes to manage their condition in the long term, for example.
- *Universal health prevention:* Focuses on providing information, knowledge, and skills to a whole population to prevent lifestyles or promote lifestyles that affect health and health outcomes.
- *Selective health prevention:* In learning disability public health nursing practice, selective health prevention activities may involve working with individuals and groups at risk of developing specific health problems, for example, providing screening services for early onset of dementia for people with Down syndrome.
- *Indicated health prevention:* This activity involves screening programmes targeting specific individuals who exhibit early signs of specific illnesses or diseases.

Factors that influence intellectual disability nurses' public health practice

Public health role clarity

As discussed earlier, public health practice is multi-professional and multi-agency in nature; it is, therefore, important that intellectual disability nurses are clear about their public health roles within their area of practice (Wick, 2007). Public health role clarity is an important foundation of how intellectual disability nurses engage with public health practice to meet the public health needs of people with intellectual disabilities (Mafuba, 2013).

Agreed-upon dialogical definition of public health practice

As discussed earlier, the concept of public health is contentious (Dawson and Verweij, 2007). Intellectual disability nursing students and intellectual disability nurses need to be aware of a lack of *'shared knowledge'* and *'shared categorisations'* of public health problems that people with intellectual disabilities experience. The impact of this is likely to be organisational variations in the public health services provided to people with intellectual disabilities. To prevent variations in interpretation of what *'public health'* means in practice, intellectual disability nurses and collaborating professionals and agencies need to agree on what public health means in their area of practice.

Demographic intelligence

In the United Kingdom, there is no unified central database of the population of people with intellectual disabilities. Local registers exist, and as previously discussed, these are important in highlighting the extent of the known and unknown health needs of the population of people with intellectual disabilities (Emerson and McGrother, 2010). Current, validated, and accurate registers are vital in the implementation of public health initiatives for people with intellectual disabilities by intellectual disability nurses (Turner and Robinson, 2010). Registers provide essential statistical intelligence about the populations of people with intellectual disabilities, which intellectual disability nurses require to fulfill their public health practice. Understanding the distribution of the population and morbidity rates of people with intellectual disabilities is therefore important for intellectual disability nurses to deliver targeted and appropriate public health services for people with intellectual disabilities (Mafuba, 2013). Demographic intelligence is important in the investigation and diagnosis of the epidemiological problems that affect people with intellectual disabilities. In addition, demographic intelligence is useful in facilitating the prioritisation of public health programmes for people with intellectual disabilities. Furthermore, it enables better targeting of public health initiatives. Demographic intelligence is also useful for monitoring and evaluating the impact of public health programmes and strategies on the population of people with intellectual disabilities. The work being undertaken by the Improving Health and Lives Learning Disabilities Observatory in England (now part of Public Health England) is making significant contributions to the demographic intelligence of the population of people with intellectual disabilities.

Interprofessional and interagency collaboration

Interprofessional working in the delivery of health and public health programmes has been advocated (WHO, 1999; Wildridge et al., 2004; Dion, 2004; Tope and Thomas, 2007; Mason-Angelow, 2020). The need for interprofessional working in public health cannot be overemphasised since public health problems are too complex to be met by one profession (WHO, 1999). In addition to interprofessional working, public health practice is by nature interagency (Tope and Thomas, 2007). Intellectual disability nurses need to be aware that interagency partnership working could be difficult to develop (Wildridge et al., 2004). This may result in interagency and philosophical tensions for a variety of reasons, including philosophical differences. Historically in the United Kingdom intellectual disabilities specialist services – for example, intellectual disability nurses – have practiced under the leadership of psychiatry. Psychiatry has historically prioritised psychiatric treatments rather than prevention. It is important for intellectual disability nurses to be aware that philosophical tensions are inevitable in an interprofessional environment such as public health practice (Bridges, Fitzgerald and Meyer, 2007; Robinson and Cottrell, 2005).

Leadership

In providing public health services to people with intellectual disabilities, intellectual disability nurses find themselves occupying a fine line between health and social care (Mafuba, 2009). Strategic leadership in organisations that employ intellectual disability nurses is essential for intellectual nurses to effectively meet the public health needs of people with intellectual disabilities (Mafuba, 2013). The multi-professional and inter-organisational public health environments in which intellectual disability nurses practice is complex and requires clearly defined public health leadership to meet the public health needs of people with intellectual disabilities.

Resources

The increasing divergence between public health needs and limited financial resources has led to implicit rationing of health services, including public health services in the United Kingdom (Hunter, 1995; Ham and Coulter, 2001; Eichler et al., 2004; Greer, 2004). Ham and Coulter (2001) have noted that the impact of implicit and explicit rationing of public health services contributes to exclusion of services that are at the margins of health services, such as those for people with intellectual disabilities. The consequence of this is that public health organisations that employ intellectual disability nurses tend to focus on the bigger picture.

Politics

The nature of United Kingdom health service policy is that policy formulation is very much driven from the centre (Ham, 2004; Mafuba, Gates and Cozens, 2018), with policy implementation delegated to local organisations. Political decisions by the central government constantly shift the boundaries of how intellectual disability nurses engage with public health practice. In addition, local public health priorities may not focus on the public health needs of people with intellectual disabilities (Mafuba, 2013; RCN, 2021).

BOX 4.6
CASE STUDY 4.2

Having read this chapter, read the following extract from *Healthy Lives, Healthy People: A Call to Action on Obesity in England* (DH, 2011, p. 23) and answer the questions that follow.

As our priority is now healthy weight in adults as well as children, effective and tailored support for the more than 60% of adults who are already overweight or obese is essential. Successful local strategies will need to strike a balance between 'treatment' interventions that *help individuals to reach a healthier weight and sustained preventive effort to help to make healthy weight increasingly the norm. These are not alternatives – both are vital if we are to 'shift the curve'.*

Many local areas already commission weight management services and a range of providers are already delivering and developing evidence-based services aimed at different population groups. The commissioning of weight management services will remain the responsibility of local areas, but we will provide support to build local capability and support evidence-based approaches.

Box 4.7
Student Activity 4.2

Why is the Ottawa Charter important and what are its central themes?

What is the difference between health education and health promotion?

What role do empowerment and self-advocacy play in health promotion? Reflect on an example from your experience of working with a person with an intellectual disability.

Identify at least five professionals who could be involved in promoting the health and well-being of people with intellectual disabilities, explaining the potential roles such professionals could play.

Reflect on what you have learnt here and how this will assist you in meeting the professional requirements for your course.

Conclusion

Whereas the health and life expectancy of the people in the United Kingdom has improved in recent decades, the health and life expectancy of people with intellectual disabilities has not improved at the same rate. People with intellectual disabilities still experience significant inequalities in health and health outcomes. Preventive health is pivotal in improving the health and health experience of people with intellectual disabilities. This means intellectual and learning disability nurses will need to assimilate new public health roles and engage with public health practice in new ways to improve the health and life expectancy of people with intellectual disabilities.

Because of their daily contact with people with intellectual disabilities, intellectual disability nurses will increasingly play a pivotal role in enabling people with intellectual disabilities to live healthy lives, reduce preventive mortality, and influence the implementation of public health policy for people with intellectual disabilities. The Royal College of Nursing and '*All Our Health*' has provided a template for the development of the public health roles of intellectual disability nurses (RCN, 2012). This requires:

■ All nurses, regardless of their work environment, are required to know and understand the health needs of their local population and provide meaningful and tailored public health interventions that are holistic and patient-centred.

■ The identification of defined populations that would enable healthcare teams to target individuals who would most benefit from upstream approaches.

■ Working in partnership with other members of health and social care organisations to influence the work on tackling the wider determinants of health.

■ Engaging local people and groups, including those who are not working, in upstream awareness and action to manage their own health and their community's well-being.

■ Nurses engaging in proactive work to be informed, aware, and responsive to disease outbreaks and other threats to health, nurses using public health evidence in everyday practice, not just evidence for treating illness.

■ To measure and disseminate the impact that changes to models of care, to inform commissioning services and others who would benefit from this knowledge.

■ Nurses working to a public health knowledge and skills framework based on the 'novice to expert' criteria (RCN, 2012, p. 12).

References

Abbott, S. (2007) Leadership across boundaries: A qualitative study of the nurse consultant role in English primary care. *Journal of Nursing Management*, 15(7), pp. 703–710.

Acheson, D. (1988) *Independent inquiry into inequalities report*. London: TSO.

Baggott, R. (2011) *Public health policy and politics* (2nd edition). London: Palgrave Macmillan.

Barr, O. (2006) The evolving role of community nurses for people with learning disabilities: Changes over an 11-year period. *Journal of Clinical Nursing*, 15, pp. 72–82.

Barr, O., *et al.* (1999) Health screening for people with learning disabilities by a community learning disabilities nursing service in Northern Ireland. *Journal of Advanced Nursing*, 29(6), pp. 1482–1491.

Bevan, G. (2006) Setting targets for healthcare performance – lessons from a case study of the English NHS. *National Institute Economic Review*, 197(1), pp. 67–79.

Blaxter, M. (2004) *Health*. Cambridge: Polity.

Boarder, J.H. (2002) The perceptions of experienced community learning disability nurses of their roles and ways of working. *Journal of Learning Disabilities*, 6(3), pp. 281–296.

Bridges, J., Fitzgerald, M. and Meyer, J. (2007) New workforce roles in healthcare: Exploring the longer-term journey of organisational innovations. *Journal of Health Organisation and Management*, 21(4–5), pp. 381–392.

Brown, M., *et al.* (2011) Learning disability liaison nursing services in south-east Scotland: A mixed-methods impact and outcome study. *Journal of Intellectual Disability Research*,56(12), pp. 1164–1171.

Buckles, J., Luckasson, R. and Keefe, E. (2013) A systematic review of the prevalence of psychiatric disorders in adults with intellectual disability, 2003–2010. *Journal of Mental Health Research in Intellectual Disabilities*, 6(3), pp. 181–207.

Carey, I.M., *et al.* (2017) Do health checks for adults with intellectual disability reduce emergency hospital admissions? Evaluation of a natural experiment. *Epidemiology and Community Health*, 71(1), pp. 52–58.

Chapman, H. (2018) Nursing theories 4: Adherence and concordance. *Nursing Times*, 114(2), p. 50 [online].

Chauhan, U., *et al.* (2012) *Impact of the English directly enhanced service (DES) for learning disability*. Manchester: University of Manchester.

Cope, G. and Shaw, T. (2019) *Celebrate me: Capturing the voices of learning disability nurses and people who use services*. London: Foundation of Nursing Studies.

Coyle, E. (2007) Public health in Wales. In Griffiths, S. and Hunter, D. (Eds.), *New perspectives in public health*. London: Routledge, pp. 37–44.

Dawson, A. and Verweij, M. (2007) The meaning of 'public' in 'public health'. In Dawson, A. and Verweij, M. (Eds.), *Ethics prevention and public health*. New York: Oxford University Press, pp. 13–29.

Department of Health (2007) *The Bamford review of mental health and learning disability (Northern Ireland)*. Available at: https://www.health-ni.gov.uk/sites/default/files/publications/dhssps/legal-issue-comprehensive-framework.pdf (Accessed 24 November 2022).

DH (1990) *NHS and community care act*. London: HMSO.

DH (1992) *The health of the nation: A strategy for health in England*. London: HMSO.

DH (1995) *The health of the nation: A strategy for people with learning disabilities*. London: HMSO.

DH (2001) *Valuing people: A new strategy for the 21st century*. London: TSO.

DH (2002) *Action for health: Health action plans and health facilitation*. London: Department of Health.

DH (2007a) *Tackling health inequalities*. London: Department of Health.

DH (2007b) *Good practice guide in learning disabilities Nursing*. London: Department of Health.

DH (2007c) *Promoting equality*. London: Department of Health.

DH (2009a) *Health action planning and health facilitation for people with learning disabilities: Good practice guidance*. London: Department of Health.

DH (2009b) *Valuing people now: A new three-year strategy for people with learning disabilities*. London: Department of Health.

DH (2010) *Healthy lives, healthy people: Our strategy for public health in England*. London: Department of Health.

DH (2011) *Healthy lives, healthy people: A call to action on obesity in England*. London: Department of Health.

DH (2013) *Six lives progress report on healthcare for people with learning disabilities.* London: Department of Health.

DHSSNI (1996) *Health and wellbeing: Towards the new millennium.* Belfast: DHSSNI.

DHSSNI (1997) *Well in 2000.* Belfast: DHSSNI.

DHSSPS (2004) *A healthier future.* Belfast: DHSSPSNI.

DHSSPSNI (2002) *Investing for health.* Belfast: DHSSPSNI.

DHSSPSNI (2014) *Making life better: A whole system strategic framework for public health 2013–2023.* Belfast: DHSSPSNI.

Dion, X. (2004) A multi-disciplinary team approach to public health working. *British Journal of Community Nursing*, 9(4), pp. 149–154.

Doherty, A.J., *et al.* (2020) Barriers and facilitators to primary health care for people with intellectual disabilities and/or autism: An integrative review. *BJGP Open*, 4(3). doi: 10.3399/bjgpopen20X101030.

Doody, O., Lyons, R. and Ryan, R. (2019) The experiences of adults with intellectual disability in the involvement of nursing care planning in health services. *British Journal of Learning Disabilities*, 47(4), pp. 233–240.

DRC (2006) Equal Treatment: Closing the Gap. Stratford upon Avon: Disability Rights Commission.

Eichler, H., *et al.* (2004) Use of cost-effective analysis in healthcare resource allocation decision making: How are cost effective thresholds expected to emerge? *Value in Health*, 7(5), pp. 518–528.

Elliot-Cannon, C. (1981) Do the mentally handicapped need specialist community nursing? *Nursing Times*, 77(27), pp. 77–80.

Emerson, E., Copeland, A. and Glover, G. (2011) *The uptake of health checks for adults with learning disabilities: 2008/9 to 2010/11.* Available at: www.karentysonspage.org/Emerson%202011%20Health%20Checks%20for%20People%20with%20Learning%20Disabilities%202008-9%20%202010-11.pdf (Accessed 28 July 2022).

Emerson, E. and Glover, G. (2010) *Health checks for people with learning disabilities 2008/9 & 2009/10.* Available at: www.karentysonspage.org/Emerson%202011%20Health%20Checks%20for%20People%20with%20Learning%20Disabilities%202008-9%20%202010-11.pdf (Accessed 28 July 2022).

Emerson, E. and McGrother, C. (2010) *The use of pooled data for learning disabilities registers: A scoping review.* Available at: www.choiceforum.org/docs/vid.pdf (Accessed 28 July 2022).

Faculty of Public Health (2019) *UK faculty of public health strategy 2019–2025.* Available at: www.fph.org.uk/media/2582/fph-publichealthstrategy-2019to2025-v5.pdf (Accessed 12 April 2022).

Faculty of Public Health (2020) *Functions and standards of a public health system.* Available at: www.fph.org.uk/media/3031/fph_systems_and_function-final-v2.pdf (Accessed 12 April 2022).

Gates, B. (1994) *Advocacy: A nurses' guide.* London: Scutari Press.

Glover, G., *et al.* (2017) Mortality in people with intellectual disabilities in England. *Journal of Intellectual Disability Research*, 61(1), pp. 62–74.

Greer, S.L. (2009) *Territorial politics and health policy.* Manchester: Manchester University Press.

Greer, S.L. (2004) *Territorial politics and health policy: UK health policy in comparative perspective.* Manchester: Manchester University Press.

Gregson, N.C., Randle-Phillips, C. and Hillman, S. (2022) People with intellectual disabilities' experiences of primary care health checks, screenings and gp consultations: A systematic review and meta-ethnography. *International Journal of Developmental Disabilities*. doi:10.1080/20473869.2022.2056402.

Griffiths, R. (1988) *Community care: Agenda for action. Report for the secretary of state for social services.* London: HMSO.

Griffiths, S. and Hunter, D. (1999) *Perspectives in public health*. Oxford: Radical Medical Press.

Griffiths, S., Jewell, T. and Donelly, P. (2005) Public health in practice: The three domains of public health. *Public Health*, 119(10), pp. 907–913.

Ham, C. (2004) *Health policy in Britain: The politics and organisation of the national health service* (5th edition). Basingstoke: Palgrave Macmillan.

Ham, C. and Coulter, A. (2001) Explicit and implicit rationing: Taking responsibility and avoiding blame for healthcare choices. *Journal of Health Services Research and Policy*, 6(3), pp. 163–169.

Hemm, C., Dagnan, D. and Meyer, T.D. (2015) Identifying training needs for mainstream healthcare professionals, to prepare them for working with individuals with intellectual disabilities: A systematic review. *Journal of Applied Research in Intellectual Disabilities*, 28(2), pp. 98–110.

Heslop, P., *et al.* (2013) *Confidential inquiry into premature deaths of people with learning disabilities (CIPOLD)*. Bristol: Norah Fry Research Centre-University of Bristol.

Holloway, D. (2004) Ethical dilemmas in community learning disabilities nursing: What helps nurses resolve ethical dilemmas that result from choices made by people with learning disabilities? *Journal of Learning Disabilities*, 8(3), pp. 283–298.

Hott, B.L. and Flores, M.M. (2021) Introduction to learning disability quarterly special series on single-case research design: Part one of two. *Learning Disability Quarterly*, 0(0). https://doi.org/10.1177/07319487211040493.

Hsieh, K., Rimmer, J.H. and Heller, T. (2014) Obesity and associated factors in adults with intellectual disability. *Journal of Intellectual Disability Research*, 58(9), pp. 851–863.

Hughes-McCormack, L., *et al.* (2017) Prevalence of mental health conditions and relationship with general health in a whole-country population of people with intellectual disabilities compared with the general population. *BJPsych Open*, 3(5), pp. 243–248.

Hunter, D.J. (1995) Rationing healthcare: The political perspective. *British Medical Bulletin*, 51(4), pp. 876–884.

Iacono, T., *et al.* (2014) A systematic review of hospital experiences of people with intellectual disability. *BMC Health Services Research*, 14(505). doi:10.1186/s12913-014-0505-5.

Institute of Public Health (2020) *What is public health*. Available at: https://publichealth.ie/what-is-public-health/ (Accessed 22 April 2022).

Jukes, M. (1994) A response to the statement on learning disability nursing. *British Journal of Nursing*, 3(11), p. 543.

Kaiser, S. and Mackenbach, J.P. (2008) Public health in eight European countries: An international comparison of terminology. *Public Health*, 122(2), pp. 211–216.

Kiani, R. and Miller, H. (2010) Sensory impairment and intellectual disability. *Advances in Psychiatric Treatment*, 16(3), pp. 228–235.

Lennox, N., Beange, H. and Edwards, N. (2000) The health needs of people with intellectual disability. *Medical Journal of Australia*, 173(6), pp. 328–330.

Llewellyn, P. and Northway, R. (2007) The views and experiences of learning disability nurses concerning their advocacy education. *Nurse Education Today*, 27(8), pp. 955–963.

Mafuba, K. (2009) The public health role of learning disability nurses: A review of the literature. *Learning Disability Practice*, 12(4), pp. 33–37.

Mafuba, K. (2013) *Public health: Community learning disability nurses' perception and experience of their role*. Unpublished PhD thesis. London: University of West London.

Mafuba, K. and Gates, B. (2013) An investigation into the public health roles of community learning disability nurses. *British Journal Learning Disability*, 43(1), pp. 1–7.

Mafuba, K., Gates, B. and Cozens, M. (2018) Community intellectual disability nurses' public health roles in the United Kingdom: An exploratory documentary analysis. *Journal of Intellectual Disabilities*, 22(1), pp. 61–73.

Marshall, D. and Moore, G. (2003) Obesity in people with intellectual disabilities: The impact of nurse-led health screenings and health promotion activities. *Journal of Advanced Nursing*, 41(2), pp. 147–153.

Mason-Angelow, V. (2020) *This is us – this is what we do: A report to inform the future of learning disability nursing*. Booklet. Bath: National Development Team for Inclusion.

McCarron, M., *et al.* (2015) Mortality rates in the general irish population compared to those with an intellectual disability from 2003 to 2012. *Journal of Applied Research in Intellectual Disabilities*, 28(5), pp. 406–413.

McCarron, M., *et al.* (2018) *Shaping the future of intellectual disability nursing in Ireland*. Dublin: Health Services Executive.

McConkey, R., Moore, G. and Marshall, D. (2002) Changes in the attitudes of GP's to the health screening of people with learning disabilities. *Journal of Learning Disabilities*, 6(4), pp. 373–384.

McConkey, R., Taggart, L. and Kane, M. (2015) Optimizing the uptake of health checks for people with intellectual disabilities. *Journal of Intellectual Disabilities*, 19(3), pp. 205–214.

McGarry, J. and Arthur, A. (2001) Informal caring in late life: A qualitative study of the experiences of older carers. *Journal of Advanced Nursing*, 33(2), pp. 182–189.

McMahon, M. and Hatton, C. (2021) A comparison of the prevalence of health problems among adults with and without intellectual disability: A total administrative population study. *Journal of Applied Research in Intellectual Disabilities*, 34(1), pp. 316–325.

Mencap (2004) *Treat me right! Better health for people with learning disabilities*. London: Mencap.

Mencap (2007) *Death by indifference: Following up the treat me right report*. London: Mencap.

Mencap (2012) *Death by indifference: 74 deaths and counting*. London: Mencap.

Mencap (2020) *My health, my life: Barriers to healthcare for people with a learning disability during the pandemic*. London: Mencap.

Michael, J. (2008) *Healthcare for all: Report of the independent inquiry into access to healthcare for people with learning disabilities*. London: Department of Health.

Mobbs, C., *et al.* (2002) An exploration of the role of the community nurse, learning disability, in England. *British Journal of Learning Disabilities*, 30(1), pp. 13–18.

NafW (2001) *Improving health in Wales*. Cardiff: National Assembly for Wales.

National Learning Disability Professional Senate (2015) *Delivering effective specialist community learning disabilities health team support to people with learning disabilities and their families or carers*. Available at: www.bild.org.uk/wp-content/uploads/2020/01/National-LD-Professional-Senate-Guidelines-for-CLDT-Specialist-Health-Services-final-4-Jan-2019-with-references.pdf (Accessed 29 July 2022).

NHS England (2019) *The NHS long term plan*. Available at: www.longtermplan.nhs.uk (Accessed 1 August 2022).

NHS England (2021) *Learning from lives and deaths – people with a learning disability and autistic people (LeDeR) policy 2021*. Available at: www.england.nhs.uk/publication/learning-from-lives-and-deaths-people-with-a-learning-disability-and-autistic-people-leder-policy-2021/ (Accessed 29 July 2022).

NHS England (2022) *Network contract directed enhanced service (DES)*. Available at: www.england.nhs.uk/gp/investment/gp-contract/network-contract-directed-enhanced-service-des/ (Accessed 1 August 2022).

NHS Executive (1998) *Signposts for success in commissioning and providing health services for people with learning disabilities.* London: DH.

NHS Health Scotland (2004) *Health needs assessment report – summary - people with learning disabilities in Scotland.* Glasgow: NHS Health Scotland.

NI Executive (2008) *Programme for government.* Belfast: NIE.

NMC (2018) *The code: Professional standards of practice and behaviour for nurses, midwives and nursing associates.* London: Nursing and Midwifery Council.

Norah Fry Research Centre (2021) *The learning disabilities mortality review (LeDeR): Annual report.* Bristol: University of Bristol.

Nursing and Midwifery Board of Ireland (2016) *Nurse registration programmes standards and requirements* (4th edition). Dublin: Nursing and Midwifery Board of Ireland.

Nursing and Midwifery Council (2018) *Future nurse: Standards of proficiency for registered nurses.* London: NMC.

Parliamentary and Health Service Ombudsman and Social Services Ombudsman (2009) *Six lives: The provision of public services to people with learning disabilities.* London: TSO.

Powell, H., Murray, G. and McKenzie, K. (2004) Staff perceptions of community learning disability nurses' role. *Nursing Times*, 100(19), pp. 40–42.

Public Health England (2016 updated 2020) *Reasonable adjustments: A legal duty.* Available at: www.gov.uk/government/publications/reasonable-adjustments-a-legal-duty/reasonable-adjustments-a-legal-duty (Accessed 1 August 2022).

Public Health England (2018) *Learning disabilities: Applying all our health.* Available at: www.gov.uk/government/publications/learning-disability-applying-all-our-health/learning-disabilities-applying-all-our-health#core-principles-for-health-professionals (Accessed 25 March 2022).

Ramsey, L., *et al.* (2022) Systemic safety inequities for people with learning disabilities: A qualitative integrative analysis of the experiences of English health and social care for people with learning disabilities, their families and carers. *International Journal for Equity in Health*, 21(13). doi:10.1186/s12939-021-01612-1.

RCN (2012) *Going upstream: Nursing's contribution to public health: Prevent, promote and protect.* London: Royal College of Nursing.

RCN (2021) *Connecting for change: For the future of learning disability nursing.* London: RCN.

Robertson, J., *et al.* (2011) The impact of health checks for people with intellectual disabilities: A systematic review of evidence. *Journal of Intellectual Disability Research*, 55(11), pp. 1009–1019.

Robertson, J., *et al.* (2014) The impact of health checks for people with intellectual disabilities: An updated systematic review of evidence. *Research in Developmental Disabilities*, 35(10), pp. 2450–2462.

Robertson, J., *et al.* (2015) Prevalence of epilepsy among people with intellectual disabilities: A systematic review. *Seizure*, 29, pp. 46–62.

Robinson, M. and Cottrell, D. (2005) Health professionals in multi-disciplinary and multi-agency teams: Changing professional practice. *Journal of Interprofessional Care*, 19(6), pp. 547–560.

Roll, A.E. (2018) Health promotion for people with intellectual disabilities – a concept analysis. *Scandinavian Journal of Caring Science*, 32(1), pp. 422–429.

Ruddick, L. (2005) Health of people with intellectual disabilities: A review of factors influencing access to healthcare. *British Journal of Health Psychology*, 10(4), pp. 559–570.

Ryan, J., *et al.* (2021) Overweight/obesity and chronic health conditions in older people with intellectual disability in Ireland. *Journal of Intellectual Disability Research*, 65(12), pp. 1097–1109.

Scottish Executive (2000a) *Our national health: A plan for action, a plan for change.* Edinburgh: Scottish Executive.

Scottish Executive (2000b) *The same as you.* Edinburgh: Scottish Executive.

Scottish Executive (2003) *Improving health in Scotland.* Edinburgh: Scottish Executive.

Scottish Government (2007) *Better health better care: Action plan.* Edinburgh: Scottish Government.

Scottish Government (2008) *Equally well.* Edinburgh: Scottish Government.

Scottish Government (2021) *Learning/intellectual disability and autism: Transformation plan.* Edinburgh: Scottish Government.

Scottish Office (1992) *Scotland's health: A challenge to us all.* Edinburgh: HMSO.

Taggart, L., *et al.* (2018) Pilot feasibility study examining a structured self-management diabetes education programme, DESMOND-ID, targeting HbA1c in adults with intellectual disabilities. *Diabetic Medicine,* 35(1), pp. 137–146.

Tope, R. and Thomas, E. (2007) *Creating an interprofessional workforce.* London: DH.

Tromans, S., *et al.* (2020) Priority concerns for people with intellectual and developmental disabilities during the COVID-19 pandemic. *BJPsych Open,* 6, p. e128. doi:10.1192/bjo.2020.122.

Tuffrey-Wijne, I., *et al.* (2013) Identifying the factors affecting the implementation of strategies to promote a safer environment for patients with learning disabilities in NHS hospitals: A mixed-methods study. *NIHR Journals Library.* doi:10.1136/bmjopen-2013-004606.

Tuffrey-Wijne, I., *et al.* (2014) The barriers to and enablers of providing reasonably adjusted health services to people with intellectual disabilities in acute hospitals: Evidence from a mixed-methods study. *BMJ Open,* 4(4), p. e004606.

Turner, S., Giraud-Saunders, A. and Marriott, A. (2013) *Improving the uptake of screening services by people with learning disabilities across the Southwest Peninsula – a strategy and toolkit.* Bath: National Development Team for Inclusion.

Turner, S. and Robinson, C. (2010) *Health checks for people with learning disabilities: Implications and actions for commissioners.* Durham: Improving Health and Lives, Learning Disabilities Observatory.

Welsh Assembly Government (2002) *Well-being in Wales.* Cardiff: Welsh Assembly Government.

Welsh Assembly Government (2003) *Wales: A better country.* Cardiff: Welsh Assembly Government.

Welsh Assembly Government (2005) *Designed for life: Creating world class health and social care for Wales in the 21st century.* Cardiff: Welsh Assembly Government.

Welsh Government (2018) *Learning disability improving lives programme.* Cardiff: Welsh Government, June.

Welsh Government (2022) *Learning disability strategic action plan 2022 to 2026: Our plan for developing and implementing learning disability policy from 2022 to 2026.* Available at: https://gov.wales/learning-disability-strategic-action-plan-2022–2026-html (Accessed 28 July 2022).

Welsh Office (1998) *Strategic framework: Better health better Wales.* Cardiff: Welsh Office.

Welsh Office NHS Directorate (1989) *Welsh health planning forum: Strategic intent and direction for the NHS in Wales.* Cardiff: Welsh Office.

Welsh Office NHS Directorate (1992) *Caring for the future.* Cardiff: Welsh Office.

Whitehead, M. (1992) The concepts and principles of equity and health. *International Journal of Health Services,* 22(3), pp. 429–445.

WHO (1986) *First conference on health promotion: Ottawa charter for health promotion 17–21 November.* Ottawa: WHO, Health and Welfare Canada, Canadian Association for Public Health.

WHO (1999) *Health 21: The health for all policy framework for the WHO European region: European health for all – series no. 6.* Copenhagen: World Health Organisation.

WHO (2012) *European action plan for strengthening public health capacities and services.* Malta: WHO.

WHO (2022) *The 10 essential public health operations.* Available at: www.euro.who.int/en/health-topics/Health-systems/public-health-services/policy/the-10-essential-public-health-operations (Accessed 28 July 2022).

Wick, C.J. (2007) Setting the stage: Writing job descriptions that work. *Executive Housekeeping Today*, 29(7), pp. 9–11.

Wilde, J. (2007) Public health in a changing Ireland: An all-Ireland perspective. In Griffiths, S. and Hunter, D. (Eds.), *New perspectives in public health*. London: Routledge, pp. 45–54.

Wildridge, V., *et al.* (2004) How to create successful partnerships: A review of the literature. *Health Information and Libraries Journal*, 21(1), pp. 3–19.

Winslow, C. (1920) The untilled fields of public health. *Modern Medicine*, 2, pp. 183–191.

Further Reading

NMC (2018) *The code: Professional standards of practice and behaviour for nurses, midwives and nursing associates.* London: Nursing and Midwifery Council.

Nursing and Midwifery Board of Ireland (2016) *Nurse registration programmes standards and requirements* (4th edition). Dublin: Nursing and Midwifery Board of Ireland.

RCN (2012) *Going upstream: Nursing's contribution to public health: Prevent promote and protect.* London: Royal College of Nursing.

Useful Resources

BILD: www.bild.org.uk/

Contact: https://contact.org.uk/ **Enable Scotland:** www.enable.org.uk/

Foundation for People with Learning Disabilities: www.learningdisabilities.org.uk/

General Medical Council: www.gmc-uk.org/learningdisabilities/

Inclusion Ireland: www.inclusionireland.ie/

Intellectual Disability Info Web Pages: www.intellectualdisability.info/

Learning Disabilities Observatory: www.improvinghealthandlives.org.uk

Mencap: www.mencap.org.uk/

Mencap Northern Ireland: www.mencap.org.uk/northern-ireland

Mencap Wales: www.mencap.org.uk/wales

Nursing and Midwifery Board of Ireland: www.nmbi.ie/Home

Nursing and Midwifery Council: www.nmc.org.uk/

O'Neill, S., Heenan, D. and Betts, J. (2019) *Review of Mental Health Policies in Northern Ireland: Making Parity a Reality.* Ulster University. Available at: www.ulster.ac.uk/__data/assets/pdf_file/0004/452155/Final-Draft-Mental-Health-Review-web.pdf

CHAPTER 5

Vicky Sandy-Davis and Linda Steven

Intellectual disability nursing and mental health

Introduction

It is known that people with intellectual disabilities are at greater risk of developing mental health problems than is the wider population. Because of the high prevalence of mental ill health and its impact on the quality of life of this population, an understanding of mental ill health and its manifestations is vital to prepare intellectual disability nurses so that they understand mental well-being, in order that this can be promoted and maintained for those who are vulnerable (Barr and Gates, 2019). To be explored in this chapter are the nature and manifestations of good mental health, as well as manifestations of mental ill health, assessment tools used in nursing practice, and how to conduct a mental state examination. A range of treatment approaches will be outlined, including the Care Program Approach and its function in the coordination of care packages for those with complex mental health needs. Finally, relevant mental health legislation including the Mental Capacity Act, assessment of mental capacity and the role of the Independent Mental Capacity Advocate (IMCA) will be outlined. There will also be an explanation of the function and purpose of the Deprivation of Liberty Safeguards.

Since the introduction of the White Paper *Valuing People*, which placed responsibility on the NHS to ensure that *'all mainstream services are accessible to people with intellectual disability'* (DH, 2001), many commissioners of health services have pursued mainstream mental health service provision for people with intellectual disabilities, with services

being primarily driven by policies such as *The Five Year Forward View for Mental Health* (NHS England, 2016) and *Modernising the Mental Health Act: Increasing choice, reducing compulsion,* (Gov.UK, 2018). These policies hold particular importance in the context of the recent Coronavirus pandemic because it is anticipated to cause an increase in new mental health issues (Perkins, 2020), with people with intellectual disabilities potentially being at greater risk of mental health deterioration than the wider population (Tromans *et al.*, 2022).

It is vital therefore, that a coordinated approach is provided across health and social care services. However, the interface between mental health services and specialist intellectual disability services remains fragmented. Whereas there is a shift towards the integration of intellectual disability and mainstream services in the UK, there is concern that mainstream services are failing to meet the needs of those with intellectual disabilities (Kaushal *et al.*, 2020). Of further concern is a finding by Ee, Kroese, and Rose (2021) that professionals who do not work in intellectual disability services do not feel comfortable working with this group because of a lack of knowledge and understanding. The role of intellectual disability nurses in developing therapeutic relationships with individuals with intellectual disabilities is therefore crucial (Crotty and Doody, 2015).

This chapter will focus on the knowledge and practical skills that intellectual disability nurses will need to meet the mental health needs of people with

DOI: 10.4324/9781003296461-5

intellectual disabilities, and this will be contextu- alised within the *Future nurse: Standards of profi- ciency for registered nurses* (Nursing and Midwifery Council (NMC), 2018), and the *Nursing registration programmes and requirements* (Nursing and Mid- wifery Board of Ireland (NMBI), 2016).

Box 5.1 This chapter will focus on the following issues:

- Introduction
- The nature of mental health and well-being
- Manifestations of mental ill health
  - Affective disorders
  - Depression
  - Bipolar disorder
  - Anxiety
  - Suicide and Self-harm
  - Schizophrenia
  - Obsessive compulsive disorders
  - Eating disorders
  - Personality disorder
  - Substance misuse
- General observations and recording: assessment tools for mental health
  - General observations and recording
  - Mood
  - Sleep charts
  - Weight charts
  - ABC charts
- Mental State Examination (MSE)
  - Appearance
  - Behaviour
  - Cognition
  - Experiences
  - Mood and affect
  - Speech
  - Thought content

- Specific mental health assessment tools
    - Assessment of dual diagnosis (ADD)
    - Learning disability version of the cardinal needs schedule (LDCNS)
    - Psychiatric Assessment Schedules for Adults with Developmental Disabilities (PAS-ADD)
    - The Hamilton Rating Scale for Depression (HRSD)
    - Beck Anxiety Inventory (BAI)
    - Schedule for Affective Disorders and Schizophrenia (SADS)
- Treatments
    - Medication
    - Talking therapies
    - Electroconvulsive therapy (ECT)
    - Other approaches
- The Care Programme Approach
- The Mental Health Act 1983
    - Involuntary admission: Assessment
    - Part II of the Mental Health Act
    - Part III of the Mental Health Act
    - Assessment or treatment
    - Admission for assessment under MHA 1983
    - Part II: Compulsory admission to hospital and guardianship
    - Part X: Miscellaneous and supplementary
    - Part III: Patients concerned in criminal proceedings or under sentence
    - Admission for Treatment MHA 1983
    - Part II: Compulsory admission to hospital and guardianship
    - Part III: Patients concerned in criminal proceedings or under sentence
    - Appropriate treatment test
    - Assessment of mental capacity: IMCAs and DOLS

Box 5.2 Competences

Nursing and Midwifery Council (2018) Proficiencies

Platform 2: Promoting health and preventing ill health – 2.1, 2.2, 2.3, 2.4, 2.5, 2.6, 2.7, 2.10, 2.11, 2.12

Platform 3: Assessing needs and planning care – 3.6, 3.15

Platform 5: Leading and managing nursing care and working in teams – 5.12

Platform 7: Coordinating care – 7.1, 7.2, 7.3, 7.4

Nursing and Midwifery Board of Ireland (2016) Competences

Domain 2: Nursing practice and clinical decision-making competences – 2.1, 2.2, 2.3, 2.4, 2.5

Domain 3: Knowledge and cognitive competences – 3.1, 3.2

Domain 4: Communication and interpersonal competences – 4.1, 4.2

Domain 6: Leadership potential and professional scholarship competences – 6.1

The nature of mental health and well-being

The same range of mental health problems are experienced by people with intellectual disabilities when compared to the wider population, however, prevalence is higher (Sheerin *et al.*, 2019). The Adult Psychiatric Morbidity Survey (2016) has estimated that 25% of people with lower intellectual functioning presented with symptoms of common mental health issues and that this number decreased in line with an increase in intellectual functioning, and this compares to one in six of the wider population (McManus *et al.*, 2016). In 2017/18 severe mental illness was 8.4 times more common in people with an intellectual disability than those without.

Until relatively recently, health services in the United Kingdom for people with intellectual disabilities resided within Psychiatry (Kaushal *et al.*, 2020), and this gave rise to separate services for this population. This is still in part the case, particularly around their mental health needs. Until the 1970s this was not challenged, but the growth of the concept of normalisation, in conjunction with the development of the social model of disability, led to philosophical changes in clinical commissioning of intellectual disability services away from *'separateness'* toward *'inclusion'*. This resulted in the almost complete closure of all long-stay intellectual disability hospitals during the 1980s and 1990s, and a move to so-called community-based services. These services strive for integration and inclusion into mainstream activities that range from employment to health, as outlined in the government's white paper *Valuing People* (DH, 2001), and the subsequent 'refresh' *Valuing People Now* (DH, 2009). Other more general mental health policy is temporally in keeping with this shift, and can be seen, for example, in the *Five Year Forward View for Mental Health* (NHS England, 2016), which seeks to ensure that mental health services are accessible and available to all. However, Kaushal *et al.* (2020) have stated that Psychiatrists without specialist training in intellectual disabilities may not have adequate knowledge to assess and manage mental ill health for this group of patients. Guidance put forward by the National Institute for Health and Care Excellence (NICE) outlines the responsibilities of specialist intellectual disability services to ensure that the needs of those who fall into this category are met, and this therefore recognises the specific presentation and support needs of people with intellectual disabilities with mental ill health (NICE, 2016).

Current developments in policy and legislation place a focus on increased choice in service development, with the co-production model ensuring that people with intellectual disabilities can make a valued contribution to their own treatment, as outlined in *Modernising the Mental Health Act, increasing choice, reducing compulsion* (2018), and the *Five year Forward View for Mental Health* (2016). The need for the specialist skills of the intellectual disability nursing workforce is therefore vital in meeting the needs of this population across the breadth of service provision. This is further clarified by Crotty and Doody (2015) who have stated that the person-centred approach offered by intellectual disability nurses can be pivotal in the provision of high quality and individualised care.

There is much more to good health than simply being physically healthy; any notion of health must also incorporate a healthy mind (see Chapter 4). Someone who has a healthy mind should be able to think (relatively) clearly and respond to and be able to deal with the everyday challenges of living. Additionally, that person should be able to make and sustain good relationships with his or her friends and the colleagues with whom he or she works, as well as his or her own immediate family. Finally, he or she should feel some sense of inner peace and be able to enjoy life and share a feeling of well-being with others in the community. When these things are present, the individual may be considered to have good mental health.

Achieving mental well-being is every bit as challenging as achieving good physical health. Every year, approximately one in six adults in the United Kingdom will experience a mental health problem, with General Anxiety Disorder (GAD) and depression being the most common (McManus *et al.*, 2016; Cooper *et al.*, 2007). Mrayyan, Eberhard, and Ahlstrom (2019) have stated that the prevalence of depression and anxiety are more common in people with intellectual disabilities, and that prevalence increases with age. There has been an increase in access to treatment for common mental health disorders, with a sharp increase in the use of antipsychotics being identified (Mental Health Foundation, 2016).

However, it should be acknowledged that there are difficulties in measuring the prevalence of mental ill health in people with intellectual disabilities on this basis. An estimation by Public Health England (2016) purports that in 2015, between 30,000 and 35,000 adults with an intellectual disability were prescribed an antipsychotic, an anti-depressant or both without any clinical justification. Whilst antipsychotics and benzodiazepines were prescribed to a significantly larger percentage of people with intellectual disabilities between 2016 and 2021, this percentage has fallen. However, the percentage of people with intellectual disability *without* an active diagnosis of depression who were prescribed anti-depressants rose by 0.8% in the same period (NHS Digital, 2021).

Mental health problems include eating disorders, obsessive compulsive disorder, dependency on drugs and alcohol, personality disorder, bipolar disorder, and schizophrenia. There is a good and wide range of treatment options for mental ill health and psychological disorders, and these include medication, psychotherapy, or other treatments (Mental Health Foundation, 2016). It must be borne in mind that a mental illness is a medical condition where a person's thinking, feeling, mood, ability to relate to others, and daily functioning can all be disrupted. In just the same way as physical illnesses can affect someone's life, mental illnesses are medical conditions that often result in a diminished capacity for coping with the ordinary demands of life. In general terms, mental illness is a complex condition of altered mental health, but one where recovery is possible. Mental illnesses can affect anyone, regardless of age, race, religion, or income (although these factors may have a predisposing influence), and it must also be borne in mind that mental illness is not the result of some personal weakness, nor is it a reflection of some flaw in an individual's persona, nor an indication of the way in which someone has been brought up, although significant childhood events can lead to a lack of resilience in adulthood. Most importantly, it should be remembered that mental illnesses are treatable (Mental Health Foundation, 2016). In other words, mental ill health is something that could, and does, affect all kinds of people and from all walks of life. This is an important thing for any nurse or health and social care professional to try and help others understand and could do much to reduce or positively inform the negative stereotyping and ignorance that has surrounded mental ill health for centuries. Most people who are diagnosed with a serious mental illness can experience relief from their symptoms through shared decision-making, and this includes people with intellectual disabilities. This has the added benefit of improving the quality of care provided as well as, importantly, patient outcomes and healthcare efficiency (NICE, 2019; DH, 2012).

Manifestations of mental ill health

In the past, presentation of psychiatric disorder was broadly divided into two major types of mental illness, and these types were based upon manifestation of symptomology.

Neuroses was a term historically used to refer to a range of mental illnesses that encompassed symptoms that were extreme manifestations of the normal range of emotional experiences, and they typically included disorders such as depression, anxiety, or panic attacks. Generally, neuroses tend to be more amenable to treatment, and were often said to be characterised by *'insight'* by the person experiencing the illness into both their condition and the presenting symptoms. These illnesses are now more frequently called common mental health problems. However, it should be remembered that this will not necessarily mean the illnesses are less severe than those with psychotic symptoms.

Psychoses was a term historically used to describe a range of mental illnesses with symptoms that interfered with a person's perception of reality and typically included hallucinations, delusions, or paranoia, with the person seeing, hearing, smelling, feeling, or believing things that no one else does is able to perceive or understand. In the past this group was further subdivided into organic disorders (for example, vascular dementia), metabolic disorders (for example, porphyria), functional disorders (for example, schizophrenia), and affective disorders (for example, manic depressive psychosis, which is now referred to as bipolar disorder). Generally, they tend to be more challenging to treat than neuroses and were often said to be characterised by a *'lack of insight'* by the person experiencing the illness both about their condition and symptoms, that to a lesser or greater extent are characterised by thought disorder/s, hallucinations, and delusions. These illnesses are now more often referred to as severe mental health problems.

This following section identifies a range of common and severe mental health problems that adults and children with intellectual disabilities may experience. Such problems include affective disorders, anxiety, suicide, and deliberate self-harm (DSH), schizophrenia, obsessive compulsive disorders, eating disorders, personality disorder, and, finally, alcohol and drug dependency.

Affective disorders

Affective disorders refer to a wide range of mental disorders that are all characterised by dramatic changes or extremes of mood. Affective disorders can include mania (elevated, expansive, or irritable mood with hyperactivity, pressured speech, and inflated self-esteem) or depressed (dejected mood with little interest in life, sleep disturbance, agitation, and feelings of worthlessness or guilt) episodes, and often the two are combined. People with an affective disorder may or may not have psychotic symptoms such as delusions, hallucinations, or a loss of contact with reality. The prevalence rate of affective disorders in people with intellectual disability is known to be higher than the wider population and increases with age. Mrayyan, Eberhard, and Ahlstrom (2019) have reported that 5.9% of older adults with intellectual disability have at least one type of affective disorder, compared to 4.5% of the wider population. How affective disorders vary between people with mild and severe intellectual disabilities is poorly understood.

Depression

Depression is a mood disorder and is characterised by feelings of sadness, emptiness or irritability, or a loss of pleasure accompanied by additional cognitive or behavioural symptoms that significantly affect the ability to function (ICD-11,

2022). In psychiatry, two main types of depression are proposed. These are *'endogenous'* and *'exogenous'*. The former is more severe and perhaps explained by biological factors, and often not associated with external triggers to depression. The latter, sometimes referred to as reactive depression, is less severe, milder, can sometimes be explained by external *'triggers'* of significant life events such as loss, and will sometimes manifest itself with an overlapping anxiety.

Historically, it was believed that people with intellectual disabilities were unaffected by depression. However, it is now recognised that those with mild to moderate intellectual disabilities have insight and understanding of their emotional responses and are also aware of the social factors that increase their vulnerability. Jahoda (2020) has asserted that this includes commonly recognised issues such as poverty, marginalisation, a limited peer group, and lack of social activity.

People with mild intellectual disabilities often present with well-developed communication skills, and therefore are more likely to have the ability not only to recognise but also to articulate their emotions. This means that assessing their level of mood can be undertaken using a standard assessment method, with the involvement of the individual being assessed where possible. This is supported by Mileviciute and Hartley (2015) who found that there were significant differences in symptoms reported by supporting staff compared to self-report from individuals with mild intellectual disabilities. It was found that affective and cognitive symptoms can be identified through self-reporting that are difficult to recognise externally. People with moderate, severe, or profound intellectual disabilities with complex needs often have limited communication ability and are therefore unable to report or articulate their emotions effectively. In these cases, the intellectual disability nurse often must rely on reports from carers and supporters of overt changes in behaviour to successfully undertake assessment.

Weight loss is a common symptom of depression, but people with intellectual disabilities may also atypically present with an increased appetite, and therefore significant weight gain (RCN, 2010). An intellectual disability nurse should be acutely aware of other signs or symptoms, such as social withdrawal, because they could well be indicative of depression. It is also important to directly look for, or indirectly seek carers' reports about changes in other aspects of someone's behaviour. For example, behavioural changes to look out for include changes in personal hygiene and appearance; of note is diurnal mood variation, where the mood is worse on waking but improves as the day proceeds. Again, all these presentations can be indicative of depression.

It is worth noting that depression is one of the most frequently diagnosed psychiatric disorders in people with intellectual disabilities (Jahoda, 2020) and is at least double the prevalence rate compared to the wider population (Perera *et al.*, 2019; Sheerin *et al.*, 2019; Cooper *et al.*, 2007). Depression is also a particular risk to those with Downs Syndrome and many studies have highlighted a significantly increased prevalence in this population (Walton and Kerr, 2015; Walker *et al.*, 2011; Poumeaud *et al.*, 2021).

Bipolar disorder

Bipolar disorder was known in the past as manic-depressive psychosis, and it is a condition that is characterised principally by its effect on mood and which in classical presentation swings from the extreme of mania to that of depression. It is defined in the ICD-11 as:

an episodic mood disorder defined by the occurrence of one or more manic or mixed episodes.

(World Health Organisation, 2022)

Bipolar disorder is relatively common, with around one person in 100 in the general population being diagnosed with this condition. It can occur at any age, though it tends to develop more commonly between 18 and 24 years of age, and rarely after the age of 40, and it affects men and women equally. There are different types of bipolar disorder (see Table 5.1).

The pattern of mood swings in bipolar disorder is known to vary widely between people. For example, some will only have only a few bipolar episodes in their lifetimes, and will be stable in between, whereas others may experience many episodes. During an episode, depression is typically experienced where the person feels very low and lethargic, and then mania where they will feel very high and overactive. This may manifest in a lesser nature and is then referred to as hypomania. The symptoms of bipolar disorder will, therefore, depend on the presenting mood being experienced. And, unlike normal mood swings, which we may all experience at some time in our lives – for example, elation at winning a competition or great sadness at losing a family pet – the mood swings in bipolar disorder are extreme, and some episodes of disorder may last for many weeks or even months. Some people may report that they do not experience a *'normal'* mood very often, and that the changes in their moods may not be associated with any life event or experience that may account for such a mood swing. During the manic phase of this disorder, symptoms commonly reported include

Bipolar I

Here there has been at least one 'high' or manic episode lasting longer than one week. Some people with bipolar I will have only manic episodes – most will also have periods of depression. Untreated, manic episodes generally last between three and six months. Depressive episodes last longer: 6 to 12 months without treatment.

Bipolar II

Here there has been more than one episode of severe depression, but only mild manic episodes. These are called 'hypomania'.

Rapid cycling

This is characterised by more than 4 mood swings in a 12-month period. This affects around 1 in 10 people with bipolar disorder, happens with both types I and II, and is more common in people with learning disabilities.

Cyclothymia

Here, mood swings are not as severe as those in full bipolar disorder but can last longer and develop into full bipolar disorder.

Source: Royal College of Psychiatrists, 2020. Available at www.rcpsych.ac.uk/mental-health/problems-disorders/bipolar-disorder.

Table 5.1 Typology of bipolar disorders

elevated mood, delusions (characteristically some of these can be grandiose), being overly talkative (pressure of speech), ideas that seem to jump (flight of ideas), the use of rhyming language (clang association), and possibly overactive, and at times uninhibited, behaviour.

BOX 5.3
CASE STUDY 5.1

John is in his late 30s, and until recently had a good appetite and was described by support staff as being very happy and content. He is known to his local community team for people with learning disabilities (CTPLD) because several years ago he was diagnosed by his general practitioner with depression following the traumatic death of his father from a cerebral vascular accident (stroke). John lives in supported living, and since the recent closure of his day service that he had been attending for many years, it has been noticed that he has become somewhat withdrawn. John now works two days a week at a local Mencap charity shop. He has a very close relationship with his brother, who calls round every week to take John out to a local pub on a Wednesday evening, where they are both members of a local darts team. He receives little help where he lives, with only a support worker calling in once a day, twice a week, in the mornings, just to make sure he is up, washed, and ready to go to work part-time in a charity shop, where he works from 9:30 a.m. until 3:30 p.m. John's brother has noticed that he has recently lost a lot of weight, and reports *'that his clothes just hang off him'*. John's brother has called the charity shop to see how John is getting on there, and they say that he seems very quiet and that almost as soon as he arrives, he spends most of the day asking if it is time to go home. John's brother has also left a letter for the support worker asking her to phone him because he is a little worried about his brother. The support worker says she does not know John very well, because she has only been supporting him for a few weeks, but that she has noticed when she calls round at 8:00 a.m. John is nearly always asleep; he is very difficult to rouse, saying that he has been awake since very early and he is now tired. He often says he doesn't want breakfast because he feels sick. John's brother decides to ask John if he thinks he should go to the doctor to check that all is well. Initially, John said no because he was frightened of his doctor. This was surprising to John's brother, who knows that John's GP is very supportive of John; eventually he agrees.

Box 5.4
Learning Activity 5.1

John and his brother visit the GP. The GP diagnoses depression. He prescribes Citalopram (Cipramil) 20 mg in the morning and suggests that the CTLD might be able to offer John some help, as they did before, including looking for more things to do during the week, and he subsequently makes a referral. The GP has asked John's brother to come along with John in three weeks' time just to see how things are, and in the meantime make a referral to your CTLD. You are asked to visit John at home where his brother will be present.

What kinds of things are you, as a community intellectual disability nurse, able to offer John?

John and his brother tell you that he has been on the tablets for a week now and that he does not feel better. What explanation might you offer him?

John says that he has real problems with a dry mouth, and that he feels very sleepy all the time. What explanation and advice might you offer him?

How do you think the GP made his diagnosis? What things would he have been looking for? Would he have used any tools to help him in his assessment? Why has he been prescribed this medicine?

It has been found that there is a significantly higher incidence of bipolar disorder in adults with intellectual disabilities, with a study undertaken by Cooper *et al.* (2018) finding a lifetime prevalence rate of 2.3%, which is double that of the general population. It is also thought that the gender ratio of bipolar disorder is similar in people with intellectual disabilities compared to the general population. Typically, changes in levels of activity, appetite, and sleep can be observed in people with intellectual disabilities, but grandiose delusions, which can often be characteristic of mania, are said to be less capacious in people with intellectual disabilities. It is also suggested that *'rapid cycling'* bipolar disorder is more common in people with intellectual disabilities (moving from depression to mania and vice versa), and that this is associated with brain injury and abnormal electroencephalogram (EEG) readings (RCN, 2010).

It should be noted that people with severe or profound intellectual disabilities and accompanying behavioural issues may present with an increase in challenging behaviour in response to environmental factors, and this can sometimes mistakenly be attributed to a diagnosis of bipolar disorder (Cooper *et al.*, 2018). A detailed holistic assessment is therefore vital in identifying underlying causes of adverse behavioural presentation.

Anxiety

This disorder is characterised by an almost unbearable emotional state that combines fear, a sense of impending doom, and a range of accompanying physical symptoms such as palpitations, tachycardia, sweating, dizziness, derealisation, dyspnoea, and generalised discomfort. It should be noted that anxiety is a normal phenomenon often experienced as a response to a range of external stressors in most, if not all, people. However, some people will experience anxiety without an external stressor being present, and when this happens, and it becomes debilitating, it is known as a disorder. It can be experienced as part of a phobic disorder such as agoraphobia or depression, or as a generalised anxiety disorder (GAD).

There is considerable variation in the reported prevalence rates of anxiety disorders, although some claim that the rate is higher in the population of people with intellectual disabilities when compared with the wider population. Cooper *et al.* (2007) reported a rate of 3.8% and this is supported by Reid, Smiley and Cooper (2011) whose research produced similar results. Whilst this suggests that prevalence has remained stable over this short period, Reid, Smiley and Cooper (2011) have suggested that there has been little research carried out prior to this and it is therefore difficult to make a longitudinal comparison. Maïano *et al.* (2018), in their study of the prevalence of anxiety disorders in youth with intellectual disabilities, found that the prevalence increased to 5.4% when individuals self-reported their symptoms. It is also suggested that anxiety disorders manifest themselves equally in males and females with intellectual disabilities when compared with the wider population, where incidence is said to be higher in women (RCN, 2010).

It is suggested that the presentation of anxiety disorders may differ within the population of people with intellectual disabilities from that of the wider population, and research findings indicate that this is true across all age groups (RCN, 2010; Austin *et al.*, 2018; Mrayyan, Eberhard and Ahlstrom, 2019). Some people with intellectual disabilities are unable to describe their internal thinking as possible symptoms of anything other than physical discomfort, and this may result in them describing experiences of mental distress as manifestations of physical illness. So, for example, an acute anxiety attack may be reported as a stomachache or headache or as feeling sick. So, as is the case with depression in people with intellectual disabilities, where no accurate self-report is likely to be forthcoming, the intellectual disability nurse must directly, or indirectly through carers or supporters, seek evidence of behavioural signs of acute anxiety and/or sleep disturbance. It is advisable to consider the provision of additional, proactive support should evidence of anxiety emerge (Reid, Smiley and Cooper, 2011) and every effort should be made to enable the individual to contribute to assessment and subsequent therapeutic intervention.

Suicide and self-harm

Whilst there are numerous definitions of suicide, it is widely accepted that in the case of a suicidal act, the individual will have had the intention and understanding that their actions would directly result in their death. Research into suicide statistics in people with intellectual disabilities is scarce, however, a review of literature carried out by Nagraj and Omar in 2017 found that the risk of suicide in adolescents with intellectual or physical disabilities is increased relative to those in the neurotypical population. There is also a higher likelihood of exposure to risk factors in the community for people with intellectual disabilities, including issues such as bereavement, deprivation, and unemployment. Contrary to some commonly held beliefs about a lack of understanding of the consequences of suicidal behaviours in people with intellectual disabilities, there is clear evidence that many people in this population can conceptualise and discuss suicidal ideation (thoughts or ideas about suicide) and have the capacity to act on suicidal thoughts. It is important to note that despite the evidence, there is a lack of tools for supporting staff to proactively discuss these issues with the people that they support (Wark *et al.*, 2018).

The Cross-Government Suicide Prevention Workplan (HM Government, 2019) highlights the need for suicide awareness training across all public sectors including healthcare settings, and to this end a series of self-harm and suicide competence frameworks has been developed by Health Education England (HEE, 2017) to develop knowledge and skills for professionals in all areas of practice. The professional responsibility of intellectual disability nurses to develop the skills needed to carry out person-centred assessments for signs and symptoms of self-harm and/or suicidal ideation, is outlined in the *Future nurse: Standards of proficiency for registered nurses* (Annexe B: 1.1.6, 2018). It is clear therefore, that intellectual disability nurses should be equipped with the skills and knowledge to enable them both to talk about suicide with the people that they support, and to assess and plan for the risk of suicidal thoughts or intention.

Self-harm, or self-injurious behaviour (SIB) is defined by van den Bogaard *et al.* (2018, p. 708) as:

> *behaviour in which a person harms (or attempts to harm) oneself deliberately and physically.*

This includes examples such as biting, burning, and scratching oneself, swallowing toxic or inedible objects, inserting objects into the body, and head banging. It is important to recognise that self-harming behaviours offer temporary relief and that underlying causes are not resolved through the act of self-harming (Mental Health Foundation, 2022). It should also be noted that whereas there is a risk of accidental death through self-harming behaviour, there is a distinction between individuals who present with self-harming behaviour who do not intend to die, and those that self-harm with suicidal intention. Whilst it was previously believed that self-harm was a separate issue to suicidal behaviour, more recent research has found that the risk of suicide is significantly increased in a person with a history of self-harming behaviour (Royal College of Psychiatrists, 2020).

Evidence suggests that self-harm is a means to manage emotional distress. The use of talking therapies such as cognitive behaviour therapy has been demonstrated to be a useful approach in the management of self-harm, with evidence suggesting that the development of problem-solving skills can reduce the number of incidents in people with intellectual disabilities (Rees and Langdon, 2016; Moses, 2018).

There have been misconceptions about the underlying causes of self-harm and self-injury in people with intellectual disabilities compared with the wider population, with a distinction often being made between people with intellectual disabilities and those without, but with mental ill health (Lovell, 2007). Whilst there has been a significant focus on the causes of self-injurious behaviour in people with intellectual disabilities, Rees and Langdon (2016) have put forward the likelihood of self-harming behaviours as having a shared etiology with the wider population. Causes can include genetic, social, psychological, and environmental factors including stressful life events, bereavement, social isolation, and impaired social communication, mental or physical ill health, and alcohol or drug misuse. Sensory processing issues in those with autism, severe or profound intellectual disabilities or communication difficulties can also lead to self-harming behaviours, and it is thought that operant conditioning can reinforce self-injurious behaviours and lead to consistent self-harming behaviour in the longer term (van den Bogaard *et al.*, 2018; Courtemanche, Lloyd and Tapp, 2018; NICE, 2022).

Self-harming behaviour can be very distressing, not only for the person with an intellectual disability, but also for those who are supporting them. Whilst there is sometimes still a misconception that one of the causes of self-harming behaviour is *'attention seeking'*, there is now a wealth of knowledge about the potential causes and effective management of self-harm. Intellectual disability nurses need to ensure that they, as well as others, treat people with dignity, respect, and compassion. Punitive actions or negative attitudes from supporting staff can be distressing for people who have self-harmed and can lead to further and often more severe incidents of self-harming behaviour and this can result in the avoidance of medical attention (NICE, 2022) as well as a potential breakdown in therapeutic relationships and communication with supporting staff. It is therefore imperative that intellectual disability nurses have the knowledge and skills to able carry out effective person-centred assessment and to offer non-judgmental, respectful, and compassionate support to individuals who self-harm or express suicidal ideation or intent.

Schizophrenia

Schizophrenia is a serious mental illness that can impair all areas of the life of an individual and can cause severe distress for them and those around them. It is described in the ICD-11 (2022) as characterised by disturbances in thinking, perception, and behaviour. It is the most common form of psychosis, with prevalence in the population of people with intellectual disabilities thought to be at least three times that of the general population. Estimates range from 2.6% to 4.4% in people with intellectual disabilities (McCorkindale, Fleming and Martin, 2017), compared with 1 in 300 people or 0.45% of the world population (WHO, 2022). It has been widely established that delayed motor delay and late developmental milestones indicate a higher risk of adult-onset schizophrenia, and whilst some studies suggest earlier onset in people with intellectual disabilities, it has more recently been suggested that the age of onset is similar across the population, with a rapid escalation in teenage years which decreases significantly after the mid-twenties (Stochl *et al.*, 2019).

As is the case in other mental illnesses, in people with severe or profound intellectual disabilities with complex needs, diagnosing this condition can be difficult. Also, in the population of people with intellectual disabilities, some of the cardinal symptoms such as delusions are suggested to be more simplistic than those that might ordinarily be found in the wider population (RCN, 2010), perhaps because delusions in people with intellectual disabilities are a construct of their potentially limited life experiences. So, for example, a delusion found in someone from the general population believing that the police and secret service are regularly screening all their telephone calls and mail might manifest itself in someone with intellectual disabilities as all people are talking about them. It is also said that people with intellectual disabilities are less likely to have thought echo, second-person hallucinations, and running commentary; essentially this involves someone hearing their own thoughts, as opposed to them being externally located.

It is important that a clear distinction is made between delusional beliefs and those that stem from real experiences. For example, it is known that people with intellectual disabilities are now the subject of both *'hate'* and *'mate'* crime, with an estimated 52,000 incidents of disability-motivated crimes against adults every year, and incidents of both sexual assault and domestic abuse reported to be at least three times higher in disabled adults compared to those without disabilities (Office for National Statistics, 2019). It is therefore vital that a robust, person-centred assessment should always be undertaken in response to the presentation of delusional beliefs in order that an appropriate response and additional support is provided.

It should be remembered that any potential decline in social functioning or self-help skills may be masked by the support a person with intellectual disabilities receives from support workers or carers. Conversely, another form of masking can occur when poor social functioning or self-help skills are attributed to their intellectual and learning disabilities, as opposed to being symptomatic of a major mental illness such as schizophrenia.

It should also be remembered that some behaviours seen in people on the spectrum of autistic conditions might be like those seen in schizophrenia. For example, neologisms (the making of new words) are also commonly seen in autism as well as bizarre motor mannerisms. It has been suggested that many people with intellectual disabilities do not demonstrate a sufficient range of symptoms to meet the standard criteria (ICD-11) for schizophrenia, so often a diagnosis of *'psychotic episode'* is reported.

Obsessive-compulsive disorders

It is suggested that obsessive-compulsive disorder (OCD) is a relatively common form of anxiety that is characterised by obsessive thinking concomitant with compulsive behaviour. These obsessions can be very distressing, and those with this condition typically present with repetitive thoughts, which they may freely articulate as completely irrational but state that they cannot be disregarded. Compulsions are ritual actions that people feel compelled to repeat to relieve concomitant anxiety or alternatively, to prevent obsessive thoughts. It is as if the rituals have some magical property. For example, a very common compulsion is someone believing that his or her hands are dirty, so he or she will wash them repeatedly, often resulting in dry and cracked skin that may become sore and infected. This is a symbolic ritual that has significant meaning, and instances can be found in literature and history: Pontius Pilate and Jesus of Nazareth and Jaggers the solicitor in *Great Expectations* by Charles Dickens. It has been found that OCD affects around 1 in every 50 people at some point during their lifetime (Royal College of Psychiatrists, 2021). The prevalence of OCD in people with intellectual disabilities is thought to be 3.5% (Al-Abdulla *et al.*, 2022). It is difficult to give a clear diagnosis of OCD without being clear that a patient can articulate how they might fight not to engage in compulsive behaviour. It is also difficult in some circumstances to differentiate between true compulsions, and some stereotypical movements, mannerisms, or even complex spasms. Finally, it is also the case that compulsions and stereotypic behaviour are not uncommon in people with autistic spectrum conditions, and this may make diagnosis difficult.

Eating disorders

Eating disorders are typically characterised by an abnormal attitude toward food that causes someone to significantly change his or her eating habits and behaviour. It is common for someone with an eating disorder to focus his or her thinking disproportionately on his or her weight and bodily appearance, and this can lead to making unhealthy choices about food, with subsequent damage to his or her health and well-being. Common eating disorders include anorexia nervosa and bulimia and binge eating. Anorexia nervosa and bulimia are said to be less common in people with intellectual disabilities than is the case in the wider population, but hyperphagia (excessive hunger or increased appetite) and pica (persistent ingestion of non-nutritive substances) are more prevalent. However, in people with mild intellectual disabilities, prevalence rates of eating disorders may be like those seen in the wider population. Weight loss may not always be indicative of an eating disorder, and may be symptomatic of another mental health problem, such as depression, or a physical health problem. It is important to note that any diagnosis of bulimia or anorexia nervosa will need to be based upon an individual being able to report his or her thinking of distorted body image, which will require relatively well-developed and sophisticated verbal skills. Of relevance to eating disorders is overeating, and this is particularly associated with Prader-Willi syndrome.

Box 5.5
Learning Activity 5.2

Research Prader-Willi syndrome and identify how the constant desire to eat food, driven by a permanent feeling of hunger, which can lead to dangerous weight gains, can best be managed.

Personality disorder

Personality disorder has been the subject of much debate and is often regarded as a contentious and unhelpful diagnostic label. It is a term that is used to describe a constellation of difficulties relating to the development of personality. It has been suggested that use of the term is an attempt to avoid applying the medical model to what is essentially a cluster of personality traits that can have a detrimental effect on the well-being of an individual and those around them. Personality disorder is not diagnosed before the age of 18 years, and this is in recognition of the development and flexibility of the personality during childhood. There have been many attempts at encapsulating an appropriate definition of personality disorder, and most recently, the following definition is put forward in The International Classification of Mental and Behavioural Disorders (ICD-11) (WHO, 2022):

> *A syndrome characterized by a persistent personality disturbance that represents a change from the individual's previous characteristic personality pattern that is*

*judged to be a direct pathophysiological consequence of a health condition not clas-
sified under Mental and behavioural disorders, based on evidence from the history,
physical examination, or laboratory findings.*

Attempts have been made to classify types of personality disorder and these are
often based on presenting characteristics of the individual. Webb (2014), for
example, has put forward five types or clusters, including odd/eccentric; dra-
matic/erratic; anxious/fearful and *'other'* which refers to an individual who does
not fit into any of the other categories. It should be remembered that the intricacies of personality development result in a vast range of presentations which
affect the myriad characteristics of personality, either singularly or across several
overlapping characteristics. Webb puts forward a simplified way of viewing differences in personality presentation as follows in Figure 5.1.

There is a paucity of research into the prevalence of personality disorders in
the wider population and estimates vary between 4% and 15% (Webb, 2014;
Volkert, Gablonski and Rabung, 2018). Research into personality disorder in
people with intellectual disabilities is rare, and it is suggested that establishing
prevalence is *'impossible'*, with estimates varying from <1% to 91% in community settings and 22% to 92% in hospital settings (Alexander and Cooray, 2003
in Williams and Rose, 2020, p. 768). This is thought to be a result of difficulties in presentation and assessment of people with intellectual disabilities and
accompanying communication difficulties (Williams and Rose, 2020).

Contrary to the lack of research into prevalence, there are an abundance of
findings relating to the causes of personality disorder and this has largely focused
on dysfunctional childhood attachment, trauma, and the effects of abuse including sexual abuse on the development of the personality (Boucher *et al.*, 2017;
Wojciechowski, 2019; Mainali, Rai and Rutofsky, 2020). It can be asserted that
this is also the case with individuals with intellectual disabilities, who have been
consistently found to be more susceptible to trauma and adverse life experiences,
higher incidents of abuse, institutionalisation and limited skills and opportunity
to navigate difficult situations with repeated experiences of failure (Webb, 2014;
Byrne, 2020; Mason-Roberts *et al.*, 2018; Williams and Rose, 2020). Historically,
it was believed that personality disorder was untreatable, however, recent findings demonstrate that psychological, psychosocial, and behavioural interventions with additional pharmacological treatment can be successful. A consistent
and individualised approach in a stable environment is integral.

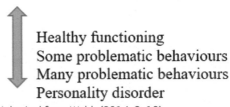

Figure 5.1 *Source:* Adapted from Webb (2014, 9. 10)

Differences in personality presentation.

People with intellectual disabilities and accompanying personality disorder have been repeatedly reported to be challenging to work with because of mis-understanding of the causes of adverse behaviours, with staff attributing these to personality traits rather than situational issues (Lee and Kiemle, 2015). However, with effective training, the skills and knowledge of intellectual disability nurses place them in an optimum position to offer high quality and individual-ised care in this specialised area of practice.

Substance Misuse

It has been theorised that the de-institutionalisation and integration into the community, whilst being a positive move forward for people with intellectual disabilities, has increased their exposure to alcohol and other illicit substances (Sharma and Lakhan, 2017; Huxley et al., 2019; Robertson et al., 2020). Contemporary research is scarce, and findings vary, however, an increase in the use of alcohol and illicit drugs is indicated, and whilst the prevalence is lower than the neuro-typical population, this is an emerging problem (Huxley et al., 2019; Robertson et al., 2020). There are several risk factors associated with the use of illicit substances that are particular to individuals with intellectual disabilities. This includes a lack of access to health facilities which can result in a reluctance to seek help for problematic alcohol and drug use, as well as adverse interactions with medication for co-morbidities; a specific issue for people with intellectual disabilities (Huxley et al., 2019; Sharma and Lakhan, 2017). It has also been asserted that health promotion and prevention, and screening tools designed to raise awareness and reduce incidents of substance misuse are rarely designed with people with intellectual disabilities in mind, instead targeting those without intellectual disabilities (Sharma and Lakhan, 2017).

It has also been identified that people with intellectual disabilities who are in contact with the Criminal Justice System for drug related offences are at increased risk of entering back into similar behaviours on their release, because of a lack of safe accommodation or income, and this can result in further incarceration and significantly poor health outcomes (Bhandari et al., 2015).

The relationship of 'mate crime' with increased misuse of substances by people with intellectual disabilities should not be overlooked. Mate crime is described as a form of hate crime in which the victim is known to the perpetrator and involves 'exploitation, manipulation and cruelty' (Forster and Pearson, 2020, p. 1103). There have been several examples of people with intellectual disabilities who have been victims of mate crime reported in the media over the past decade or so and many of these have involved the usage, storing, selling, and trafficking of illicit drugs and alcohol (Landman, 2014; BBC News, 2011).

It is important that intellectual disability nurses are aware of the risks of substance misuse and can identify signs of exposure to, and use of illicit substances in the people that they support. An awareness of mate crime is also important to identify victims of criminal behaviour and respond appropriately. With additional training, individualised support and access to the most appropriate services are vital, and it is the role of the intellectual disability nurse to ensure that the right support is offered from the most appropriate services.

General observations and recording: assessment tools for mental health

There are numerous approaches and tools that can be used to assess mental health or mental ill health. Some of these approaches or tools have been designed specifically for people with intellectual disabilities, whereas the wider population has designed others for use. And of the latter, some of these are less helpful for people with intellectual disabilities. No matter which approach or tool is used to identify a mental health disorder, a diagnosis can be made more easily if the assessment is supported with good observational skills to corroborate any diagnosis. These observations are of particular use to people with intellectual disabilities who may not report changes to their mental well-being, and this could be for several reasons. For example, they may not be able to recognise the significance of changes in their thoughts and feelings or their symptoms may be cloaked by the kinds of support they may be in receipt of. When this is the case then either through the direct and/or indirect input from the intellectual disability nurse they should seek to elicit observations from family and/or care staff. This makes it of critical importance for the intellectual disability nurse to make sure that they direct carers and support staff as to what to record, as well as how to document their observations in a range of areas such as changes to mood or sleep disturbance/s or sudden and unexplained changes in weight or behaviour.

General observations and recording

As a precursor to undertaking a MSE or using a specific mental health assessment tool, general observations and recording can be used to establish the likelihood of an underlying mental health problem. This process of titration of approach along with tools used is helpful and can prevent unnecessary distress or wasting valuable resources – of which time tends to be the most important. The following observations are useful.

Mood

Whereas mood is variable in all people, sustained changes to someone's *'normal'* mood might be indicative of an underlying psychopathology. The intellectual disability nurse can help carers develop an easy-to-use record that captures an individual's mood over a pre-determined period. One way to do this might be to divide the day up into sections and use a series of visual keys to record mood, such as smiley or sad faces.

Sleep charts

If an individual presents with significant changes in his or her sleeping patterns, this may be symptomatic of a range of mental health disorders. For example, waking up early in the morning or even sleeping in very late may be signs of depression. Alternatively, lack of sleep may be a sign of hypomania. Once again, maintaining a record, where possible, can be helpful.

Weight charts

Given that weight gain, or loss, is classically associated with evidence about how people are looking after themselves, careful observations of weight could elicit useful information; lack of, or increased appetite, may be a sign of an underlying mental health problem. This is simply recorded by maintaining weight charts that can be completed on a weekly or monthly basis and making ongoing judgments.

ABC charts

The use of antecedent/behaviour/consequence (ABC) charts is well established in the field of learning disabilities (see Chapter 9). Their use is to provide a structured record of behaviours that might be described as distressed or challenging. They offer an opportunity to identify why particular behaviour/s might occur by recording behaviour/s before, during, and after a particular behavioural incident. As well as potentially identifying triggers for, and functions of, that behaviour, they also enable us to hypothesise or predict how an incident might best be managed or resolved in the future.

Mental State Examination (MSE)

People with intellectual disabilities are at higher risk of experiencing a range of biological (e.g., physical illness; epilepsy; sensory impairments), psychological (e.g., trauma; low self-efficacy/self-esteem) and social factors (e.g., poverty; social exclusion) which increase their vulnerability to the development and maintenance of mental health problems (Gates, Fearns and Welch, 2015). Situating a mental health assessment within a biopsychosocial framework takes account of the complex interplay between these factors. The intended aim in using this framework is to develop a formulation of the person's mental health problem which can then subsequently inform an individualised intervention and support plan. This includes understanding the nature of the problem and how it developed, the precipitating factors that have led it to become a problem at the present time, and the perpetuating factors that maintain the problem. Identification of protective factors, or positives in the person's life, is also crucial and reflects a strength-based approach to care.

To conduct a thorough and comprehensive assessment the information gathering process should be as rich as possible and from a range of sources. Obtaining multiple perspectives enables a more robust picture of the issues the person is experiencing (Pickard and Rye, 2018). Current guidelines recommend the assessment to be coordinated by a professional with expertise in mental health problems in people with intellectual disabilities and should involve:

■ The person with the mental health problem, in a place familiar to them if possible, providing any help they may need to prepare for the assessment

- Family members, carers and care workers, and others the person may want involved in their assessment
- Other professionals, if needed
- The opportunity for the person to speak on their own to find out if they have any concerns, including safeguarding concerns, that they do not want to talk about in front of family members, carers or care workers.

(NICE, 2016)

The assessment should include the person's background history, including any trauma or adverse life events; their physical health; past mental health history; current mental health; and an assessment of their social circumstances. Current presentation can be evaluated using the Mental State Examination (MSE). The MSE is much more thorough than a general overview of how someone appears to be functioning and provides a systematic structure to help understand and evaluate the person's mental health at a given point in time (Assadi, 2020). MSEs are an incredibly helpful and fundamental component of mental health assessment and one that intellectual disability nurses should be well versed in. The structure of an MSE should be like that used within the wider population, but practitioners need to be cognizant of an individual's level of communication and cognitive capacity, and this may determine how questions are framed or reframed. It should also be noted that people with intellectual disabilities may acquiesce, especially if they do not fully understand what is being asked of them (Standen, Clifford and Jeenkeri, 2017). It is important that a full history, including, where possible, that of the family, is made before conducting the MSE proper; this can assist in making sense of presenting behaviour and comparing this with that of their *'normal'* behaviour. When an MSE is undertaken by an intellectual disability nurse, they will need to be informed by the following areas, which are of central importance to assessing someone's mental state.

Appearance

When assessing appearance, the intellectual disability nurse should focus on general health, manner, presenting persona, cleanliness, how the person is dressed, facial expression/s, or general demeanor. This may give an indication of the person's mood as well as their ability to care for themselves. Whilst these observations can be helpful, they need to be made within the context of someone having an intellectual disability and what is typical for the person.

Behaviour

An overall impression needs to be formed as to the parameters of the person with an intellectual disability and their presenting behaviour/s, and whether this can be described broadly as normal for that person. For some people with intellectual disabilities, this may be more difficult to do than imagined. Some people with intellectual disabilities may present, for example, with behaviours appropriate to their developmental stage, however, this behaviour may be wrongly thought of as being due to symptoms of mental illness. The issue here is one of making a judgment based on relative *'norms'*, so a distinction will need to be made between behaviour that appears to suggest someone is depressed, with the knowledge that this person is normally very quiet and subdued. What is being looked for in this assessment are significant deviations of behaviour that materially and substantially move away from how the person typically behaves. Distinctions need to be drawn between perceived behaviour and behaviour that might be explained by other, already known and diagnosed conditions such as autism. But this should not stop the clinician from looking for signs of restlessness or agitation or its opposite psycho-motor retardation, and observe for level of eye contact, level of engagement, and facial expression. It is also important to remember that signs of mental illness may manifest atypically in some people with intellectual disabilities; for example, screaming or biting, particularly as the level of intellectual disability increases.

Cognition

Cognition refers to the mental actions or process of acquiring knowledge and understanding through thought, experience, and the senses. It includes perception, discernment, awareness, apprehension, learning, understanding, comprehension, enlightenment, insight, intelligence, reason, reasoning, thinking, and (conscious) thought. Clearly any assessment of cognitive processes will vary because of someone's level of ability and their level of concentration, orientation, and memory may all be compromised. This component of the MSE may be particularly compromised where dementia is suspected, which may be the case particularly in people with Down syndrome. Any questions asked to assess cognition must be constructed in an accessible and meaningful way cognizant with someone's developmental level. So, questions need to be relevant and straightforward, such as 'What is your brother's name?', 'Where do you live?', and 'When do you go to the pub?' These questions can be used to expand the assessment and to come to a decision, if possible, about a person's cognitive state.

Experiences

Hallucinations occur when someone sees, hears, smells, tastes, or feels things that don't exist outside of their mind; they can involve any of the senses. Hallucinations tend to be common in people with schizophrenia and are often experienced as hearing voices. They can be frightening because they may be unexpected or unwanted. More frequently than not, an identifiable cause can be isolated. They can, for example, occur because of taking drugs or alcohol, or as already stated, as part of a mental illness. Hallucinations can also occur because of extreme tiredness or recent bereavement. However, these are rare occurrences. It should be borne in mind that hallucinations can be very difficult to isolate in people with intellectual disabilities. One area of potential confusion may occur in olfactory, gustatory, or visual hallucinations, where their manifestation is commonly accounted for by the aura of a seizure (refer to Chapter 6). The person with intellectual disabilities may not be able to articulate their experiences verbally, or the nurse may observe signs in their behaviour, for example, talking to people that no one else can see or grimacing as though tasting something foul.

Mood and affect

It is helpful to seek an individual's subjective experiences or mood, before making a judgment about his or her observed manifestation of emotion/s or affect. This should be surmised through careful and sensitive questioning and prompts. Pictures can help people with intellectual disabilities locate their feelings, and images such as those from the *Books Beyond Words* series, for example, *Ron's Feeling Blue*, or *Sonia's Feeling Sad* (Hollins, Banks and Curran, 2011) are useful in identifying the different emotions they might be experiencing. Some individuals may have problems in reporting their emotional state for several reasons (for example, difficulty in understanding emotions). In these instances, intellectual disability nurses' observations will play a greater role in helping to diagnose a mood disorder. As before, in the general observations, seek input from a person's carer if they have one, or alternatively family and/or friends. It is also important to consider biological indicators of mood problems, such as change in appetite or sleep disturbance.

Speech

Depending on the person's verbal communication skills, aspects of speech should be considered within the assessment. For example, rate of speech (is the person talking more rapidly than they usually would? Is their speech pressured?), volume, tone, and flow of ideas.

Thought content

It is important that any individual's presentation is placed within the context of his or her normal range of functioning. That said, changes in thinking might be one of the strongest indications of a mental health problem. The range of thought disorders include *flight of ideas*, which refers to language that may be difficult to understand when it jumps from one seemingly unrelated idea to another; *circumstantiality*, which refers to language that may be difficult to understand or is long-winded and convoluted; *word salad*, which is seen when words that are strung together resulting in gibberish; *neologisms*, meaning *new words* -- whereas it is common in children, it is considered indicative of brain damage or a thought disorder (such as schizophrenia) when present in adults; *thought insertion*, which is a delusional thought that things are being placed into a person's mind by someone or an external source, and is often a symptom of schizophrenia; and, finally, *Knight's move* thinking, which is a phenomenon similar to derailment of thought or loosening of associations, and is characterised by strange associations and directions between ideas; the name for this disorder derives from the move used by the knight in the game of chess. Given the complexity and sometimes subtle nature of thought disorder, it is important in people with intellectual disabilities to be sure that thinking is really disordered and not merely an artefact of their developmental level. It would be relatively easy to interpret someone's thought content as delusional if he or she is not able to articulate a rational explanation for something they may say. Assessing risk is a fundamental component of any mental health assessment. Any thoughts of harming themselves or others should be fully explored when considering thought content.

Standardised rating scales

Standardised tools can be used as part of the overall assessment process to provide baseline data about aspects of the person's mental health. They are also useful in monitoring changes over time and evaluating the effectiveness of any interventions. For some people with intellectual disabilities, using standard mental health assessment tools may not be appropriate, for example due to the language used and caution required when interpreting results (NICE, 2016). Recommendations advise using tools which have been specifically designed for people with intellectual disabilities, four examples of which are outlined as follows.

Learning Disability version of the Cardinal Needs Schedule (LDCNS) (Raghavan et al., 2004)

The LDCNS is based on the systematic assessment of needs using the Cardinal Needs Schedule (CNS) (Marshall, Hogg and Gath, 1995). This provides a model of needs assessment that includes assessment of functioning of the individual's symptoms, behaviour problems, and personal and social skills in several areas of functioning, determining whether problems exist in any of these areas, applying a set of criteria to establish the appropriateness of addressing an identified problem, and finally, determining the need for appropriate intervention in the areas of functioning where problems have been identified.

Psychiatric Assessment Schedules for Adults with Developmental Disabilities (PAS-ADD) (Moss et al., 1998)

This is the generic name for a series of mental health assessment tools originally developed for people with intellectual disabilities. Most recently, this system has incorporated children and adolescents (including those with and without intellectual disability), making child mental health assessments more reliable and valid throughout generic children's services. Whereas the PAS-ADD system maximises the contribution of the individual, and, where possible, the individual's family carers, frontline staff, and a range of professionals, its clinical emphasis provides structured frameworks for assessment. PAS-ADD is presented in different formats; there is a semi-structured interview for professional staff that assesses mental state and a checklist version for carers and support staff of potential indicators of mental health problems.

Other widely used tools are the Glasgow Anxiety Scale for People with an Intellectual disability (GAS-ID) (Mindham and Espie, 2003) and the Glasgow Depression Scale for People with a Learning Disability (GDS-LD) (Cuthill, Espie and Cooper, 2003). These rating scales have been validated for use with people with intellectual disabilities and show reliability and validity. Both consist of several self-report measures which explore specific emotions experienced in the previous week. Each item is measured on a three-point Likert scale (no/never; sometimes; a lot/always).

Interventions for mental health problems

A range of possible interventions are available to manage mental health problems and promote psychological well-being. These typically include medication, psychological therapies (sometimes known as *'talking therapies'*), social interventions and personal management strategies. Often a combination of approaches will be required which reflect the multi-factorial, biopsychosocial nature of the development and maintenance of mental health problems. This requires creativity and flexibility on the part of the nurse in facilitating the development of a care plan which has the person's values, wishes, and needs at the centre.

Psychotropic medication

Psychotropic medication is a broad term referring to drugs that act on the brain and affect behaviour, mood, thoughts, and perception. These drugs are widely used amongst people with intellectual disabilities (McMahon, Hatton and Bowring, 2020) and include antipsychotics, antidepressants, mood stabilisers, anxiolytics, and anti-epileptic medication. When used carefully, antipsychotic medication can reduce the distress associated with mental illness in people with intellectual disabilities (Royal College of Psychiatrists, 2016).

Antipsychotics

Antipsychotic medication is used to reduce and manage the symptoms of acute psychosis and as a maintenance treatment to prevent future relapse. Antipsychotics are generally divided into two classes: the older *'typical'*, *'first generation'* agents, the neuroleptics, and the newer *'atypical'*, or *'second generation'* agents; these have been developed since the 1990s.

Typical antipsychotics include Chlorpromazine (Largactil), Haloperidol (Haldol), and Trifluoperazine (Stelazine). Problems with the typical agents include extensive and often distressing adverse effects that include stiffness and shakiness (extrapyramidal side effects), often called pseudo-Parkinson's disease, sluggish and slow thinking, restlessness (akathisia), lowering of blood pressure (postural hypotension), and sexual dysfunction. The pseudo-Parkinson's condition can be controlled with anticholinergic drugs – orphenadrine (Disipal) and procyclidine (Kemadrin) are two commonly used anticholinergics.

A longer-term problem with typical antipsychotics is tardive dyskinesia (TD). TD is difficult to treat, and, more often, an incurable form of dyskinesia, where involuntary, repetitive body movements of the mouth, tongue, and jaw occur.

Atypical antipsychotics are usually described as having less neuromuscular adverse effects although this does not mean they have no adverse effect on body movement (Taylor, Paton and Kapur, 2015). They can also be more likely to cause metabolic effects such as weight gain, hyperlipidaemia, and altered blood sugar levels. Other adverse effects include sexual dysfunction and extrapyramidal effects. Examples of atypical antipsychotics include Amisulpride (Solian), Aripiprazole (Abilify), and Olanzapine (Zypadhera). Clozapine (clozaril) is an atypical antipsychotic used in treatment resistant schizophrenia. NICE (2015) guidance has recommended its use only when two other antipsychotics have first been used. Clozapine carries the highest risk of the rare but potentially life-threatening adverse effects of neutropenia and agranulocytosis (extremely low levels of white blood cells) which requires regular blood monitoring before and during treatment (Mwebe, 2021). Use of this medicine requires the consent of the person which can be a key consideration in deciding whether clozapine is used.

Depot injections

Some antipsychotic drugs can be given by depot injection intramuscularly where a delivered *'reservoir'* of medicine slowly releases itself into the bloodstream. This is useful for patients who may not remember to take their medicine or who may have poor concordance with oral medication (McFadden, 2019). The injection is given every one to four weeks, depending on the dose required. The medication is slowly released into the body over several weeks. The benefits and side effects of the depot injection are much the same as if it were taken orally. Examples include Modecate (fluphenazine decanoate), Depixol (flupenthixol decanoate), and Clopixol (zuclopenthixol decanoate).

> **Box 5.6**
> **Learning Activity 5.3**
>
> Look up each of these antidepressants and make careful notes about their side effects. You will find that some of them are very similar, whereas others have very specific side effects that you as an intellectual disability nurse will need to know.

Antidepressants

Antidepressants are very commonly prescribed for depression. Generally, modern management of depression indicates that antidepressants are not recommended for the initial treatment of mild depression; it is the case that the risks may outweigh the benefits. Current practice is based upon using self-guided cognitive behaviour therapy (CBT), or short courses of cognitive therapy with a therapist. Whereas for severe depression, a combination of antidepressants along with individual CBT should be considered, this combination is thought to be more cost effective than either treatment approach on its own.

The main groups of antidepressants are:

Selective Serotonin Reuptake Inhibitors (SSRIs)

SSRIs are often the first choice of medication for depression because they have fewer side-effects than other antidepressants. Examples include Fluoxetine (Prozac), citalopram (Cipramil) paroxetine (Seroxat), and sertraline (Lustral).

Serotonin-adrenaline Reuptake Inhibitors (SNRIs)

SNRIs are like SSRIs and include Duloxetine (Cymbalta and Yentreve) and venlafaxine (Efexor).

Tricyclic Antidepressants (TCAs)

TCAs are an older type of antidepressant medication and are associated with increased side effects compared to the SSRIs/SNRIs. Examples include Amitriptyline (Tryptizol), Clomipramine (Anafranil), and Imipramine (Tofranil).

Hypnotic and anxiolytic medication

Minor tranquillisers and hypnotics, primarily benzodiazepines, are used to treat anxiety and sleep problems. They are usually prescribed only on a short-term basis because of their addictive nature. These include benzodiazepines such as Diazepam, Lorazepam, and Alprazolam. Other examples include nitrazepam (Mogadon), and zopiclone (Imovane).

Mood stabilisers

Mood-stabilising medications are used to treat bipolar disorder. They are usually taken long term, even when a person is not experiencing an episode of mania, hypomania, or depression. The oldest mood stabiliser is Lithium; anticonvulsant drugs developed to treat epilepsy are now often used as mood stabilisers. Additionally, some antipsychotic medications also appear to be effective as mood stabilisers. Examples of medicines used as mood stabilisers include Lithium, Sodium Valproate (Epilim), Carbamazapine (Tegretol), and Lamotrigine (Lamictal), where dosage is introduced based on concurrent medication. It is advisable to refer to the latest edition of the British National Formulary for further information and guidance.

Despite their clinical utility when used appropriately, there is a growing body of evidence which highlights concerns about the overuse of psychotropic medication in people with intellectual disabilities. It is frequently the case that antipsychotics are prescribed on a long-term basis in the absence of a diagnosed mental illness (Sheehan et al., 2015). A systematic review by Sheehan and

Hassiotis (2017) found that antipsychotics could be reduced or discontinued in a substantial proportion of adults who are prescribed them for perceived challenging behaviour. In response to concerns, NHS England initiated the 'STOMP' project: 'Stopping the Over-Medication of People with an intellectual disability, autism or both'. The extent to which the STOMP project has impacted on the use of apsychotropic medication in people with intellectual and learning disabilities is yet to be evaluated (Branford *et al.*, 2019).

Talking therapies

Talking therapies, also known as psychological therapies, are frequently used to help people better understand their thoughts and feelings, and to assist them in making connections between their behaviours, moods, and psychological well-being. Such interventions can help people find important ways to change their lives by encouraging them to act and think in a more positive way. It should be noted that these therapies are not always suitable for all people with intellectual disabilities, and as a rule are more suited to those with mild intellectual disabilities. There is a distinct lack of evidence for the effectiveness of interventions (either psychological or pharmacological) within children and adults with severe intellectual disabilities (Vereenooghe *et al.*, 2018).

Talking therapies are best understood when organised under the general heading of psychotherapy and include:

- Re-educative therapies, such as behaviour therapy or cognitive behaviour therapy (CBT)
- Reconstructive therapies, such as psychoanalysis with the Jungian or Kleinian approaches.

There is a growing body of research that supports the use of psychological interventions in people with intellectual and learning disabilities, however, studies are often small scale and evidence is limited overall. Studies by Lindsay *et al.* (2015) and Hartley *et al.* (2015) have shown effectiveness of CBT for people with mild to moderate intellectual disabilities in depression; CBT remains the intervention of choice with the most supporting evidence for use with this population.

Psychodynamic psychotherapy focuses on the relationship between therapist and client, providing an opportunity to explore and analyse emotions. A systematic review by Shepherd and Beail (2017) found emerging evidence to support the use of psychodynamic and psychoanalytic therapy in reducing psychological distress in people with intellectual disabilities but concluded that more robust research was needed.

Behavioural activation (BA) is a psychological therapy with a strong evidence base for the treatment of depression in people without intellectual disabilities (Gega and Norman, 2018). BA aims to counteract depression by increasing involvement in positive activities and engagement in everyday tasks the person may have been avoiding. An adapted version of BA for people with mild to moderate intellectual disabilities (BEAT-IT) was the focus of a recent randomised controlled trial (Jahoda *et al.*, 2017). The study compared the adapted BA with a guided self-help intervention. Although no differences were found within the two groups, significant improvement in depressive symptoms was found with each intervention. Changes were maintained at 12-month follow-up and results provide a foundation for future practice and research.

Electroconvulsive Therapy (ECT)

The National Institute for Health and Clinical Excellence recommends that electroconvulsive therapy (ECT) should only be used for the treatment of severe depressive illness, or a prolonged or severe episode of mania or catatonia, to gain fast and short-term improvement of severe symptoms. There is a consensus that ECT should be used only after all other treatment options have failed, or when the situation is thought to be life threatening.

It should be noted that the 2007 addendum to the Mental Health Act 1983 provided greater protection for detained patients who are prescribed the use of ECT for mental disorders. Whilst ECT could previously be provided compulsorily, the addendum dictates that those with capacity can choose whether to receive ECT, whilst those with an advanced decision who are opposed to ECT can only receive this intervention in an emergency. ECT is no longer permitted for patients under the age of 18 years without approval from a second opinion doctor.

Other approaches

Other important factors to consider in the overall management of mental ill health, and for the maintenance of good mental health and well-being, include:

- *Support from family and friends:* To relate to others is important to one's mental health and well-being. Helping people stay in touch with family and friends is something that the intellectual and learning disability nurse can do for a patient.

- *Undertaking something worthwhile to do during the day:* Since the demise of most day services in England, many people with intellectual disabilities find themselves with little meaningful daytime occupation. This means it is important to assist people to access part-time work, voluntary work, interest groups, reading groups at libraries, and walking groups.

- *Peer support*: When our mental health is compromised, it is sometimes helpful to be able to speak with others who have had similar experiences. This can be achieved through support groups. Intellectual disability nurses must be cognizant of all resources in their locality that they can help people with intellectual disabilities access. Community intellectual disability nurses might consider setting up small groups for people if such groups do not already exist.

- *Complementary therapies:* Consider, for example, relaxation exercises, reflexology, massage, meditation, and yoga. These all have the potential to bring about a sense of well-being and relaxation.

■ *Hobbies:* Having a hobby is a good way to maintain an interest in something that may have nothing to do with jobs or our normal routines; we undertake hobbies solely because we enjoy the activity. It is also a way of meeting like-minded people. Hobbies include car booting, model building, needlework, and knitting. Most people enjoy being able to spend time on a favourite hobby, and people with intellectual disabilities are no different.

■ *Physical exercise:* Maintaining a good level of physical activity is known to increase a sense of well-being, and this is something to be particularly aware of as people with intellectual and learning disabilities can lead very sedentary lives.

■ *Spirituality and religion:* This has the potential to bring peace and a sense of order and meaning to people's lives. It is important that intellectual disability nurses ensure that attention is given to the religious and spiritual needs of all those with whom they work.

Fletcher *et al.* (2020) have further explored a range of lifestyle and environmental factors which can promote psychological well-being in people with intellectual disabilities. Finally, a straightforward way of explaining how to maintain good mental health to people with intellectual disabilities is to use the example 'five-a-day' (see Figure 5.2).

Walk: Get outside and get the sun on your face; walking and getting out in the sunlight, even if it's cloudy, is good for you.
Talk: Spend time talking and listening to others. It's good to spend time making friends; it's good to say and hear kind things.
Plan: Plan your day. It's good to have a structure to your day, so that you have some routine, and have things to look forward to. Make plans for the weekend, like meeting up with a friend or going to the park or for a swim – whatever it is you enjoy.
Laugh: There's an old saying: *'Laughter is the best medicine'*. It's always good to have a laugh and it's even better if it's with other people or friends. Remember to have a sense of humour!

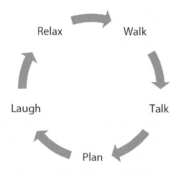

Figure 5.2

The 'five-a-day' way to good mental health.

Relax: Do things that help you to relax, listen to music, read a book, go for a walk, have a nice hot bath, or do yoga! Whatever works for you! The most important thing is to find the 'five-a-day' that works for you and keep at it every day if you can!

The care programme approach

The Care Programme Approach (CPA) is addressed comprehensively in Chapter 7; therefore, its inclusion here is simply to place it into a context of supporting someone with intellectual disabilities with complex mental health needs. CPA is a particular way of assessing, planning, and reviewing someone's mental healthcare needs and represents a comprehensive, person-centred, systematic, and integrated approach to multiagency care planning that simultaneously involves managing risk. It provides a way of supervising people known to mental health services and who have been previously sectioned under the Mental Health Act. To receive CPA an individual must be assessed against a list of criteria, and the following is a list of the criteria that will be of relevance to someone with intellectual disabilities and a severe mental illness who has been discharged into the community:

■ Severe mental disorder (including personality disorder) with a high degree of clinical complexity.

■ Current or potential risk(s) of suicide, self-harm, harm to others, relapse history requiring urgent response, disinhibition, physical/emotional abuse, cognitive impairment, child protection issues.

■ Current or significant history of severe distress/instability or disengagement.

■ The presence of intellectual disability.

■ Current/recent detention under the Mental Health Act.

■ Multiple service provision from different agencies including criminal justice.

The Mental Health Act 1983

Background

The Mental Health Act seeks, where necessary, to compel people with mental disorders to be assessed and treated for that disorder. The Mental Health Act of 1983 was amended in 2007. The amendments to the Act were intended to limit the impact of mental disorders on the individual and society, including safeguards against the abuse of process, and access to independent review. The nature and scope of these amendments are comprehensively dealt with in Chapter 7. It should also be noted that the Act's principal scope is limited to England and Wales; Scotland, Northern Ireland and the Republic of Ireland all have different, but nonetheless similar, mental health legislation.

Involuntary admission for assessment

Involuntary admission to hospital must take place only if a person is suffering from a mental disorder within the meaning of the Mental Health Act (MHA), and where detention in a hospital is deemed necessary for a person's health and safety or the protection of others. Within the Act, mental disorder refers to any disorder or disability of the mind. Of particular importance is that a person with intellectual disabilities cannot be suffering from a mental disorder, within the meaning of the Act, unless his or her disability is associated with abnormally aggressive or seriously irresponsible conduct. There are 10 parts to the Act. In the 10th part there are supplemental provisions that include its application to Scotland, Northern Ireland, and the Isles of Scilly; there are also six schedules. For the purposes of this chapter, parts II and III are possibly the most significant in relation to mental ill health in people with intellectual disabilities, but other parts are also referred to.

Part II of the Mental Health Act

Part II of the MHA makes civil provision as well as arrangements for compulsory admission to hospital and guardianship. Most people who are admitted involuntarily to hospital for assessment or treatment of mental disorders are admitted under Part II of the Act.

Part III of the Mental Health Act

Part III of the Act makes provision and arrangements for patients who are concerned with criminal proceedings, or under sentence to be detained to hospital for assessment or treatment of a mental disorder.

Assessment or treatment

Sometimes it can be unclear whether a patient who needs to be detained should be admitted for assessment or treatment. People with intellectual disabilities who are admitted for assessment will often need to receive treatment, and the same is true of patients who are admitted for treatment; they will need to be assessed as part of the treatment process.

Admission for assessment MHA 1983

The primary reason for assessment for most people with intellectual disabilities will be to obtain an understanding of problematic or offending behaviour associated with a mental disorder, as well as any relationship between their intellectual disabilities and their behaviour that might result in harm to themselves or harm to others.

Indications for assessment

■ A person with intellectual disabilities has never previously been admitted to hospital or has not been in regular contact with specialist services.

- The diagnosis or cause of the patient's problems is unclear. Previously established treatment or interventions may need to be re-formulated, and this may include an assessment of the need for informal treatment.
- The presenting needs or condition are judged to have changed since an earlier involuntary admission.

Part II: Compulsory admission to hospital and guardianship

Section 2: Admission for assessment. This is for up to 28 days and requires evidence of mental disorder, and this cannot be achieved without detention.

Section 4: Admission for assessment in an emergency. This is for up to 72 hours and is used out of urgent necessity, and with a view to admission for assessment under Section 2.

Section 5: (2) This is commonly referred to as a doctor's holding power, which is for up to 72 hours. The patient should already be receiving treatment for a mental disorder as an inpatient, and there should be a view to admission for assessment under Section 2.

Section 5: (4) This is commonly referred to as a nurse's holding power; this is for a period of up to six hours. There must be evidence of immediate risk of harm. The use of this section requires a need to secure attendance of a responsible approved clinician as soon as possible.

Part X: Miscellaneous and supplementary

Section 135: This permits a warrant for the police to search for, and remove, a patient to place of safety for a mental health assessment; this is for a period of up to 72 hours. The use of this section requires evidence to suggest mental disorder, as well as a need for a mental health assessment.

Section 136: This provides for police power to remove a person from a public place to a place of safety for a mental health assessment; this is for a period of up to 72 hours. The use of this section requires evidence to suggest a mental disorder, as well as a need for a mental health assessment.

Part III: Patients concerned in criminal proceedings or under sentence

Section 35: Remand to hospital for report on an accused's mental condition. This is for up to three periods of 28 days, but this must not exceed 12 weeks in total. It requires evidence to suggest that an accused person, who is to be remanded awaiting trial or sentence, is suffering from a mental disorder and requires assessment in hospital.

Admission for treatment under MHA 1983

Treatment for many people with intellectual disabilities who are involuntarily admitted to a hospital will be focused on addressing the *'abnormally aggressive'* and *'seriously irresponsible conduct'* that resulted in their detention. In the context of forensic nursing treatment, treatment measures may include:

- Behavioural interventions, such as the development or implementation of effective behavioural support and management plans that can be generalised to other settings or manage risk.

- Offence-specific treatment, such as sex offender treatment programmes, treatment of arson behaviour, or treatment of violent offending.

- Related treatment, such as anger management, anxiety management, problem solving, and cognitive skills programmes.

- Interventions to improve day-to-day functioning, such as social skills programmes, activities for daily living skills programmes, and interpersonal skills training.

Some people who are admitted involuntarily for treatment will also require specific treatments for mental illnesses, such as schizophrenia or bipolar disorder.

Part II: Compulsory admission to hospital and guardianship

Section 3: Admission for treatment. This is for periods of six months and then renewable annually. This requires evidence of suffering from a mental disorder that needs treatment in hospital and cannot be treated without detention.

Part III: Patients concerned in criminal proceedings or under sentence

Section 36: Remand of accused person to hospital for treatment. This is for up to three periods of 28 days, not exceeding 12 weeks in total. This requires evidence that the accused person who is to be remanded awaiting trial or sentence is suffering from a mental disorder that requires treatment in hospital.

Section 37: This can be with or without a restriction order (Section 41). It is also known as a hospital order; this gives courts the power to order hospital admission for treatment. This may include Ministry of Justice restrictions in discharge (Section 41). This is for two periods of six months and then renewable annually. This is used where a conviction for an imprisonment offence requires treatment in a hospital for mental disorder; the hospital order replaces the sentence.

Section 38: This is known as an interim hospital order. This is for periods of 28 days; it is renewable by the court for a total period not exceeding one year. This is used where a conviction for an imprisonment offence requires a period of treatment in a hospital to allow assessment regarding the appropriateness of Section 37.

Section 47 with or without a restriction order (S.49): This section covers the transfer to a hospital of a person serving a prison sentence. This may include Ministry of Justice restrictions in discharge (Section 49) until the restriction order expires. This is used when the person serving a sentence of imprisonment requires treatment for a mental disorder in hospital.

Appropriate treatment test

Finally, the availability of appropriate treatment is a requirement of detention in a hospital for treatment of a mental disorder. Treatment must be appropriate, considering the nature and degree of the person's mental disorder and all the other circumstances of the person's case. The revised MHA 1983 code of practice provides extensive guidance regarding this appropriate treatment test.

Future changes to the Mental Health Act

At the time of writing, the Mental Health Act is undergoing significant change. Following an extensive independent review (Department of Health and Social Care, 2018), and building on the *Five Forward View for Mental Health* (NHS England, 2016) which put forward 58 recommendations to develop and improve mental health service provision, a government white paper was produced in August 2021 outlining proposals to make changes to the Mental Health Act. The proposal aims to introduce new principles, both to improve patient experience and to ensure that the act is only used when necessary. The principles on which the changes to the act will be embedded include choice and autonomy, least restriction, therapeutic benefit, and the person as an individual.

The Act proposes to improve the provision for people with intellectual disabilities and autistic people and the way that they are treated in law, with less dependence on specialist inpatient services and a move towards appropriate community provision. In addition, the focus on autonomy and choice will aim to ensure that people in this group are able to make an increased contribution to their care. There will also be provision within the proposed changes to ensure that involuntary detention can only take place on the condition that there is therapeutic benefit.

Assessment of mental capacity: IMCAs and DOLS

Under the Mental Capacity Act (2005), people are presumed to be able to make their own decisions *'unless all practical steps to help him (or her) to make a decision have been taken without success'*. Thus, all people, and that includes those with intellectual disabilities, are presumed to be able to make their own decisions. Decisions can only be made for others if all practical steps to help them make a decision have been taken and without success. It must be remembered that incapacity is not based on the ability to make wise or sensible decisions; if that were the case, most of us would be deemed to be lacking capacity. To assess for incapacity, consideration needs to be given to whether the person being supported can understand the specific issue the person is deciding about. Due consideration needs to be given to whether there is:

- An impairment or disturbance in the functioning of the mind or brain.
- An inability to make decisions.

A person is only deemed unable to decide if he or she cannot:

- Understand the information relevant to the decision.
- Retain that information.
- Use or weigh that information as part of the process of making the decision.
- Communicate the decision.

If an individual is unable to decide, and therefore give his or her consent, and in this context, we are looking at decisions around treatment for mental health, then a 'best interests' decision will need to be made. When this is the case, all involved should be mindful that they should

- Not make assumptions based on the person's age, appearance, condition, or behaviour.
- Ensure that they consider all the relevant circumstances.
- Make sure that they have assessed and considered whether or when the person has capacity to make the decision.
- Ensure that the person's participation is supported in any acts or decisions made for him or her.
- Ensure that they do not decide about life-sustaining treatment.
- Make sure that they consider the person's expressed wishes and feelings, beliefs, and values.
- Take care to account for the views of others with an interest in the person's welfare, his or her carers, and those appointed to act on the person's behalf.

Most organisations provide policies governing how this should be managed. It is strongly advised that reference is made to all requirements, and these are strictly adhered to.

Also under the Mental Capacity Act, a new service was created: the Independent Mental Capacity Advocate (IMCA) service. The purpose of this service was to help vulnerable people who lack capacity and have no one to appropriately consult regarding certain important decisions that will affect them. Such decisions include medical treatment where a local authority is proposing to arrange accommodation for someone for longer than eight weeks, or where the NHS is proposing to arrange accommodation for someone for longer than 28 days. More recently, Local Authorities and the NHS are required to instruct an IMCA in certain cases that involve care reviews and adult protection cases. The NHS and Local Authorities have a duty to consult an IMCA about decisions that involve people who have no family or friends, or when it is not appropriate to consult these parties. For example, it could be that a family member or friend is unwilling to be consulted about a decision in the best interest. It is the case that family members or friends may be unwell or elderly and therefore not able to contribute to any consultation. Also, there may be other reasons that make it impractical to consult with a family member or friend; for example, he or she lives some distance away, or sometimes a family member may refuse to be consulted. Additionally, there may be issues of known abuse by family members or friends.

There are several benefits of the IMCA Service for someone who lacks capacity, including having an independent person to review significant decisions being proposed, and having someone who is articulate and knowledgeable about legislation and an individual's rights, as well as health and social care systems. It is also important to have someone skilled in supporting people who may have difficulties in communicating their views. Having an independent person who can support someone and represent them when serious decisions are being made, and when they have nobody else who can be consulted, is critical. There are also enormous benefits for statutory bodies making or proposing such life-changing decisions. This can be particularly so for practitioners working in such organisations and agencies who may find that IMCAs may assist them in making decisions. Complex decisions can be made with somewhat more confidence, and in many cases more quickly, because of the involvement of an IMCA. This leads to a consideration of deprivation of liberty, an issue that has contemporaneously risen to the top of the intellectual disability agenda.

From 2007 new procedural safeguards, known as *'Deprivation of Liberty Safeguards'* (DOLS) were introduced to protect individuals from unlawful deprivation of their liberty. These new procedures were introduced at the same time as the amendment to the Mental Health Act in 2007, and in conjunction with the Mental Capacity Act. They were developed as a long-needed response to what has become known as *'the Bournewood gap'*, an apparent *'gap'* in the law that relates to deprivation of liberty that was identified in a case involving Bournewood Hospital, England.[1] This gap arose because it was found that there was no law that effectively prevented the restriction of an individual's liberty outside of the Mental Health Act. In the case of Bournewood, it was considered that the individual in question would have been unsafe to leave the clinical environment but did not meet the criteria for detention under the Mental Health Act. The introduction of the Deprivation of Liberty Safeguards therefore resulted in the legal justification of restrictions on the liberty of an individual provided that:

- Reasonable steps are taken to establish that the individual lacks capacity in relation to the matter in question.
- It is reasonably believed that the individual does lack capacity in relation to the matter in question.
- It is in the best interests of that individual to implement an intervention that deprives them of their liberty.
- It is reasonably believed that intervention is necessary to prevent harm to that individual.
- The act in question is a proportionate response to the likelihood of the individual suffering harm.
- The act in question is a proportionate response to the seriousness of that harm.

However, making a distinction between restraining, restricting, and depriving of liberty can be problematic. It should be remembered that it is possible to *'deprive someone of their liberty'* not only through physical confinement but also by levels of control that are applied to an individual's movements. Such deprivations of liberty are also possible by using other high levels of control over an individual, such as who can visit them, and controlling when they can undertake activities, the cumulative effect being that someone is being deprived of his or her liberty. By way of contrast, an individual who, for example, resides in a locked unit during the night for his or her own safety is unlikely to be thought of as being deprived of his or her liberty, because broader contextual issues need to be taken into any assessment. Therefore, concepts of restraint, restriction, and deprivation of liberty are probably best understood as existing on a *'spectrum of control'*, with deprivation of liberty involving a higher degree or intensity of control over an individual.

Ultimately, the concept is one to be interpreted in view of the specific circumstances of that individual. That is why DoLS procedures were introduced: to *'safeguard'* the liberty of the individuals by ensuring that rigorous and transparent procedures were followed prior to any deprivation of liberty. The DoLS procedure aims to ensure that those caring for, or involved with, individuals can engage with the decision-making process whenever questions about the liberty of an individual are being explored. The DoLS procedure also aims to ensure that such decision-making is conducted carefully and is subject to independent scrutiny. The procedure designates two types of bodies: the managing authorities and supervisory bodies. The hospital or care home that is, or will become, responsible for an individual's care is referred to as the *'managing authority'*. When the Primary Care Trusts (PCTs) ceased to exist in 2013, their supervisory body responsibilities under the Deprivation of Liberty Safeguards relating to hospitals passed to local authorities, so it is they who are the *'supervisory body'*. It should be noted that the Regulations in England and Wales that govern the application and assessment procedure are different, so it is important that the correct regulations are followed.

Conclusion

This chapter has explored the high incidence of mental ill health in people with intellectual disabilities compared with the wider population. It has been established that prevalence of mental ill health remains largely unchanged, with mental health diagnoses remaining comparatively high in this population. The importance of the specialist skills and knowledge of intellectual disability nurses have been discussed in detail in relation to the ongoing need for specialist support, and the promotion of mental well-being in people with intellectual disabilities.

The nature and manifestations of mental ill health have been considered and discussed, as well as characteristics of good mental health and well-being. A range of assessment tools have been put forward and guidance on the process of a mental state examination has been detailed. An outline of examples of treatment approaches has also been put forward.

Finally, relevant legislation has been discussed, including the Mental Health Act and the Care Programme Approach, The Mental Capacity Act, and the role of the Mental Capacity Advocate (IMCA), and the Deprivation of Liberty Safeguards.

Acknowledgment

Grateful thanks to Briege Gates, (Previously) Clinical Nurse Manager, Manchester University NHS Foundation Trust for the use of the five-a-day model for the maintenance of good mental health.

Note

1 This case concerned a young man who was taken to Bournewood hospital and detained there. Originally, he had been admitted informally in his 'best interests' – solicitors were engaged to pursue a case of unlawful detention.

References

Al-Abdulla, Z., *et al.* (2022) Obsessive-compulsive symptoms in an adolescent with intellectual disability. *Case Reports in Psychiatry*, p. 4943485. Doi:10.1155/2022/4943485. PMID: 35360258; PMCID: PMC8964226.

Alexander, R. and Cooray, S. (2003) Nonpharmacological treatment for individuals with intellectual disability and 'personality disorder'. *Journal of Applied Research in Intellectual Disabilities*, 33(4), pp. 767–778.

Assadi, G. (2020) The mental state examination. *British Journal of Nursing*, 29(22), pp. 1328–1322.

Austin, K.L., *et al.* (2018) Depression and anxiety symptoms during the transition to early adulthood for people with intellectual disabilities. *Journal of Intellectual Disability Research*, 62(5), pp. 407–421.

Barr, O. and Gates, B. (2019) *Oxford handbook of learning and intellectual disability nursing*. Oxford: Oxford University Press.

BBC News (2011) Gemma Hayter murder: Three jailed for life. *BBC News*. Available at: www.bbc.co.uk/news/uk-england-coventry-warwickshire-14885830 (Accessed 24 June 2022).

Bhandari, A., *et al.* (2015) Comparison of social circumstances, substance use and substance-related harm in soon-to-be-released prisoners with a and without intellectual disability *Journal of Intellectual Disability Research*, 59(6), pp. 571–579.

Boucher, M.E., *et al.* (2017) Parent-child relationship associated with the development of borderline personality disorder: A systematic review. *Personality and Mental Health*, 11(4), pp. 229–255.

Branford, D., *et al.* (2019) Stopping over-medication of people with an intellectual disability, autism or both (STOMP) in England part 2- the story so far. *Advances in Mental Health and Intellectual Disabilities*, 13(1), pp. 41–51.

Byrne, G. (2020) A systematic review of treatment interventions for individuals with intellectual disability and trauma symptoms: A review of the recent literature. *Trauma, Violence and Abuse*, 23(2), pp. 541–554.

Cooper, S.A., *et al.* (2007) An epidemiological investigation of affective disorders with a population-based cohort of 1023 adults with intellectual disabilities. *Psychological Medicine*, 37(6), pp. 873–882.

Cooper, S.A., *et al.* (2018) Incidence of unipolar and bipolar depression, and mania in adults with intellectual disabilities: Prospective cohort study. *The British Journal of Psychiatry*, 212(2), pp. 295–300.

Courtemanche, A.B., Lloyd, B.P. and Tapp, J.T. (2018) A descriptive analysis of self-injury in community settings: Exploring behaviour-behaviour contingencies. *Journal of Intellectual Disability Research*, 62(12), pp. 1097–1107.

Crotty, G. and Doody, O. (2015) Therapeutic relationships in intellectual disability nursing practice. *Learning Disability Nursing Practice*, 18(7), pp. 25–29.

Cuthill, F.M., Espie, C.A. and Cooper, S-A. (2003) Development and psychometric properties of the Glasgow depression scale for people with a learning disability: Individual and carer supplement versions. *British Journal of Psychiatry*, 182, pp. 347–353.

DH (2001) *Valuing people: A new strategy for learning disability for the 21st century*. London: Department of Health.

DH (2009) *Valuing people: Now*. London: The Stationery Office.

DH (2012) *Liberating the NHS: No decision about me, without me*. London: Department of Health.

Department of Health and Social Care (2018) *Modernising the mental health act, increasing choice, reducing compulsion*. London: Department of Health and Social Care.

Ee, J., Kroese, B.S. and Rose, J. (2021) A systematic review of the knowledge, attitudes and perceptions of health and social care professionals towards people with learning disabilities and mental health problems. *British Journal of Learning Disabilities*, pp. 1–17. Doi:10.1111/bld.12401.

Fletcher, J., et al. (2020) Staying healthy. In Heslop, P. and Hebron, C. (Eds.), *Promoting the health and well-being of people with learning disabilities*. Cham, Switzerland: Springer, pp. 125–138.

Forster, S. and Pearson, A. (2020) 'Bullies tend to be obvious': Autistic adults perceptions of friendship and the concept of 'mate crime'. *Disability and Society*, 35(7), pp. 1103–1123.

Gates, B., Fearns, D. and Welch, J. (2015) *Learning disability nursing at a glance*. Chichester: John Wiley & Sons.

Gega, L. and Norman, I. (2018) Brief cognitive behaviour therapy interventions for nursing practice. In Norman, I. and Ryrie, I. (Eds.), *The art and science of mental health nursing: Principles and practice* (4th edition). London: McGraw-Hill, pp. 449–471.

Gov.UK (2018) *Modernising the mental health act: Increasing choice, reducing compulsion*. Available at: https://assets.publishing.service.gov.uk/government/uploads/system/uploads/attachment_data/file/778897/Modernising_the_Mental_Health_Act_-_increasing_choice__reducing_compulsion.pdf (Accessed 24 November 2022).

Hartley, S.L., et al. (2015) Cognitive behavioral therapy for depressed adults with mild intellectual disability: A pilot study. *Journal of Mental Health Research in Intellectual Disabilities*, 8(2), pp. 72–97.

HEE (2017) *Self-harm and suicide prevention*. Available at: https://www.hee.nhs.uk/our-work/mental-health/self-harm-suicide-prevention (Accessed 24 November 2022).

HM Government (2019) *Cross-government suicide prevention workplan*. London: Crown.

Hollins, S., Banks, R. and Curran, J. (2011) *Ron's feeling blue*. London: Books Beyond Words and Royal College of Psychiatrists.

Huxley, A., et al. (2019) Prevalence of alcohol, smoking, illicit drug use amongst people with intellectual disabilities: Review. *Drugs: Education, Prevention and Policy*, 26(5), pp. 365–384.

Jahoda, A. (2020) Depression and people with a learning disability: A way forward. *Tizard Learning Disability Review*, 25(1), pp. 13–21.

Jahoda, A., et al. (2017) Comparison of behavioural activation with guided self-help for treatment of depression in adults with intellectual disabilities: A randomized controlled trial. *The Lancet Psychiatry*, 4(12), pp. 909–919.

Kaushal, P., et al. (2020) Training and service provision for people with intellectual disability and mental illness: The views of psychiatrists. *International Journal of Developmental Disabilities*, 66(1), pp. 67–74.

Landman, R.A. (2014) 'A counterfeit friendship': Mate crime and people with learning disabilities. *The Journal of Adult Protection*, 16(6), pp. 355–366.

Lee, A. and Kiemle, G. (2015) 'It's one of the hardest jobs in the world': The experience and understanding of qualified nurses who work with individuals diagnosed with both learning disability and personality disorder. *Journal of Applied Research in Intellectual Disabilities*, 28(3), pp. 238–248.

Lindsay, W.R., *et al.* (2015) A preliminary controlled trial of a trans-diagnostic programme for cognitive behaviour therapy with adults with intellectual disability. *Journal of Intellectual Disability Research*, 59(4), pp. 360–369.

Lovell, A. (2007) The relationship between problem solving ability and self-harm amongst people with mild intellectual disabilities. *Journal of Applied Research in Intellectual Disabilities*, 29, pp. 387–393.

Maïano, C., *et al.* (2018) Prevalence of anxiety and depressive disorders among youth with intellectual disabilities: A systematic review and meta-analysis. *Journal of Affective Disorders*, 236, pp. 230–242.

Mainali, P., Rai, T. and Rutofsky, I. (2020) From child abuse to developing borderline personality disorder into adulthood: Exploring the neuromorphological and epigenetic pathway. *Cureus*, 12(7), p. e9474. Doi:10.7759/cureus.9474.

Marshall, M., Hogg, L. and Gath, D. (1995) The cardinal needs schedule – a modified version of the MRC needs for care assessment schedule. *Psychological Medicine*, 25(3), pp. 605–617.

Mason-Roberts, S., *et al.* (2018) Multiple traumatisation and subsequent psychopathology in people with intellectual disabilities and DSM-5 PTSD: A preliminary study. *Journal of Intellectual Disability Research*, 62(8), pp. 730–736.

McCorkindale, S., Fleming, M.P. and Martin, C.R. (2017) Perceptions of learning disability nurses and support staff towards people with a diagnosis of schizophrenia. *Journal of Psychiatric and Mental Health Nursing*, 24(5), pp. 282–292.

McFadden, R. (2019) *Introducing pharmacology: For nursing and healthcare*. Oxford: Routledge.

McMahon, M., Hatton, C. and Bowring, D.L. (2020) Polypharmacy and psychotropic polypharmacy in adults with intellectual disability: A cross-sectional total population study. *Journal of Intellectual Disability Research*, 64(11), pp. 834–851.

McManus, S., *et al.* (2016) *Mental health and wellbeing in England: Adult psychiatric morbidity survey 2014*. Leeds: NHS Digital.

Mental capacity act 2005. London: HMSO.

Mental health act 1983. London: HMSO.

Mental Health Foundation (2016) *Fundamental facts about mental health*. London: Mental Health Foundation.

Mental Health Foundation (2022) *The truth about self harm*. Available at: www.mentalhealth.org.uk/publications/truth-about-self-harm (Accessed 7 June 2022).

Mental Health Taskforce (2016) *The five year forward view for mental health*. Available at: www.england.nhs.uk/mentalhealth/taskforce (Accessed 31 May 2022).

Mileviciute, I. and Hartley, S.L. (2015) Self-reported versus informant-reported depressive symptoms in adults with mild intellectual disability. *Journal of Intellectual Disability Research*, 59(2), pp. 158–169.

Mindham, J. and Espie, C.A. (2003) Glasgow anxiety scale for people with an intellectual disability (GAS-ID) development and psychometric properties of a new measure for use with people with mild intellectual disability. *Journal of Intellectual Disability Research*, 47(1), pp. 22–30.

Moses, T. (2018) Suicide attempts among adolescents with self-reported disabilities. *Child Psychiatry and Human Development*, 49, pp. 420–433.

Moss, S., *et al.* (1998) Reliability and validity of the PAS-ADD checklist for detecting psychiatric disorders in adults with intellectual disability. *Journal of Intellectual Disability Research*, 42, pp. 173–183.

Mrayyan, N.E., Eberhard, J. and Ahlstrom, G. (2019) The occurrence of comorbidities with affective and anxiety disorders among older people with intellectual disability compared to the general population. *BMC Psychiatry*, 19(1), p. 166. Doi:10.1186/s12888-019-2151-2.

Mwebe, H. (2021) *Psychopharmacology: A mental health professional's guide to commonly used medications.* St Albans: Critical Publishing.

Nagraj, D. and Omar, H.A. (2017) Disability and suicide: A review. *International Journal of Child Health and Human Development*, 10(4), pp. 345–354.

National Institute for Health and Care Excellence (2015) *Psychosis and schizophrenia in adults: Quality standard QS80.* Available at: www.nice.org.uk/guidance/qs80/chapter/quality-statement-4-treatment-with-clozapine (Accessed 22 July 2022).

National Institute for Health and Care Excellence (2016) *Mental health problems in people with learning disabilities: Prevention, assessment and management. NICE guideline NG54.* Available at: www.nice.org.uk/guidance/ng54 (Accessed 28 July 2022).

National Institute for Health and Care Excellence (2019) *Shared decision making.* Available at: www.nice.org.uk/about/what-we-do/our-programmes/nice-guidance/nice-guidelines/shared-decision-making (Accessed 31 May 2022).

National Institute for Health and Care Excellence (2022) *Self harm: Assessment, management and preventing recurrence.* Available at: www.nice.org.uk/guidance/inde-velopment/gid-ng10148 (Accessed 7 June 2022).

NHS Digital (2021) *Health and care of people with learning disabilities experimental statistics 2016–17 to 2020–21.* Available at: https://digital.nhs.uk/data-and-information/publications/statistical/health-and-care-of-people-with-learning-disabilities (Accessed 31 May 2022).

NHS England (2016) *The five year forward view for mental health.* London: Mental Health Taskforce.

Nursing and Midwifery Board of Ireland (2016) *Nurse registration programmes standards and requirements* (4th edition). Dublin: Nursing and Midwifery Board of Ireland.

Nursing and Midwifery Council (2018) *Future nurse: Standards of proficiency for registered nurses.* London: NMC.

Office for National Statistics (2019) *Disability and crime, UK: 2019.* Available at: www.ons.gov.uk/peoplepopulationandcommunity/healthandsocialcare/disability/bulletins/disabilityandcrimeuk/2019 (Accessed 31 May 2022).

Perera, B., *et al.* (2019) Mental and physical health conditions in people with intellectual disabilities: Comparing local and national data. *British Journal of Learning Disabilities*, 48(1), pp. 19–27.

Perkins, C. (2020) *No health without mental health: Why this matters more than ever.* Available at: https://ukhsa.blog.gov.uk/2020/05/21/no-health-without-mental-health-why-this-matters-now-more-than-ever/ (Accessed 28 July 2022).

Pickard, M. and Rye, E. (2018) Assessment. In Hemmings, C. (Ed.), *Mental health in intellectual disabilities* (5th edition). East Sussex: Pavilion, pp. 23–31.

Poumeaud, F., *et al.* (2021) Deciphering the links between psychological stress and neurocognitive decline in patients with down syndrome. *Neurology of Stress*, 14, p. 100305. Doi:10.1016/j.ynstr.2021.100305.

Public Health England (2016) *Prescribing of psychotropic drugs to people with learning disabilities and/or autism by general practitioners in England.* London: Public Health England.

Raghavan, R., *et al.* (2004) Assessing the needs of people with learning disabilities and mental illness: Development of the learning disability version of the cardinal needs schedule. *Journal of Intellectual Disability Research*, 48, pp. 25–37.

Rees, R. and Langdon, P. (2016) The relationship between problem solving ability and self-harm amongst people with mild intellectual disabilities. *Journal of Applied Research in Intellectual Disabilities*, 29(4), pp. 387–393.

Reid, K.A., Smiley, E. and Cooper, S.A. (2011) Prevalence and associations of anxiety disorders in adults with intellectual disabilities. *Journal of Intellectual Disability Research*, 55(2), pp. 172–181.

Robertson, J., *et al.* (2020) Self-reported smoking, alcohol and drug use among adolescents and young adults with and without mild to moderate intellectual disability. *Journal of Intellectual & Developmental Disability*, 45(1), pp. 35–45.

Royal College of Psychiatrists (2016) *Psychotropic drug prescribing for people with intellectual disability, mental health problems and/or behaviours that challenge: Practice guidelines*. Available at: www.rcpsych.ac.uk/docs/default-source/members/faculties/intellectual-disability/id-fr-id-095701b41885e84150b11ccc989330 357c.pdf?sfvrsn=55b66f2c_4 (Accessed 24 July 2022).

Royal College of Psychiatrists (2020) *Bipolar disorder*. Available at: www.rcpsych.ac.uk/mental-health/problems-disorders/bipolar-disorder (Accessed 6 June 2022).

Royal College of Psychiatrists (2021) *Obsessive compulsive disorder (OCD)*. Available at: https://www.rcpsych.ac.uk/mental-health/problems-disorders/obsessive-compulsive-disorder (Accessed 24 November 2022).

Sharma, M. and Lakhan, R. (2017) Substance abuse among people with intellectual disabilities: Areas of future research (editorial). *Journal of Alcohol and Drug Education*, 61(2), pp. 3–6.

Sheehan, R., *et al.* (2015) Mental illness, challenging behaviour, and psychotropic drug prescribing in people with intellectual disability: UK population based cohort study. *British Medical Journal*, 351, p. h4326. Doi:10.1136/bmj.h4326.

Sheehan, R. and Hassiotis, A. (2017). Reduction or discontinuation of antipsychotics for challenging behaviour in adults with intellectual disability: a systematic review. *The Lancet - Psychiatry*, 4(3), pp.238–256. https://doi.org/10.1016/S2215-0366(16)30191-2

Sheerin, F., *et al.* (2019) Exploring mental health issues in people with an intellectual disability. *Learning Disability Practice*, 22(6), pp. 36–44.

Shepherd, C. and Beail, N. (2017) A systematic review of the effectiveness of psychoanalysis, psychoanalytic and psychodynamic psychotherapy with adults with intellectual disabilities: Progress and challenges. *Psychoanalytic Psychotherapy*, 31(1), pp. 94–117.

Standen, P.J., Clifford, A. and Jeenkeri, K. (2017) People with intellectual disabilities accessing mainstream mental health services: Some facts, features and professional considerations. *Journal of Mental Health Training, Education and Practice*, 12(4), pp. 215–223.

Stochl, J., *et al.* (2019) Association between developmental milestones and age of schizophrenia onset: Results from the Northern Finland Birth Cohort 1966. *Schizophrenia Research*, 208, pp. 228–234.

Taylor, D., Paton, C. and Kapur, S. (2015) *Prescribing guidelines in psychiatry* (12th edition). Chichester: Wiley-Blackwell.

Tromans, S., *et al.* (2022) Priority concerns for people with intellectual and developmental disabilities during the Covid-19 pandemic. *British Journal of Psychiatry*, 6(6), pp. 1–6.

van den Bogaard, K.H.M., *et al.* (2018) Self-injurious behaviour in people with intellectual disabilities and co-occurring psychopathology using the self-harm scale: A pilot study. *Journal of Developmental and Physical Disabilities*, 30(5), pp. 707–722.

Vereenooghe, L., *et al.* (2018) Interventions for mental health problems in children and adults with severe intellectual disabilities: A systematic review. *BMJ Open*, 8, p. e021911. Doi:10.1136/bmjopen-2018-021911.

Volkert, J., Gablonski, T.-C. and Rabung, S. (2018) Prevalence of personality disorders in the general adult population in Western countries: Systematic review and meta-analysis. *The British Journal of Psychiatry*, 213(6), pp. 709–715.

Walker, J.C., *et al.* (2011) Depression in down syndrome: A review of the literature. *Research in Developmental Disabilities*, 32(5), pp. 1432–1440.

Walton, C. and Kerr, M. (2015) Down syndrome: Systematic review of the prevalence and nature of presentation of unipolar depression. *Advances in Mental Health and Intellectual Disabilities*, 9(4), pp. 151–162.

Wark, S., *et al.* (2018) Suicide amongst people with intellectual disability: An Australian online study of disability support staff experiences and perceptions. *Journal of Intellectual Disability Research*, 62(1), pp. 1–9.

Webb, Z. (2014) *Intellectual disabilities and personality disorder: An integrated approach* Hove: Pavilion Publishing.

Williams, E.M. and Rose, J. (2020) Nonpharmacological treatment for individuals with intellectual disability and "personality disorder". *Journal of Applied Research in Intellectual Disabilities*, 33(4), pp. 767–778.

Wojciechowski, T.W. (2019) Post-traumatic stress disorder and having antisocial peers in adolescence are risk factors for the development of antisocial personality disorder. *Psychiatry Research*, 274, pp. 263–268.

World Health Organization (2022) *Schizophrenia*. Geneva: WHO.

Further Reading

Hemmings, C. (2018) *Mental health and intellectual disabilities* (5th edition). Hove: Pavillion.

Royal College of Nursing (2010) *Mental health nursing of adults with learning disabilities*. London: RCN.

Useful Resources

British Institute of Learning Disabilities: www.bild.org.uk

Foundation for people with learning disabilities. 2015. Improving Access to Psychological Therapies: Positive Practice Guide: www.learningdis abilities.org.uk/learning-disabilities/publications/learning-disabilities-iapt-positive-practice-guide2

Mental Welfare Commission for Scotland. 2019. Person centred care plans. Good practice guide: www.mwcscot.org.uk/sites/default/files/201908/Per sonCentredCarePlans_GoodPracticeGuide_August2019_0.pdf

National Association for the Dually Diagnosed: https://thenadd.org/

NICE. 2016. Mental health problems in people with learning disabilities: prevention, assessment and management. Guideline 54: www.nice.org. uk/guidance/ng54

Royal College of Psychiatrists (2020) Menatl health services for adults with mild intellectual disabilities CR226: www.rcpsych.ac.uk/docs/default-source/improving-care/better-mh-policy/college-reports/college-report-cr226.pdf?sfvrsn=8220109f_2

University of Hertfordshire: Intellectual Disability and Health – Mental Health: www.intellectualdisability.info/mental-health

CHAPTER 6

Catherine Bright, Steven Walden, Sam Abdulla and
Ruth Ryan

Intellectual disability nursing for people with profound intellectual disabilities and complex needs

Introduction

People with profound intellectual disabilities and complex needs are recognised as requiring intensive and extensive support needs in nearly all aspects of living across the lifespan. Historically, social exclusion, and simultaneously poorer experiences of social and healthcare services have resulted in this group of people being marginalised and discriminated against when it came to accessing services in comparison to the general population (Mansell, 2010). The role of the intellectual disability nurse in supporting, and where necessary providing, direct care for this group of people is particularly relevant because of the high levels of dependence they may have on others throughout their lives.

Nursing, or directed nursing social care, should be regarded as a way of systematically assessing, planning and documenting interventions to meet the needs of this group of people and supports the fact that they have a right to appropriate care in all aspects of their lives. This chapter will examine the intellectual disability nurse's direct and indirect roles in supporting or caring for this group of people. As in previous chapters, this will be discussed in the context of the standards and requirements for competence set by the Nursing and Midwifery Council (NMC) for the United Kingdom (2018a), and Nursing and Midwifery Board of Ireland (NMBI) (2016) competences.

DOI: 10.4324/9781003296461-6

Box 6.1 This chapter will focus on the following issues:

- Understanding profound learning disabilities and complex needs
- How many people have profound learning disabilities and complex needs?
- Attitudes toward people with profound intellectual disabilities and complex needs
- The nature of learning disability nursing interventions for people with profound learning disabilities and complex needs
- Care planning for people with profound learning disabilities and complex needs using the activities of living framework.

Box 6.2 Competences

Nursing and Midwifery Council (2018a) Proficiencies

Platform 1: Being an accountable professional – 1.14, 1.15

Platform 2: Promoting health and preventing ill health – 2.3, 2.5, 2.6, 2.8

Platform 3: Assessing needs and planning care – 3.10, 3.16

Platform 4: Providing and evaluating care – 4.10, 4.12, 4.14, 4.15, 4.16, 4.17

Nursing and Midwifery Board of Ireland (2016) Competences

Domain 2: Nursing practice and clinical decision-making competences – 2.1, 2.2, 2.3, 2.4, 2.5

Domain 5: Management and team competences – 5.1, 5.2

Understanding profound learning disabilities and complex needs

Understanding and supporting people that live with profound intellectual disabilities to live ordinary and fulfilling lives requires both theoretical and practical knowledge. Combining theory and practice has the potential to ensure that evidenced-based care underpins families, circles of support and practitioners' ways of knowing the person and delivers support and care approaches that are safe and effective. To understand profound intellectual disabilities, it is important to recognise the variation in definitions of the terms, which ultimately influences people's approach to and interaction with this group of people.

Lacey and Ouvry's (1998) definition of profound and multiple intellectual disabilities comprise the following characteristics:

■ Profound intellectual impairment (which refers to people who score below 20 on an Intelligence Quotient [IQ] test)
■ Additional disabilities, which may include sensory disabilities, physical disabilities, epilepsy autism or mental illness

Bellamy *et al.* (2010) expand on this thinking in their study of 23 carers who found that no definition can fully articulate the complexities associated with profound intellectual and multiple disabilities but emphasises that a definition should encompass all needs of the person and not necessarily IQ alone. They suggest the following represents a theoretical viewpoint of people living with profound intellectual disability experience:

> *have extremely delayed intellectual and social functioning, have limited ability to engage verbally, but respond to cues within their environment (e.g., familiar voice, touch, gestures), require those who are familiar with them to interpret their communication intent, frequently have an associated medical condition which may include neurological problems, and physical and sensory impairments. They have the chance to engage and to achieve their optimum potential in a highly structured environment with constant support and in an individualised relationship with a carer.*

> (Bellamy *et al.*, 2010, p. 233)

Bellamy's work presents a view of an individual's intellectual, physical, sensory and emotional needs and indicates ways in which mechanisms of engagement and development through recognising the need for constant support and in an individualised relationship with a carer occurs. It is within this understanding that the term profound intellectual and multiple disability shows the reciprocal and interactive nature of living for this group of people. Mencap and PMLD Network (2022) provide a definition of profound intellectual disabilities which recognises the need for support in most aspects of life:

> *Children and adults with profound and multiple learning disabilities have more than one disability, the most significant of which is a profound learning disability. All people who have profound and multiple learning disabilities will have great difficulty communicating. Many people will have additional sensory or physical disabilities, complex health needs or mental health difficulties. The combination of these needs and/or the lack of the right support may also affect behaviour. Some other people, such as those with Autism and Down's syndrome may also have profound and multiple learning disabilities. All children and adults with profound and multiple learning disabilities will need high levels of support with most aspects of daily life.*

Appreciating variation in definitions is important in understanding that people with profound intellectual disabilities and complex needs are all individuals and should not be perceived as a list of ailments (Carnaby, 2001), but as people first, capable of experiencing the same range of human experience as their fellow citizens (Davies and Evans, 2001).

Historically, several labels have been used to refer to this group of people and these have included *'severe disabilities and complex needs', 'profound learning disabilities'*, and *'the most severely disabled'* (PMLD Network, 2002). This can and often does lead to confusion, not least for parents and carers, and often leads to difficulties with accessing appropriate services. The problem with the many terms used to refer to this group of people is that such terms are associated with the *'medical model'* (Ho, 2004), which is now seen by many to have become outdated. Paradoxically, however, this group of people often present themselves with complex health problems. Notwithstanding this and for the purposes of this chapter, the term *'profound intellectual disabilities and complex needs'* will be used throughout, and its use is grounded in the definitions already provided by Lacey and Ouvry (1998) and the PMLD Network (2013).

How many people have profound intellectual disabilities and complex needs?

As outlined in Chapter 1, in the United Kingdom it has been estimated that of the three to four persons per 1,000 population with intellectual and learning disabilities, approximately 30% will present with severe or profound intellectual disabilities. Within this group it is common to find multiple disabilities that include physical or sensory impairments or disability, as well as behavioural difficulties. Based on these estimates, one can assume that there are some 230,000 to 350,000 persons with severe learning disabilities in the United Kingdom. And of this number, Emerson (2009) has estimated that there are somewhere in the region of 16,000 adults with profound intellectual disabilities and complex needs in England. In the Republic of Ireland, the National Ability Supports System (NASS) a national database records information about Health Service Executive (HSE) disability-funded services that are received or required because of an intellectual disability, developmental delay, physical, sensory, neurological, learning, speech and/or language disabilities or autism. The most frequently reported primary disability was intellectual (22,746, 62%), followed by neurological (4,201, 12%). Amongst those whose primary disability was intellectual; their level of intellectual disability was borderline (396, 2%), mild (6,825, 30%), moderate (9,760, 43%), severe (3,222, 14%), profound (810, 4%), not verified (1,702, 7%) (Casey *et al.*, 2021).

Interestingly, it has also been predicted that there will be a significant rise in the number of people living with profound intellectual disabilities, with an estimation that it will increase by something of the order of 1.8% per year until 2026. This will result in an increase in the total number of adults with profound intellectual disabilities and complex needs and may be explained by more active support and treatments in childhood. To put this in context, given a geographical area that has a population of 250,000, we would see a rise from 78 adults from 2009, to 105 by 2026, which is a rise of over 30%. The PMLD Network concurs with this prediction suggesting that it may be accounted for because of ongoing developments in medical technology, better control of epilepsy, and an increase in the use of tube feeding (PMLD Network, 2001; Brown, 2016).

Whereas people with profound intellectual disabilities and complex needs clearly represent a small section of society, it is nonetheless a highly significant and vulnerable section. This group of people requires lifelong support to carry out the full range of activities of daily living, and, like other citizens, they are entitled to access the resources that enable them to meet their health and social care needs as and when required. It must be emphasised, as in Chapter 1, intellectual disability is a lifelong condition – therefore, when we talk about people with profound intellectual disabilities and complex needs, we are referring to both children and adults, as well as older people. As has been described in Chapter 3, intellectual disability nursing contributes to the health and well-being of people with intellectual disabilities across the entire age spectrum (U.K. Chief Nursing Officers, 2012).

Attitudes toward people with profound intellectual disabilities and complex needs

There remains a considerable lack of knowledge not only in the public, but also in health and social care professions working with people with profound intellectual disabilities and complex needs. Consider the following statements about their experiences from parents of people with intellectual disabilities:

'You shouldn't have to look after someone like that. He should be in an institution', 'If you will keep her at home what do you expect?' and, 'At the end of the day people thought my sons were worthless, utterly worthless, and we were too. I thought they were very special'.

(Mencap, 2001, p. 5)

And in relation to healthcare professionals, parents reported on disturbing attitudes being expressed:

I overheard the doctor say: that's not coming in my room. It will destroy the equipment – we had to stay with Anthony from 10am to 10pm because no one was feeding him.

(Mencap, 2004)

Victoria was rushed to hospital after a series of seizures. She needed to be put on a ventilator. The Doctor came up and spoke to us. He was suggesting that it wasn't worth trying to save her.

(Mencap, 2004)

To be told that your child is a cabbage and that you will lose all your friends if you don't place them in institutional care is inhuman. To be told without empathy for your situation reinforces the damage – and it still happens. Fortunately, we have learned to ignore experts.

(Mansell, 2010)

Mansell (2010) has supported such concerns over attitudes, and questions why this persists. He noted:

Why is it that people with profound intellectual and multiple disabilities have such difficulty in getting help? The evidence from families themselves is that prejudice, discrimination and low expectations underlie their plight.

(Mansell, 2010, p. 5)

To evidence Mansell's view, consider the publication from Mencap England, *Death by Indifference* (Mencap, 2007). In this harrowing report, Mencap reported that people with intellectual disabilities had died unnecessarily due to institutional discrimination while in NHS (National Health Service) care. This prompted the then Secretary of State for Health, Patricia Hewitt, to establish an independent inquiry, chaired by Sir Jonathan Michael, into access to healthcare for people with intellectual disabilities. The inquiry took evidence from the public, people with intellectual disabilities, carers, and professionals in the fields of health and social care. It was clear from the inquiry that this group of people was being failed by healthcare services (Michael, 2008). The inquiry reported that people with intellectual disabilities were facing suffering and sometimes even death because current legislation designed to give them access to healthcare was not being adhered to. The report also concluded that there was not a case for new legislation as it was already in place – so the challenge was then, as it remains now, to make effective use of existing legislation. The report identified examples of good practice but noted that these were '*patchy*', and often the result of committed individuals, and made 10 recommendations, which were:

1. *That all undergraduate and postgraduate clinical training must ensure that curricula include training in learning disabilities.*
2. *That all health care organisations collect data to allow people with learning disabilities to be identified by the health service so their pathways of care can be tracked.*
3. *That family and other carers should be involved in the provision of treatment and care, unless good reason is given, and that Trust Boards should ensure reasonable adjustments are made to enable them to do this effectively.*

4. *That Primary Care Trusts should identify and assess the needs of people with learning disabilities and their carers as part of their Joint Strategic Needs Assessment.*
5. *That awareness training is needed in the health service of the risk of premature avoidable death, and the Department of Health should establish a learning disabilities Public Health Observatory.*
6. *That the government directs the Department of Health to immediately amend Core Standards for Better Health, to include an explicit reference to the requirement to make 'reasonable adjustments'.*
7. *That inspectors and regulators of the health service develop and extend their monitoring of the standard of general health services provided for people with learning disabilities.*
8. *That the Department of Health should direct Primary Care Trusts (PCTs) to commission enhanced primary care services, which include regular health checks provided by general practitioners (GP) practices, and improve data, communication, and cross-boundary partnership working. This should include liaison staff that work with primary care services to improve the overall quality of health care for people with learning disabilities across the spectrum of care.*
9. *That all Trust Boards should ensure that the views and interests of people with learning disabilities and their carers are included.*
10. *That all Trust Boards should demonstrate in routine public reports that they have effective systems in place to deliver effective, 'reasonably adjusted' health services, including advocacy services, for those people who happen to have a learning disability.*

(see Box 6.1 as to progress since the Michael Report; Michael, 2008, pp. 54–56)

And yet even more recently, in the Confidential Inquiry into the premature deaths of people with learning disabilities (CIPOLD), Heslop *et al.* (2013) have identified that the mean age of death of people with intellectual disabilities (65 years for men; 63 years for women) is significantly less than that for the UK population (78 years for men and 83 for women). Subsequently men with intellectual disabilities are dying, on average, 13 years sooner than men in the general population and women with intellectual disabilities are dying, on average, 20 years younger than women in the general population. The CIPOLD team (Heslop *et al.*, 2013) found the most frequent reasons for premature deaths were delays or problems with diagnosis or treatment and difficulties with identifying needs and providing appropriate care in response to changing needs. In addition, the CIPOLD report highlighted a lack of reasonable adjustments made to facilitate healthcare for people with intellectual disabilities, when accessing clinics for appointments and investigations. These were found to be a contributory factor in several of the deaths investigated (Heslop *et al.*, 2013). Also known is that this vulnerability is of relevance and concern for those with profound learning and intellectual disabilities and complex needs using General Hospitals (Garrard *et al.*, 2010).

Box 6.3 Progress since the Michael Report

What has changed since the Michael Report? On the January 3, 2013, *The Guardian* newspaper in the United Kingdom reported on the avoidable deaths of 74 more people with learning disabilities who had died while in the care of the NHS (Bawden and Campbell, 2012); it also highlighted a further 17 serious incidents. Families were continuing to allege that hospital blunders, poorly trained staff, and indifference were to blame. This newspaper, in collaboration with Mencap, had been continuing to campaign to stop people with learning disabilities from receiving unequal healthcare. Of the cases highlighted in the report, 59 took place within a five-year period. In *The Times* newspaper, Barrow (2012) reported on an interview with Sir Jonathan Michael, who said that four years after his report, he still doubted '*that all lives were seen to be equally valuable*' across the health service. This article reports how Sir Jonathan recalled being shocked by what he found in 2008, saying that there are still concerns about attitudes toward the lives of patients with severe mental illness. Hospitals and GPs were failing to make essential adjustments to ensure that vulnerable patients received the highest standard of care. Sir Jonathan said:

> The number of patients with learning disabilities is relatively small in number but we felt then, as I do now, that if the NHS can't look after the most vulnerable, there is something fundamentally wrong.

(Barrow, 2012)

It is not unusual to hear people say that they have never seen or met a person with profound intellectual disabilities and complex needs (PMLD Network, 2002). One explanation for this in the past might have been that many of these people were historically '*shut away*' from the communities in which they had previously lived in institutional settings. Even today, many children with profound intellectual disabilities and complex needs still attend special schools resulting in fewer opportunities to interact with the wider community (Foreman *et al.*, 2004). In the past, many people with profound intellectual disabilities and complex needs lived as '*inpatients*' in long-stay hospitals for the '*mentally handicapped*', as they were known then, where they were cared for by nursing and medical staff. Almost all these hospitals have now closed, and what were the '*patients*' now live in community-based settings where they are rightly regarded as '*clients*' or '*service users*' or '*citizens*'. Because of these hospital closures many children and adults now live in their family home or in a small residential home or supported living, where they are often supported by relatives or unqualified social care staff. Therefore, to advise or assist them in recognising the many healthcare needs of such individuals, intellectual disability nurses must be able to work in collaboration with a wide variety of people, and this includes family members, paid carers, and professionals from other disciplines and in several environmental settings.

Since the almost universal closure of the old long-stay hospitals, and the impact of the white paper *Valuing People* (DH, 2001), and *Valuing People Now*

(DH, 2009), significant progress has been made toward the social inclusion of people with profound learning and intellectual disabilities and complex needs, but there is still a long way to go (McNally, 2004; Gooding, 2004; Mansell, 2010). The PMLD Network (2002) has long since argued that this group of people still need to be made more visible in society.

Carnaby (2001) has suggested that this group of people have been perceived as *'difficult to engage'*, *'passive'*, and an *'expensive'* demand on resources. Such negative perceptions can be damaging and must be challenged if attitudes are to improve. Klotz (2004) has argued that people with profound intellectual disabilities and complex needs can, and do, live socially meaningful lives, and furthermore within the United Kingdom, the Human Rights Act 1998 has enshrined in law that everyone has a fundamental right to life. Additionally, nurses are bound by professional codes of conduct, which has explicitly stated that all patients and clients must be treated with respect and dignity (NMC, 2018b; NMBI, 2016). These values are also central to the policies set out by the learning disabilities white paper *Valuing People* (DH, 2001, 2009), and in addition a national drive in the United Kingdom to ensure that healthcare service, particularly that of nursing care, is delivered to all with compassion and care respecting the rights and dignity of all (DH, 2012).

Respect and dignity are relatively abstract concepts that can be interpreted in many ways. For the purposes of this chapter, respect is defined as

A feeling of deep admiration for someone elicited by their qualities or achievements or due regard for the feelings or rights of other.

(Oxford English Dictionary, 2002)

Dignity has been defined as

The state or quality of being worthy of honour or respect.

(Oxford English Dictionary, 2002)

In the field of intellectual disability practice some interpretations of respect have led to ideological fanaticism that to treat people with profound intellectual disabilities and complex needs with respect, they must be treated in a way that is appropriate to their chronological age, so called *'age appropriateness'*. However, dictionary definitions of the terms *'respect'* and *'dignity'* lend support to Carnaby's view that the most respectful and dignified approach to interaction with this group of people is to be cognizant of an individual's specific abilities and disabilities (Carnaby, 2001). Notwithstanding this view treating an adult as an *'eternal child'* could be equally disrespectful, and could also hinder an individual's development (Wolverson, 2003). Therefore, all approaches to support or care must balance the necessity for developmental appropriateness on the one hand, with that of securing socially acceptable age-appropriate interactions on the other. In nursing, a contemporary vision based around six values of care compassion, courage, communication, competence, and commitment has been articulated. This vision seeks to embed these values, known as the so-called Six

Cs, in all nursing, midwifery, and care-giving settings throughout the NHS and social care to improve care for patients. The action to achieve this includes:

- Recruiting, appraising, and training staff according to values as well as technical skill
- Regularly reviewing organisational culture and evidence for staffing levels
- Doing more to assess patients' experience
- Helping staff make every contact count for improving health and well-being

(DH, 2012)

Respect for dignity, a person-centred approach and the six values approach to nursing and social care are all likely to lead to improved outcomes in this population of people.

The nature of intellectual disability nursing interventions for people with profound intellectual disabilities and complex needs

Nurses have a duty of care to patients, which means that clients are entitled to receive safe and competent care that should be informed by evidence-based practice (NMC, 2018b; NMBI, 2021). In the context of this chapter, evidence-based practice refers to a way of managing nursing interventions by making clinical decisions that use the best available research evidence to inform clinical expertise and judgment, utilising a person-centred understanding of patient preferences (Stannard, 2019). Until comparatively recently, there has been little evidence established concerning evidence-based practice for people with profound intellectual disabilities and complex needs, and therefore good practice has sometimes been based on research that has been undertaken with people with mild and moderate intellectual disabilities (Carnaby, 2001; Klotz, 2004). This might cause us to question both the validity and reliability of *'evidence'* gathered from one population and then applied to another (Gates and Wray, 2000; Gates and Atherton, 2001). Referring to and treating people with intellectual disabilities as one homogenous group is still commonplace in some settings and remains problematic (Kersten *et al.*, 2022). Recent studies using a sensory-dialogical approach to facilitate inclusive participatory research with people with profound and multiple intellectual disabilities as reviewed by Gjermestad, Skarsaune and Bartlett (2022) suggests a growing challenge to this notion. The body of evidence from which to construct an evidence-based practice for people with profound and multiple intellectual disabilities, drawing upon innovations in person-centred communication, is growing (Flick, 2017; Maes *et al.*, 2021; Nind and Strnadová, 2020).

In England *Valuing People* (DH, 2001) made little reference to the needs of people with profound intellectual disabilities and complex needs (Aylott, 2001; Cooper and Ward, 2011). The policies set out by *Valuing People* were based on the principles of rights, independence, choice, and inclusion. Putting these values into practice for people with profound intellectual disabilities and complex needs poses specific challenges. For example, some people are extremely limited in their abilities to make and communicate choices, and the ways in which these people require support will therefore be different from their peers. The PMLD Network (2001) have argued that the policies set out in *Valuing People* were of little use for this group, and in conjunction with Mencap published their own report that made recommendations that the government needed to make to address the needs of this group a priority (Mencap, 2001). This was partially addressed in *Valuing People Now* (DH, 2009).

The seminal work of Professor Jim Mansell (2010) challenged us to raise expectations for this group of people. He advocated extending good services that could be found in individualised and person-centred care, treating families as experts, focusing on the quality of relationships between staff and the disabled person, and sustaining cost-effective packages of care; this could be done by *'raising our sights'* (Mansell, 2010). He identified a number of obstacles that acted as barriers to improvement that include housing, community facilities, health, wheelchairs, communication aids and assistive technology, further education, employment and day-time activity, short breaks, training clinical procedure, and funding. With some 33 recommendations, his report provided a blueprint for improving services for people with profound intellectual disabilities and complex needs. In response to this challenge, *Supporting people with profound and multiple learning disabilities: Core and essential Services and Standards* was formulated

in order to identify a means of ensuring a stronger voice for people, at a national level, and to aim to ensure that people received good quality service and support regardless of where they lived and who was providing their support.

(Doukas *et al.*, 2017)

This comprehensive set of standards seeks to address previous charges of homogenising people with profound intellectual disabilities with complex needs with people with intellectual disabilities who had differing needs. The standards identify that people with profound intellectual disabilities and complex needs are a diverse group of people who have a complicated range of difficulties that require appropriate and responsive environments delivered for *each person* to meet their individual needs. When developing care plans for people whose contribution to its construction is potentially limited, it is critically important to include family members, people who know and care for the person, and all relevant professionals. Mansell (2010) and more recently Doukas *et al.* (2017) and Jacobs *et al.* (2021) have all stressed the importance of joint working between professionals to support comprehensive and seamless care. The appointment of a key worker has long been considered essential for joint working to be effective by promoting continuity and meaningful therapeutic relationships (Mansell, 2010; Doukas *et al.*, 2017; Jacobs *et al.*, 2021).

BOX 6.4
CASE HISTORY 6.1

Clara has profound intellectual disabilities and complex health needs. She is 16 years old and lives in her family home with her parents and two younger brothers. Clara has cerebral palsy and is unable to walk, sit up unaided, or control the movements of her limbs and hands. Clara spends her days in a wheelchair, which she relies on others to maneuver. She also relies on others to wash, dress, and support her nutritional intake. Clara relies on non-verbal communication, and she primarily does this through eye contact, facial expressions, and vocalisations. Clara has a BMI of 16 which is significantly underweight. Clara experiences several health problems, including:

■ Epilepsy – poorly controlled generalised tonic-clonic seizures

■ Being underweight

■ Constipation

■ Frequent chest infections (hypostatic pneumonia) due to impaired chest motility

■ Repeatedly developing pressure ulcers on her ankles, elbows, and sacral area

■ Visual impairment

■ Frequently experiences menorrhagia

Clara attends a local school for young people with special educational needs. She has respite care for two nights per month at a unit for young people with profound intellectual disabilities and complex health needs.

Learning activity 1

Take some time to think about some of the people who might be involved directly or indirectly in Clara's care. Construct a realistic list, and then compare your list with items identified in Box 6.4.

Box 6.5 People who might be involved in Clara's care

1. Family, immediate and extended
2. Friends
3. Consultants– intellectual disability, respiratory or neurology
4. GP
5. Epilepsy – specialist nurse
6. Community nurse – intellectual disability
7. Speech and language therapist
8. Physiotherapist
9. Occupational therapist
10. Continence nurse
11. Dietician
12. Advocate

13. School teacher
14. School nurse
15. Transition worker
16. Respite care staff

In case history 6.2, Clara is presented as someone with profound intellectual disabilities and complex needs. Clara is an adolescent who presents herself with potential threats and challenges to her health, which include epilepsy, nutritional problems, chest infections, constipation, pressure ulcers, and visual impairments.

Are there any people, professionals, or other informal carers listed in Box 6.4 that you have not thought of? Or have you listed people that we have not identified? Either way, it might be worth spending some time thinking about this list, and accounting for any differences with a colleague.

Care planning for people with profound intellectual disabilities and complex needs

There is increasing recognition of the importance of providing quality healthcare to meet the biopsychosocial needs of all people including those with intellectual disabilities. Formulating structured care plans, based on the nursing process of assessment, planning, implementation and evaluation has proven to provide individualised, coherent and safe care. As with all care plans, these must be constructed in a person-centred way, and this is especially important for those with profound and multiple intellectual disabilities and complex needs. The care plan should focus on the wants and needs of the individual and ensuring that they are included and empowered to make decisions regarding their care plan at every stage of the process.

The need for structured nursing care plans and communication of care is essential for this group of people because they are usually dependent on a range of people offering care and support, and this can extend to nearly all aspects of that person's life. They may need assistance with eating and drinking (or with enteral nutrition); personal care and washing (including meeting continence needs); transfer and repositioning; and taking medication. Any or all of these may require the use of specialist equipment ranging from the need to use enteral syringes to administer medication to a person with a percutaneous endoscopic gastroscopy, to the use of a tracking hoist to transfer a person from a bed to a wheelchair, to give just two examples of many.

Person-centred care planning can be used effectively with people who rely on (often idiosyncratic) non-verbal communication if a *circle of support* is in place to support the planning process (Esteban *et al.*, 2021; Martin *et al.*, 2022). A circle of support in this context is a group of people who know and care about the person and have a comprehensive understanding of their needs and preferences that can be used to plan for and advocate services that might improve the person's quality of life (Araten-Bergman and Bigby, 2020). Involving the person themselves in all aspects of the care plan is imperative, however, the empirical evidence presented in an integrative review (Doody and Bailey, 2019) has demonstrated that the experiences of adults with intellectual disabilities involvement in care planning within health services are absent within the literature. It is important to note that nursing care plans are person-centred, and outline individual goals as well as evaluation of these goals.

Care plans must be written and co-produced in such a way that all people providing direct care can understand and follow them (Clegg, 2020). For people with profound intellectual disabilities and complex needs, their support workers may often be the people they rely on most, and along with their families, may know them the best. This makes them invaluable partners in the co-production of effective person-centred care planning (Jacobs *et al.*, 2021). It is also important that care plans are constructed in such a way that they can be readily understood by care staff from a variety of backgrounds, who bring various prior experiences and knowledge with them. Consistency of care is important in terms of effective outcomes, but so too is fostering a sense of security and predictability for the person with profound intellectual disabilities and complex needs. Ideally, day or education services, residential care, and family carers should all be consistently following the same care plans and hospital passports or health profiles across all care settings (Northway *et al.*, 2017). To maintain confidentiality, care plans must contain information and be shared on a professional basis with those who need to know, to ensure that patients are best supported by the wider health and social care team. As the NMC (2018b) and The NMBI (2021) have said, nurses must:

- *act in partnership with those receiving care, helping them to access relevant health and social care, information and support when they need it [and] act as an advocate for the vulnerable, challenging poor practice and discriminatory attitudes and behaviour relating to their care.*

(NMC, 2018b)

- *communicate and work with colleagues to provide safe, quality healthcare to patients. You must consult with the patient and refer them to the appropriate healthcare professional for further treatment if this is required. This should be done in a timely manner to ensure continuity of care.*

(NMBI, 2021)

People with profound intellectual disabilities present a wide range of complex health needs. Focusing on one area of need can potentially result in the neglect of other areas of care and contributes to an increased risk of diagnostic overshadowing – for instance, if an idiosyncratic non-verbal expression of pain or discomfort is attributed to the person's disability or behaviour rather than to an underlying health issue that needs to be addressed and is misinterpreted, then that health need, potentially urgent in nature, goes unmet (Javaid, Nakata and Michael, 2019).

Similarly, Male (1996) found that at a special school for people with profound intellectual disabilities and complex needs, high levels of personal and health-care support reduced opportunities for social and educational activities, a view still echoed by Sanderson, Bumble and Kuntz (2020) some twenty-four years later; care plans must therefore ensure that the full range of needs is addressed.

There is also a risk of needs being neglected when all aspects of life take place in one location (Mansell, 2010; Simmons, 2021). Most people experience work, leisure, and relaxation activities in very different places. For people with profound intellectual disabilities and complex needs, it is possible that many of these activities could all take place within or very near the person's familial or specialist residential home. This is likely to lead to a risk of social exclusion. Access to a number and variety of environments would provide wider social, leisure, and educational opportunities, and therefore a more inclusive lifestyle but this must be promoted and advocated for by family and/or staff members who know the person well and are committed to providing this access (Mansell, 2010; Palmer and Walmsley, 2020).

Arguably, neither a medical nor social model of care can adequately meet the very complex care needs of this group. Current ideas about nursing emphasise the importance of holistic care; Cocquyt (2018) notes that the *'whole'* is truly greater than the sum of its parts in terms of multidisciplinary team working for this group, yet wider health and social care commitments to the complex needs of people with profound intellectual disabilities have not yet resulted in the drive for change in areas such as behaviours that challenge and mental health. The challenge for nurses who are planning care for people with profound intel-lectual disabilities and complex needs is to balance complex physical health, mental health and spiritual needs. It is generally accepted that all these domains intersect to affect quality of life (Cocquyt, 2018; Flynn *et al.*, 2017; Calveley, 2017) but psychological and spiritual needs tend to be lower in the order of perceived priorities (Forster, 2020).

Nursing models have been devised to help organise both the planning and provision of care. One way of ensuring the provision of holistic learning disability nursing care is to adopt a nursing model. Using a nursing model has been proven to improve consistency of care, reduce conflict, and guide decision-making, goal setting and even recruitment. It can help patients and other professionals understand the role of the nurse, enable teams to provide continuity of care and ensure all service users receive the same high standard of person-centred and evidence-based nursing care (Moulster *et al.*, 2019). The remainder of this chapter discusses care planning using the Moulster and Griffiths model of Learning Disability nursing, which is applied to the case his-tory of Clara (See Case History 6.1). This model was chosen because it is well known and widely used within intellectual disability nursing. Nurses might find other models equally useful and find that with experience they rely less on a model for care planning and more on their own knowledge, skills, and understanding.

The model has practical utility because it focuses on understanding the needs of people in terms of the activities they perform. The model embraces the idea that independence and dependence operate along a continuum relating to each activity of living separately (Moulster *et al.*, 2019). This is consistent with the generally accepted idea that the level of skills of people with intellectual disabilities can and do vary across different domains (Schalock, Luckasson and Tassé, 2021).

The model can be put into practice in a systematic way by mapping the four stages of the nursing process – assessment, planning, implementation, and evaluation – against four key principles of intellectual disabilities nursing: person-centredness, evidence-based approach, a focus on outcomes, and reflective practice that allows for the health inequalities that people with profound and multiple intellectual disabilities often face (Moulster *et al.*, 2019). This is outlined in the following table from Moulster *et al.* (2019).

The first stage, assessment, needs to be person-centred and mapped against a health equality framework baseline; it involves determining an individual's ability to carry out or participate in activities of living along with his or her healthcare needs and challenges. In the care planning stage problems are identified and documented, along with the goals that aim to address these problems. In relation to people with profound intellectual disabilities and complex needs, improvements are likely to be small and goals identified should reflect this. Care plans can include specific and direct nursing interventions or indirect actions and supports recommended by the nurse, but the emphasis must always be on the person and the nurse, carer, or supporter working together toward the goals and to overcome identified health inequalities. Both the nursing process and Moulster and Griffiths' model advocate that care plans should be implemented within normal daily routines as much as possible (Moulster, Ames and Griffiths, 2012). Consider Table 6.2, think about how Clara would need support, and who she might need to support from to participate in basic, instrumental and advanced activities of daily living such as those shown.

STAGES		Additional elements offered by the model
Nursing process	**Moulster and Griffiths model**	
1. Assessment	1. Person-centred screen 2. Nursing assessment 3. Health Equality Framework baseline	o Reflection
2. Planning	4. Nursing care plan	o Evidence base o Reflection
3. Implementation	5. Nursing implementation of care plan	o Reflection
4. Evaluation	6. Health Equality Framework 7. Care plan evaluation	o Reflection o Evidence for practice

Table 6.1 The nursing process (Adapted from Moulster *et al.*, 2019)

Activities of Daily Living		
Basic	**Instrumental**	**Advanced**
Basic psychological and self-maintenance needs like eating, toileting and getting dressed.	Necessary to maintain independent and community life living like managing finances, shopping and using public transport.	Voluntary and complex, but not essential for independence, like technology, going on holidays and practising hobbies.

Table 6.2 Activities of daily living (Adapted from Muñoz-Neira et al., 2012)

Box 6.6 Some of the people who might be involved in the direct implementation of Clara's care plan

1. Family
2. School teacher
3. Respite care staff
4. Physiotherapist (some aspects)
5. Neurologist/consultant/psychiatrist/gastroenterologist/ paediatrician
6. Speech and language therapist
7. Certain aspects of the care plan such as communication should be used by all those who encounter Clara
8. Community nurse – intellectual disabilities – indirectly

The final stage of the nursing process, evaluation, is an ongoing process in which the individual's ability to carry out the activities of daily living and health challenges should be re-examined to see if the goals have been met. When applying the Moulster and Griffiths model, evaluation of care planning should be reflective and should revisit and reevaluate the evidence-based practice that has been implemented. Due to the severity and enduring nature of profound learning and intellectual disabilities and complex needs, an appropriate goal, for example, might be to maintain a condition or prevent its deterioration. Care plans should be adjusted according to the outcome of evaluation, and this can be performed by using the nursing process in a problem-solving oriented way.

To use the Moulster and Griffiths model effectively, nurses must understand biopsychosocial factors that influence the activities of living. See Figure 6.1 – think about how these apply to Clara by referring to her case history (Engel, 1981; Haslam et al., 2021).

Table 6.2 and Figure 6.1 provide some examples of how the model and the factors that influence the activities of living might be used to develop a care plan for Clara.

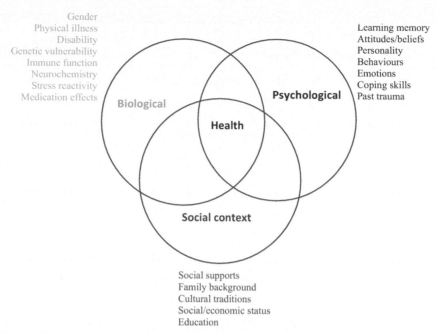

Gender
Physical illness
Disability
Genetic vulnerability
Immune function
Neurochemistry
Stress reactivity
Medication effects

Learning memory
Attitudes/beliefs
Personality
Behaviours
Emotions
Coping skills
Past trauma

Biological

Psychological

Health

Social context

Social supports
Family background
Cultural traditions
Social/economic status
Education

Figure 6.1

Biopsychosocial approach to understanding health.

Having considered how these factors may influence the activities of daily living, the following sections discuss each of these activities of living in turn. The case illustration of Clara is used throughout to consider how care planning might be carried out. Some of the more general issues that may arise when applying this model to the care and support more generally to people with profound learning and intellectual disabilities and complex needs are also considered.

Maintaining a safe environment

Many people with profound learning and intellectual disabilities and complex needs have epilepsy (Beghi, 2020). The prevalence of comorbid epilepsy is positively correlated with the severity of intellectual disability ranging from approximately 10% of people diagnosed with a mild intellectual disability to over 30% of people diagnosed with profound and multiple intellectual disabilities (Robertson *et al.*, 2015; Beghi, 2020).

Maintaining a safe environment in its widest sense is an important issue to consider for people with epilepsy. Reflect on the risks associated with bathing, falls, swimming, medicines compliance, and climbing ladders, and consider the need for a medic alert bracelet or perhaps using plastic glasses. For people with profound intellectual disabilities, audio, visual or pressure sensor monitoring, and more recently wearable monitors for seizure activity may also need to be considered, particularly by night where the person may not have a carer within their immediate vicinity (Rukasha, Woolley and Collins, 2020). The use of such equipment must be considered with regards to balancing the person's best interests with their right to privacy (Devinsky, Friedman and Besag, 2018). The risks of sudden unexpected death in epilepsy (SUDEP) are higher in people with learning and intellectual disabilities (Sun *et al.*, 2020) and are increased further by seizures from sleep, male sex or poorly controlled epilepsy, in these circumstances monitoring may significantly outweigh the risks to privacy in any best interests decision.

Carers play a vital role in monitoring and managing epilepsy and ensuring that people with profound intellectual disabilities diagnosed with epilepsy receive appropriate care from specialist health services and that they maintain a safe environment is critical. Carers are the most likely people to witness seizures, and it is vital that they can record a thorough description of seizures, because this can help medical professionals to make an accurate diagnosis as well as help manage the environment around them to reduce possible harm. An epilepsy profile detailing the person's seizure typology, triggers, and recovery trajectory should be completed in conjunction with a person-centred care plan outlining required actions and any anti-epileptic medication the person is taking. A rescue medication care plan (e.g., for the administration of buccal midazolam) should be in place if needed, signed off by the appropriate consultant and epilepsy specialist nurse. All seizure activity should be thoroughly documented in any care setting (Tittensor *et al.*, 2021).

A thorough knowledge of the person's medication is also essential to monitor its use and be alert to possible side effects. One key side effect to consider beyond more common incidences of headache, nausea and dizziness is the negative impact that some antiepileptic medications have on bone health leading to osteopenia. Dietary calcium supplements may be needed to mitigate this. Rescue medications of course carry the risk of respiratory depression, and postictal recovery should be closely monitored when such medications have been administered (Akyüz *et al.*, 2021; Sawhney *et al.*, 2020).

Clara has been diagnosed with generalised, tonic-clonic seizures. This type of seizure is characterised by a stiffening of the muscles, followed by rhythmical relaxing and tightening of the muscles, which causes the body to jerk and shake. During a seizure Clara's breathing becomes more difficult, and her skin turns a blue grey colour. When the jerking stops, her breathing and colour go back to normal and she usually sleeps for a few hours. There are other types of epilepsy (see Box 6.4) and for each of these different types of epilepsy there can be different antiepileptic drugs prescribed. Witnessing a seizure can be frightening, however, along with training and comprehensive care plans, this should enable carers to know how to respond in the event of a seizure; all these aspects related to the care management of epilepsy are things which the intellectual disability nurse should do (see Box 6.5).

Additionally in relation to maintaining a safe environment, another thing the intellectual disability nurse must be mindful of is the possibility of abuse. Although Clara lives at home, the potential for abuse must always be an issue that intellectual disability nurses are sensitised to, and the potential for this to happen to people with intellectual disabilities from those caring for them is well known.

This has been reported consistently in the research literature and continues to be reported, (Halladay and Harrington, 2015; Fyson and Patterson, 2020;

Richards, 2020; Collins and Murphy, 2021), and it may be institutionalised within configurations of human service delivery systems (Flynn, 2012; Phillips, 2016; Humber, 2016). It is also known that there are several factors connected with abuse toward people with intellectual disabilities and these include age and degree of disability (Martinello, 2015; Marsland, Oakes and Bright, 2015; Araten-Bergman and Bigby, 2020). Key risk indicators for abuse at a societal level that still need to be addressed include the still pervasive culture of disablism, notions of powerlessness and the issue of self-interest and conflicts of interest in care provision (Marsland, Oakes and Bright, 2015; Barden *et al.*, 2022). What is arguably still less well understood is the extent to which people with intellectual disabilities are abused, and this is for a number of reasons for this that includes inconsistent and inadequate operationalisation of the term abuse, difficulty in ensuring such abuse is reported, and suggestions of unreliability of persons with intellectual disabilities as witnesses for any potential criminal proceeding against the perpetrator/s, which is often couched in a lack of reasonable adjustments not being made for communication needs (Morrison, Bradshaw and Murphy, 2021).

This further compounds difficulties in estimating prevalence. Northway *et al.* (2013) have advocated amongst other things for people with intellectual disabilities to have greater access to personal safety and abuse awareness courses. They articulated that when people with intellectual disabilities disclose abuse, then other people must listen to them, but in relation to people with profound intellectual disabilities and complex needs this may prove difficult but is not insurmountable if astute observation and person-centred communication are implemented (Brison, 2021; Talman *et al.*, 2019).

Box 6.7
Learning activity 2

Go back to the list of people who might be involved in Clara's care. From this list, identify who is likely to be involved in the **direct** implementation of her care plans.

Box 6.8 Types of epilepsy

Focal seizures: Altered state of consciousness

Focal Aware (Simple partial) seizures

Usually originates from one area of the brain, electrical activity tends not to spread, common sensations include déja vu; if the seizure does progress this may be referred to as an aura.

Focal Impaired Awareness (Complex partial) seizures

Usually originates from one area of the brain, person loses awareness of surroundings, may follow on from a simple partial seizure, may experience automatisms (lip smacking, chewing, fiddling with buttons or clothes); the person may wander around and may be confused for some time, and as the seizure subsides the person becomes more aware of their environment.

Primary generalised seizures (non-focal): Complete loss of consciousness

Absence seizures

The commonest type of primary generalised seizure, usually found in children (rare in adults); may stare blankly, sometimes blink, person unaware they are having a seizure, may experience repeated episodes in any one day, distinguished from complex partial because there is no aura or automatisms.

Myoclonic seizures

Most common type (juvenile myoclonic epilepsy) presents often in adolescence, commences with sudden, brief muscle jerking of the limbs which occur singly or in a cluster, often early in the morning.

Tonic-clonic seizures

Represents a convulsive seizure; the person will lose consciousness and collapse to the ground. They may cry out and their body stiffens followed by rhythmical jerking (convulsion); tongue or cheek may be bitten. The seizure normally terminates after a short while, followed by drowsiness.

Tonic seizures

Sudden stiffening of the muscles, the person falls to the ground and there is a loss of consciousness.

Atonic seizures

Sudden loss of muscle tone with instantaneous collapse/person falls to the ground. Drop attack (often causing facial injuries).

* Partial seizures may progress if electrical activity spreads across the brain, and therefore does remain focal, resulting in a generalised tonic-clonic seizure, so-called focal with secondary generalisation.

Box 6.9 Elements of Clara's epilepsy care plan

Name: Clara

What happens during this type of seizure?

How long does this seizure normally last?

What to do if your seizure lasts longer than (Use this section to give instructions to others on what they should do if your seizure lasts longer than usual):

Is there anything that makes your seizures more likely?

Is there anything that needs to be done in the person's day-to-day life to manage their epilepsy and their safety with regards to this type of seizure?

If a rescue medication care plan is needed, it may look something like this:

Emergency medicine (Please fill in this section if the person has been prescribed emergency medicine.)

How much emergency medicine should be given initially?

Prescribing doctor Tel:

Carer Tel: Other Tel:

Can a second dose be given? Yes/No

When should 999 be dialed for emergency help if the full prescribed dose of emergency medicine fails to control the seizure?

After minutes (please record as appropriate):

Other (please give details):

Who needs to be told:	The exact format of care planning will be subject to local as well as national guidance (www.epilepsy.org.uk)
Maximum dose of emergency medicine to be given in a 24-hour period:	

Communication

It has been estimated that 50% to 90% of people with intellectual disabilities have difficulties with communication, and some 20% of people with intellectual disabilities have no verbal communication at all (RCSLT, 2015).

People with profound intellectual disabilities and complex needs are often unable to use formal methods of communication and may subsequently rely on others to interpret their facial expressions, and their non-verbal behaviours. However, Antonsson *et al.* (2008) has found that carers often believed that they were able to interpret needs and understand cues facial expressions, vocalisations, eye contact, and posture, but that these were not always successfully interpreted and when communication was misinterpreted, this could cause distress (Antonsson *et al.*, 2008). Thurman, Jones and Tarleton (2005) place significant importance on the role of the communication partnership for individuals with higher communication needs, suggesting that for those who may have less capability to use formal communication methods, it is the role of the communication partner, often a care giver, to interpret the informal communication. Improving communication with people who have profound intellectual disabilities and complex needs is therefore an important component of the carer's role; particular attention should be given to this aspect of care within the care planning process, and the intellectual disability nurse must be mindful of directing carers.

Clara should be, if she has not already, referred to a speech and language therapist (SALT) to conduct a communication assessment, which is a core function and skill of the speech and language therapist. Through this assessment, which should include carer consultation, the strengths, barriers and facilitators to effective communication for a person with intellectual disabilities can be identified (Chadwick, Buell and Goldbart, 2019).

For individuals with profound intellectual disabilities a communication passport can be an effective tool to support more effective communication for use across health, social care, and education services (Education Scotland, 2021). A communication passport aims to help carers understand and interpret a person by gathering information in a structured and accessible way, this might include their health needs, emergency contact information, how they communicate and how someone should communicate with them, their likes and dislikes and any other pertinent information. If the communication passport is produced in a user-friendly, accessible format it is much more likely to be used. It can also provide the individual with more opportunities to communicate effectively with a larger number of people who they may meet. Communication passports can be paper documents or can be digitalised; whatever form that they take, the document should be owned by the person with intellectual disabilities (PAMIS, 2022).

Another communication strategy that is beneficial for some people who have profound intellectual disabilities is '*Intensive Interaction*' (Nind and Hewett, 2004). Intensive Interaction involves developing the repetitive, pre-linguistic behaviours that are used routinely by the individual into a shared '*language*', which is thought to enable others to gain access to the person's world (Caldwell, 1997). In this way, it is thought that meaningful communication sequences can be experienced that are mutually enjoyable and relaxing (Hewett, 2012; Hewett *et al.*, 2012).

To perceive and understand the world, people with profound intellectual disabilities and complex needs are thought to rely more heavily on multiple sources of sensory stimulation (Ayer, 1998). However, it is common for this group to experience sensory processing difficulties that might further disadvantage their ability to communicate and experience the world (Doukas *et al.*, 2017). It is vital for regular hearing and sight assessments to identify and respond to sensory needs and changes as early as possible especially for people with profound intellectual disabilities, where these are often unnoticed (Truesdale and Brown, 2017). Appointment details should be recorded and strategies put in place to ensure that the results of assessments are disseminated to everyone involved in the person's direct care.

The opportunity and ability to make choices is recognised as a core competency of self-determination and can be an indicator of better quality of life (Brown and Brown, 2009; Agran, Storey and Krupp, 2010), however, there is evidence to suggest that the greater the level of intellectual disabilities a person has, the less often they are given the opportunity to make choices (Agran, Storey and Krupp, 2010). Choices are made within environmental contexts and these conditions should reflect an individual's needs to enable a person to understand, make and communicate an informed decision (Stancliffe, 2020). It is thought that by documenting responses to a range of choices offered, over time patterns may emerge that suggest that consistent, valid choices are being made. Aylott (2001) has used the term '*choices inventory*' to refer to this strategy. Belifore and Toro-Zambrana (1994) have developed a protocol that aims to achieve this. They drew a distinction between choice and preference whereas choice is essentially a selection of one option from several options offered, preference refers to relatively predictable behaviour. Preferences can be identified in a systematic way by observing and recording how an individual responds to various environmental stimuli. This information can help carers to support people to make higher quality choices and exercise greater self-determination and achieve a higher quality of life (Cannella-Malone and Sabielny, 2020).

Within the correct environmental conditions, over time it would be possible to establish a range of preferences for Clara, and incorporate these into her care plan, thus enabling better understanding, facilitating choice-making and increasing quality of life.

Breathing

Respiratory problems are common in people with profound intellectual disabilities and complex needs, and this group is particularly susceptible to chest infections (Standley, 2016). Some studies and reports have found that respiratory disorders were a leading cause of death for people with intellectual disabilities (Hollins *et al.*, 1998; Glover and Ayub, 2010; Heslop *et al.*, 2013; Truesdale and Brown, 2017).

For people such as Clara, who experience difficulties with breathing, a care plan might need to address methods of enhancing respiratory function. This could include instructions on:

- Postural care
- Postural drainage to remove excess sputum
- Oral and nasal suction
- Minimising the risks of aspiration (Detailing the signs and symptoms that will identify chest infections promptly and how to effectively respond to and seek support for these signs).

Carers also need to be alert to signs and symptoms of asthma, and hay fever and other seasonal respiratory conditions, which can further exacerbate breathing difficulties. More recently, the effects of Covid-19 were starkly felt by people with intellectual disabilities, with an increased rate of hospitalisation and up to an eight-fold increased risk of mortality (Courtenay and Cooper, 2021). Compliance with vaccination programmes for vulnerable groups such as people with profound intellectual disabilities can help to reduce the effect of seasonal and specific respiratory conditions.

Eating and drinking

Dysphagia is defined as a disorder of swallowing usually resulting from physical impairment or neurological disorder; it is often associated with stroke, dementia, multiple sclerosis, Parkinson's disease, head and neck cancers, acquired brain injury, and respiratory conditions (RCSLT, 2015).

Historically evidence has suggested that anything between 36% and 70% of people with intellectual disabilities may have dysphagia, however, more recent evidence would seem to suggest that the actual figure is 8% – this is likely to be an underestimate due to lack of awareness and lack of diagnosis (Public Health England, 2016).

This condition is common in people with cerebral palsy, due to motor impairment, neurological development, and may be exacerbated to gastro-esophageal reflux disorder (Yi *et al.*, 2019). Difficulties with eating and drinking can lead to malnourishment and potential dehydration, which can be prevented by monitoring food and fluid intake and weight and responding promptly if problems arise, but of most concern, poor management of dysphagia can lead to avoidable fatalities, and there is a clear need for improved knowledge of our healthcare staff for this condition (Mencap, 2007; Heslop *et al.*, 2013). Particularly problematic is that people with learning and intellectual disabilities are at great risk of developing respiratory infections caused by aspiration or reflux if they have difficulties with swallowing (Truesdale and Brown, 2017).

Being underweight poses Clara a risk to her health and well-being with an increased risk of pressure sores, fatigue and general malaise. She does not eat very much and is frequently constipated. This is concerning and indicates an urgent need for a thorough multidisciplinary assessment (Harding and Wright, 2010). A speech and language therapist, who has been specially educated and prepared in the assessment of swallowing difficulties and management, should be asked to assess Clara's specific difficulties and recommend a strategy to ensure that she receives adequate nutrition safely. A dietitian should also be involved to assess the nutritional content of Clara's diet and make recommendations for how her diet might be improved to promote appropriate weight gain.

Clara also has frequent recurring chest infections, and this may be a sign of aspiration. Aspiration, a term used to describe the inhalation of foreign bodies from the mouth and throat into the lungs, is potentially life threatening and would need to be addressed as a matter of urgency. If Clara can eat orally, her care plan would need to include details about the appropriate consistency of food, how often and how much she should be fed, the appropriate utensils to use, and how to ensure that she maintains a posture that maximises her ability to eat safely. A high risk of aspiration can indicate the need for non-oral feeding.

Even if Clara is unable to eat orally, it is important that she should not miss out on the shared mealtime experience with her family. This can be an important social time when families get together not only to eat, but also to share one another's company and conversation; her inclusion in family events is important.

Eliminating & continence care

Due to the nature of their disabilities, many people with profound intellectual disabilities and complex needs are incontinent. Continence care is an intimate intervention and must be attended to with sensitivity. Privacy and respect are vital when carrying out all aspects of personal and intimate care. This means more than simply closing the door when providing care. It means being careful not to make insensitive comments in front of other people and giving undivided attention whilst carrying out care activities. Carers should try to avoid becoming blasé about continence care even though it can become a routine part of their work.

Constipation is reported in up to 40% of people with intellectual disabilities and complex needs. A poor diet, lack of mobility, impact of medication and conditions that affect the peripheral nervous system are all known to be contributory factors (Mathew *et al.*, 2021). In the first instance, treatment options for chronic constipation may include lifestyle changes such as increasing water intake and increasing the amount high-fibre foods (Krogh *et al.*, 2017) such as vegetables, pulses, and fruits in the diet. This is a natural way of increasing bulk and fibre. For people who have difficulties chewing or swallowing, the use of *'smoothies'* can be an alternative to increase the fibre content of the diet. The use of all medications should be closely monitored and regularly reviewed as these may impact on elimination. Physical activity is also an effective intervention in the management of constipation; however, evidence suggests that people with intellectual disabilities do not regularly meet the recommended minimum physical activity levels (Mathew *et al.*, 2021). Alternative therapies such as bowel massage have also been shown to improve the condition for some people (Emly, Wilson and Darby, 2001). Should lifestyle changes be ineffective, then Clara and her carers may want to discuss prescribed medications to help manage this, however, this should be seen as a last resort where other approaches have been unsuccessful. Over the counter remedies should always be discussed with a health professional such as a nurse, pharmacist, or doctor before they are commenced.

Washing, dressing and personal hygiene

Personal and intimate care is a significant and time-consuming part of life for many people with profound learning and intellectual disabilities and complex needs. When developing a care plan for Clara, respect and dignity are of paramount importance. When providing personal care, consideration should be given to individual preferences and cultural customs. The NMC has established the need to practice with respect and dignity through educational standards and within their code of practice (NMC, 2018a, 2018b).

Safety considerations are also important for both carers and Clara. Moving and handling guidelines must be adhered to, as well as the policies in place to protect vulnerable people from abuse (Cambridge and Carnaby, 2000a). Carers and care organisations will need support to ensure they have the correct equipment and training to enable them to carry out care tasks safely.

Personal care provides a valuable opportunity for sensory experiences and one-to-one interaction (Cambridge and Carnaby, 2000b). It should not be rushed but used as a time for social interaction and the development of skills.

People with incontinence are particularly susceptible to incontinence-associated dermatitis (IAD); this is an inflammation of the skin that can affect the perinium, buttocks, hips, groin, sacrum, vulva, and scrotum (Ladha, Wagg and Dytoc, 2017). The management of IAD and protecting the skin is therefore a prime consideration when carrying out continence care planning. Firstly, appropriate continence care products should be used; Clara's care plan should detail routine preventive measures, including keeping the skin clean and dry without scrubbing, and using appropriate cleaning and moisturising products and skin barriers where appropriate, the signs of erosion/skin breakdown and a treatment plan to follow if skin breakdown does occur (Voegeli, 2018). For people with specific sensitivities the use of detergents, biological washing agents, talcum powder, and products containing lanolin or perfume should be avoided. Alternatives such as emollients, non-biological washing agents, and perfume-free products are readily available. A pharmacist, GP or specialist can give advice about the choice and use of these products to suit an individual's needs (Voegeli and Hillery, 2021).

Appropriate hygiene practices must also be considered when managing menstruation. Self-management may be possible for individuals with mild and moderate intellectual disabilities, however, individuals with profound intellectual disabilities are likely to require higher levels of support to maintain good standards of hygiene around their menstrual cycle (Rodgers and Lipscombe, 2005). It is important that individuals are offered as much education, choice, and support in the management of menstruation as their non-disabled peers would expect to receive (Tracy, Grover and Macgibbon, 2016). Recording of the regularity and presentation of periods can help to establish patterns of behaviour and the implications this might have on a person's presentation. Attention should be paid to the heaviness of menstrual flow, symptoms of pain (dysmenorrhea) changes in behaviour and for individuals with epilepsy there may be changes to the pattern of seizure activity (Tracy, Grover and Macgibbon, 2016); the use of pain relief and non-medical interventions to ease discomfort during menstruation should be considered as appropriate.

People with profound intellectual disabilities and complex needs are often reliant on others to ensure that their oral hygiene is maintained. The mouth, teeth and gums should be cleaned at least twice a day (up to three times for people who do not feed orally) and checked by the dentist every six months. However, oral care can be distressing for some people so it might be worth considering a desensitation programme, different brushes and flavoured or unflavoured toothpaste may help. If resistance to oral care is a persistent problem it is worth consulting a dentist who may prescribe toothpaste with added fluoride or mouth wash and in some areas, specialist services give advice on dental care for people with intellectual disabilities. Oral care is necessary for maintaining good health and for reducing the risk of gum disease, tooth decay and respiratory infection.

Oral care is also particularly important within the context of the use of medication to manage other health conditions which may adversely impact oral health.

Maintaining body temperature

It may be more difficult for people with profound intellectual disabilities and complex needs to maintain their body temperature due to poor circulation caused by restricted mobility. Regular monitoring of Clara's temperature is important to enable carers to respond promptly and appropriately if she develops a high or low temperature, as this may be indicative of an underlying health problem.

Should Clara be unable to communicate whether she was too hot or cold, carers must be mindful about weather conditions and ensure that she wears appropriate clothing. Such clothing might include gloves, hats, and scarves in the winter, and cool, cotton clothing in the summer. Clothing should also be comfortable and suitable for Clara's age and culture.

Sunburn and heatstroke should be prevented by applying high-factor sun cream and ensuring that Clara avoids the sun around mid-day and at particularly hot times. Carers should remember that dark skins, as well as fair skins, are susceptible to sunburn. Fluid intake should be increased when the weather is hot, to avoid dehydration. Particular attention may also need to be paid to some medicines which can also increase photosensitivity.

Mobilising and postural care

Issues of mobility and postural care are highly relevant for people who have physical disabilities, and this is often the case for those people with profound intellectual disabilities and complex needs; lack of appropriate postural care may have significant impact their health and well-being (Robertson *et al.*, 2018). Clara is completely reliant on others for her physical positioning and to ensure that the correct measures are taken to improve her posture and maintain comfort. The role of a physiotherapist would be to assess Clara's needs for orthotics, wheelchairs, seating and special footwear, and to conduct a review at prescribed intervals to determine any changes in need. This is particularly important at Clara's stage in life, as she is going through puberty and is likely to require larger equipment to account for her growth.

Clara's care plan should describe the correct use of equipment such as orthotics, hoists and specialist technology and give instructions about how to conduct interventions as recommended by the physiotherapist. Her care plan might include a series of passive exercises and the correct use of equipment, such as a standing frame, to improve or maintain her posture. Physical activity is also shown to have a positive impact on mobility, with interventions such as hydrotherapy offering a range of improved health outcomes for people with profound and multiple learning disabilities (Tbaily, 2022).

When considering issues of mobility for people with very restricted movement, carers should be mindful of the effects this might have on an individual. Located in one plane of orientation for prolonged periods of time can make sudden or extreme movements seem unpleasant and even frightening. Carers should remember that some people with profound intellectual disabilities and complex needs can, in a sense, be physically locked into their own bodies, and this may result in a lack of self-determination on their part and total reliance on others for movement.

Postural care to reduce the effect of physical changes as a result of contractures or skeletal abnormalities has become more commonplace within clinical discussion and research, with recognition that 24-hour maintenance of good positioning is vital to delay deterioration (Robertson *et al.*, 2018). As well as shape changes, it is important to remember that lack of mobility is a contributory factor to reduced bone density, which may increase an individual's fragility and increase the risk of fracture, combining this risk with the use of anti-epileptic drugs which can also lead to reduced bone density may require that Clara undergoes bone density checks as part of her regular health checks (Walsh *et al.*, 2022).

Working and playing

Providing meaningful activities to people with profound intellectual disabilities and complex needs can be challenging, and research shows that people with profound intellectual disabilities are more likely to spend increased amounts of time isolated and disengaged than their peers with less significant degrees of impairment (Beadle-Brown *et al.*, 2016). People with profound intellectual disabilities and complex needs are often reliant on others to initiate activities, and their involvement may largely be passive, and it may also be difficult to assess how meaningful the activity is for someone who has limited communication abilities. When offering activities, the individual's abilities and preferences should be considered, knowledge of which can be developed as discussed previously in this chapter. However, beyond the known preferences of activity of a person with profound intellectual disabilities, new and different activities should still be explored and facilitated (Doukas *et al.*, 2017), expanding the range of experiences at opportunities available to a person.

Multi-sensory spaces are often found in special schools, day centres, and larger residential homes. The literature suggests that multi-sensory spaces can be used for relaxation, sensory stimulation, leisure, and entertainment; the parameters for what should be included and how these facilities should be used have never been firmly established (Cameron *et al.*, 2020). Whereas there is contrasting evidence for the benefit of using multi-sensory spaces, advocates of the use of multi-sensory spaces suggest that these spaces can counterbalance the sensory deprivation that people with profound and multiple intellectual disabilities may experience, however, the dearth of evidence which can objectively measure positive outcomes for the use of multi-sensory spaces does limit our capability to consider them as an evidence-based intervention (Carter and Stephenson, 2011).

If multi-sensory rooms are to be used effectively and meaningfully then their use should be based on individual assessment and observation and someone with profound intellectual disabilities and complex needs will require the support of other people to benefit from the environment and to have a meaningful experience. Care plans should detail the anticipated purpose of the use of the multi-sensory room and be accompanied by risk assessments that detail how the room should be used safely.

Carers should not forget that the world is full of natural and man-made environments that can and do provide stimulation, enjoyment and opportunities for social interaction for this group. Person-centred active support enables people with profound and multiple disabilities to be able to participate and engage in meaningful everyday activity. Using person-centered active support to identify the appropriate level of support to include people with profound intellectual disabilities and complex needs in everyday activities has been shown to increase participation and support skills development (Beadle-Brown, Hutchinson and Whelton, 2012).

Expressing sexuality

Sexual health remains a topic surrounded by stigma and is often overlooked by nursing teams (Hendry, Snowden and Brown, 2018). The sexuality of people with intellectual disabilities is poorly understood and has often been neglected by health and social services and within research (Medina-Rico, López-Ramos and Quiñonez, 2017) and evidence shows that people with LGBTQ+ identities and disabilities face increased stigma due to these intersecting marginalised identities (O'Shea *et al.*, 2020). Over recent years, a move away from the medical model of care toward a holistic model of healthcare has led to greater recognition of the sexuality of people with intellectual disabilities, and the expression of their sexuality. Nonetheless this expression is still restricted by what are perceived to be acceptable expressions within predetermined cultural norms (Whittle and Butler, 2018).

Expressing sexuality is not limited to sexual contact but is inclusive of romance, intimacy and intimate relationships and may intersect with our expression of identity and is essential for well-being as well as being a fundamental right (Bauer *et al.*, 2014). Hendry, Snowden and Brown (2018) found that while sexuality is indeed a broad church, supported people often are not offered the opportunity to express themselves fully due to preconceived attitudes and beliefs held by caregivers. For people with profound intellectual disabilities and complex needs, care plans might include activities to encourage bodily awareness, opportunity and support with masturbation, information about how clothing and appearance can be used as an expression of sexuality and sexual identity, and how people should be supported through developmental changes such as puberty, menstruation, and menopause, the first two of these being particularly relevant to Clara.

Whilst supporting the expression of sexuality, the care plan should also reflect issues relevant to consent and capacity because many people with profound learning and intellectual disability and complex needs will be unable to consent to sexual activity.

Sleeping

The reported prevalence of sleep problems for people with intellectual disabilities ranges from 8.5% to 34.1%, with respiratory disorder, sensory impairment and medications being contributory factors (Van de Wouw *et al.*, 2012). Clara is known to be at risk of developing pressure sores on her ankles, elbows, and sacral areas, and this is thought to be caused by her positioning in bed. An assessment by a physiotherapist might recommend the use of a *'sleep system'* to enable carers to position Clara in such a way that it removes pressure from the areas prone to sores. Carers are responsible for maintaining the integrity of Clara's skin and preventing the development of pressure sores through appropriate positioning and postural support.

The time at which a person goes to bed and gets up should be determined by the individual's own sleep pattern. The amount of time people need to sleep varies. Lying in bed when not asleep may be boring and become uncomfortable, and not having enough sleep is thought to be detrimental to physical and psychological health and quality of life (Barnes and Drake, 2015). To aid restful sleep, carers should ensure that Clara's bedroom is maintained at an appropriate temperature and that environmental noise and light is reduced to a minimum.

Dying

Although life expectancy for people with intellectual disability is increasing, this group has an increased risk of early death (Hollins *et al.*, 1998; Heslop *et al.*, 2013, Truesdale and Brown, 2017).

Problems recognising and assessing symptoms of illness mean that diagnoses, and therefore access to appropriate treatment, are often delayed in this group (RCN, 2013) especially when we consider that self-reporting is often our first indicator that a person is in pain (Finlay *et al.*, 2018) and misinterpretation of communicative behaviours in people with a learning and intellectual disability can delay this. Pain is often the earliest indicator of illness, but carers and healthcare providers can have difficulties recognising that a person with profound intellectual disabilities and complex needs is in pain (Doody and Bailey, 2019), and consequently, not respond appropriately to manage the person's pain.

People with profound intellectual disabilities and complex needs are at greater risk of pain because of associated physical conditions such as cerebral palsy and gastroesophageal reflux (Truesdale and Brown, 2017). Pain management strategies, which might include the administration of analgesics and correct positioning, should be both proactive and reactive and should be detailed in a person's care plan.

When required to provide palliative care, carers should seek the support of specialist services (see Chapter 3). People with intellectual disabilities have palliative care needs that mirror those of the general population, albeit with the requirement for some reasonable adjustment and some of the issues that might need to be considered at this stage of life include pain and symptom control, consent, ways of communicating about illness and death with the individual and his or her family, and how relatives can be supported through this difficult time (Adam *et al.*, 2020). Consideration should also be given to how carers will be supported to cope with the effects of their own experience of loss and bereavement when the person dies.

In any kind of congregated living arrangement, people with profound intellectual disabilities and complex needs are also likely to be affected by the loss of another resident. Research on bereavement and people with intellectual disabilities has suggested that the experience of grief can be prolonged, and its effects can include anxiety, depression and irritability (Oswin, 1991; Hollins and Esterhuyzen, 1997; Guerin *et al.*, 2021). People with intellectual disabilities should be supported to develop their understanding of the concept of dying; this might be done through education, and they may also benefit from attending and participating in cultural ritual such as funerals and memorial activities (Guerin *et al.*, 2021).

These findings have challenged widespread beliefs that people with intellectual disabilities are incapable of experiencing grief; for more detail the reader might care to refer to Chapter 3.

Spirituality

Spirituality has been considered a significant dimension of well-being (Narayanasamy, Gates and Swinton, 2002). Hatton *et al.* (2004) have argued that meeting people's religious and spiritual needs is an essential role for services to fulfil. However, spiritual needs are probably one of the most challenging and neglected areas of care for people with profound intellectual disabilities and complex needs.

Narayanasamy, Gates and Swinton (2002) have argued that a distinction must be made between religion and spirituality. They have found that services largely failed to address spiritual needs but were better at meeting religious needs, which might have involved supporting individuals with religious activities and practices. Legere (1984) has defined spirituality as *'to give meaning and purpose'*, which might be a helpful way for carers to think about how to meet this area of human need.

Care planning and decision-making can be problematic in this area, because differences in values and beliefs between members of care staff and family members can cause tensions. Person-centred approaches offer a solution to some of these problems. By encouraging open discussion and prioritising an individual's needs above the aspirations of family and staff, decisions can be made about how to meet their religious and spiritual needs.

There are some resources that might be useful for developing care plans to address religious and spiritual needs (see Hatton *et al.*, 2004). However, these do tend to concentrate on the needs of people with mild to moderate intellectual disabilities, and our understanding about how these needs might best be met for people with profound intellectual disabilities and complex needs is still very limited.

Relationships

People with intellectual disabilities have the same need and desire to develop friendships and intimate relationships as do their peers (Box and Shaw, 2014). While concerns around safety are important considerations, the opportunity to build relationships should be facilitated and carers play a vital role in supporting people with profound intellectual disabilities and complex needs to maintain and develop relationships throughout their lives (Bates, Terry and Popple, 2017). Familial relationships can also support a sense of belonging and enhance well-being for people with intellectual disabilities (Strnadová, Johnson and Walmsley, 2018). Connection and inclusion within the context of Covid-19 has created challenges for people with intellectual disabilities due the historic digital exclusion of this group as we have moved into a more digitally connected world. It has been identified that facilitating connection and risk enabling practices can have positive outcomes for belonging as well as self-reported psychological safety and well-being for people with intellectual disabilities (Spassiani *et al.*, 2022).

The need for human touch has been well established; the use of touch is rooted within social constructions of gender appropriateness, cultural norms and social conventions (Pedrazza *et al.*, 2018) and policies in health and social services are sometimes interpreted in a way that restricts the use of touch. This is regrettable, as touch might be a person's only, or most meaningful, way of communicating and connecting with the social world and there is evidence to suggest that there is greater need for human touch during times of distress (Pedrazza *et al.*, 2018). Touch can also be used to provide sensory stimulation and to offer comfort using therapeutic touch and massage (Gale and Hegarty, 2000).

The implementation of care plans

The success of any care plan is dependent on its implementation. Care plans were never devised to be paper exercises whereby forms are filled out and '*filed away in a cabinet*' only to be retrieved at the next date for review. They should be active '*live*' documents, updated on a regular basis and used daily by those involved in providing care. The implementation phase of the care planning process is therefore the '*actioning*' of supporting health and well-being. It is in this phase where the development of the assessment and plan come together through the delivery of personal and intimate care in addition to specified social and therapeutic interventions.

Nurses and other members of the support team will provide care and support either directly or indirectly, independently or collaboratively. Each intervention included in the plan of care supports the achievement of individualised goals. Therefore, implementation comprises performing a task and essentially documenting each task. A sample framework to structure reporting the implementation phase is offered by Yoost and Crawford (2020). Supporting people living with profound intellectual disabilities and the management of multiple chronic conditions in addition to the need for social and psychological support requires a multi-disciplinary approach. Therefore, families, individual supporters and all support workers will have a part to play in this phase, both individually and collectively. All supporters of the individual need to be aware of how to carry out the activities required to implement planned interventions. This highlights the importance of communication throughout the implementation in addition to organising the actions of staff and providing evaluation and evidence of the care provided (Doody and Bailey, 2019).

As the implementation of specific interventions are performed, continuous objective and subjective data are gathered through observation and feedback from the individual, their family and support workers. As needs are attended to, the plan may be updated if required. In aspiring to support the person with profound intellectual disabilities and complex needs to live an ordinary life with support, Mattousova-Done and Gates (2006) have described the theory of '*the nature of care planning and delivery in intellectual disability nursing*' as an inter-relationship of care planning, person-centred planning, health action plan and

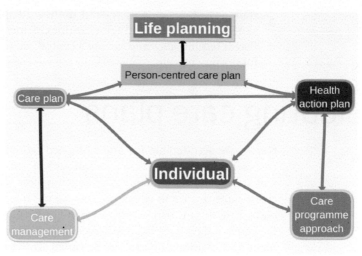

Figure 6.2

The interrelationship of care planning approaches in a person-centred model.

care approach (implying person-centred), and their description is illustrated in Figure 6.2.

Evident within this approach is the necessity that the care plan is sufficiently flexible to accommodate the inputs and outcomes of health action plans and the individual's response to care being provided. Whether care plans are stored at home, in a school or a day centre, it is imperative that agreement on how to record the effectiveness of interventions is agreed by all involved. The appropriateness and response of the individual is monitored to identify compliance with interventions and how the individual experiences the interventions. Many family carers are now active in the task of writing daily reports in care plans as it alleviates the need to recall from memory and aids communication and continuity of care (De Haas and Ryan, 2016).

The implementation phase of the nursing process is the stage where desired outcomes are observed, however, it is important to note how these desired outcomes may be hindered. Ghogomu *et al.* (2017) report on research from a Canadian perspective and whilst they refer to older adults living in residential settings, they identify common barriers and solutions to implementing optimal evidence-informed care planning for long term care residents which have similarities to the disability area. These are:

■ Common barriers were lack of staff knowledge and training, lack of communication, inconsistent and fragmented location of documentation at the provider level, lack of family involvement and communication at the resident/family level, and issues with staffing and the length of the care plan at the work environment level

■ Key strategies to overcome common barriers are noted as providing education, training and support to staff, facilitating communication between all staff, providing guidance to staff on how to approach and facilitate discussions with residents and their families, using standardised forms and consistent terminology, and having a centralised location or consistent location for documentation.

Evaluating care plans

Nurses are accountable for and obligated to measure interventions and outcomes that demonstrate how care was, or was not, delivered in a timely, competent and cost-effective manner. Evidencing these requirements is a complex and challenging process in which evaluation, the final phase of the nursing process plays a significant part. '*Outcomes*' which the individual and their family and the nurse judges have been achieved, as predetermined in the original assessment and planning phases, are recorded in the evaluation phase, and if and to what degree the support and care were successful in achieving these goals. Evaluation of interventions is often referred to as an 'appraisal' of whether the intervention worked, worked well or not, and how the individual felt about the intervention(s).

Many family carers note that it is the family who provides the consistent presence and care in a person's life, because paid carers tend to be more temporary. The family carer is often identified as an '*expert by experience*' when it comes to the care of their family member who lives with profound intellectual disabilities and complex needs. Therefore, acknowledging the intensive and extensive interactions and care that family members deliver daily in supporting their family member is important in this phase of the nursing process.

The evaluation phase measures outcomes and progression towards attainment of goals, and dreams/wishes. Ultimately, evaluation plays a major role in determining whether the individual's physical, emotional, social, intellectual and specific care needs were met and how the outcomes as identified in the initial assessment phase or as per the Individual Service Agreement between the individual and the service provider were achieved. As previously stated, care plans are seen as active documents constantly evolving in response to the formative or summative evaluation of current and past interventions, changes in the individual's needs and/or wishes, and the development of new knowledge and ideas. The evaluation process should determine the effectiveness of care, make necessary modifications, and will continuously ensure favorable client outcomes.

Measurement and outcomes play an important part in the evaluation phase of the nursing process. Physical outcomes can be routinely examined and recorded during the evaluation phase (such as body mass index, blood pressure or the frequency of seizures) and comparisons to baseline data thereby provide evidence to suggest if interventions were successful or not. Auditing social activities and social engagements is another aspect that is increasing in this group to ensure that psychosocial goals are appraised for effectiveness. In essence, these measurements demonstrate accountability for the quality, safety and satisfaction of individuals and their families in the care delivered. This means showing '*everyone*' the measurements you have made to demonstrate that you have done what you set out to do. Presentation of these outcomes therefore is an important part of the support and caring journey. Measuring abstract concepts, such as spiritual well-being or quality of life is, however, more problematic. The individual subjectivity associated with what constitutes quality of life poses a challenge for the evaluation of care plans, but ultimately supporting the individual and their close circle of support and or family in making this determination is important to acknowledge for this group of people. Therefore, the use of communication profiles as discussed previously in this chapter enables carers to develop an understanding of the success of the care plan from the individual's perspective and to report on these findings.

When caring for people living with profound intellectual disabilities and complex needs the evaluation phase of the nursing process relies on proxy reports such as subjective experiences and opinions of other people. The use of triangulation of evidence and adopting multiple perspectives is therefore essential in evaluating care and support for people with profound intellectual disabilities and complex needs. Building reflection into the evaluation phase of the process is important; reflective practice provides an opportunity to consider different perspectives and their contribution to care planning and care delivery. Nurses need to be mindful of assumptions and interpretations of behaviour (Nieuwenhuijse *et al.*, 2019).

Digitalisation and care plans

Electronic care plans (e-care plans) and electronic health records are not widely available in many disability services, however, their potential uses are increasingly being discussed. Integrating nursing care planning processes within an electronic health record offers people with intellectual disabilities the opportunity to maintain personal sensitive data in a secure single source with many benefits.

The basic Electronic Health Record (EHR) is an electronic database with information concerning a person's health records such as demographic characteristics, medical history, family history of diseases, previous hospitalisations, previous and current therapies, possible allergies and intolerances, as well as laboratory results, genetic test results, and diagnostic imaging results. In addition, it may include data about healthcare professionals and hospitals/clinics that provided previous healthcare interventions (Entzeridou, Markopoulou and Mollaki, 2018).

Other potential uses of EHR's database may be the basis for epidemiological studies or a source for comparative effectiveness research. This provides clinicians and researchers with opportunities to research processes, economics and statistical nature of care delivery. In order to facilitate better management of clinical care and welfare, most EHR systems (EHRs) that are currently used are integrated with additional functions, such as Computerised Physician Order Entry (CPOE) that allow medical professionals to enter medication orders electronically and Clinical Decision Support (CDS) that facilitate decision-making (Entzeridou, Markopoulou and Mollaki, 2018). Thus, EHRs are being implemented worldwide to improve safety, healthcare quality and efficiency (Yu and Qian, 2018).

Given the accelerated development and adoption of information technology across healthcare e-care plans are developing in nursing practice and may in time become more commonplace than traditional paper-based versions. E-care plans like EHRs offer the potential to aggregate data from multiple sources and communicate data out to other sources with more ease and efficacy than traditional paper-based versions. Software algorithms offer the potential to calculate dependency and risk scores, identify specific care requirements and create care plans to meet those needs. Additionally, e-care plans can offer the potential of standardising assessment tools and evaluation tools, or alternatively adapt to needs, which may serve well the profoundly learning and intellectually disabled population. While systems are still some way off in standardising care plans, the potential to improve accessibility of assessment tools, implementation tools, and educational tools through this approach will be an advancement in ensuring individualised safe, effective and quality care is provided to this group of people. Intellectual disability nursing can play an important role in supporting this agenda by working with our engineering and technology colleagues and data controllers to ensure standardisation and systems that meet the needs of people living with profound intellectual disabilities and their families.

Conclusion

This chapter has demonstrated how intellectual disability nursing care can be planned and delivered for people with profound intellectual disabilities and complex needs, both through direct interventions and indirectly through prescribed care plans for social care staff, health and support workers. It has been argued that this group represents one of the most marginalised groups of people in society. They are at higher risk from social exclusion and experience poorer health than does the rest of the population, often compounded by multiple physical co-morbidities. The discussion of care plans in this chapter has been presented as one way to ensure that this group of people receives systematic planning and documentation of interventions by their carers. This approach should be adopted to meet an individual's daily needs for support in all aspects of his or her life. Care plans also need to be viewed within a context of the wider multidisciplinary team because people with profound intellectual disabilities and complex needs often require input from a wide range of social and healthcare professionals throughout their lives. It has been suggested in this chapter that the use of a specific model of nursing care planning might assist person-centered care planning being undertaken in a more organised and guided way which can be used by all those involved in the person's care. This chapter has considered the central role of the intellectual disability nurse in developing person-centred robust care plans which can be the basis for the work of the wider multidisciplinary and care team. Effective care planning ensures the safe and timely delivery of all aspects of care to this complex group of people. The intellectual disability nurse fulfills many roles in this process but central to this is a detailed understanding of the person with profound intellectual disabilities and complex needs which underpins all other aspects of the nursing role in care planning and delivery for this vulnerable group of people.

References

Adam, E., *et al.* (2020) The palliative care needs of adults with intellectual disabilities and their access to palliative care services: A systematic review. *Palliative Medicine*, 34(8), pp. 1006–1018.

Agran, M., Storey, K. and Krupp, M. (2010) Choosing and choice making are not the same: Asking "what do you want for lunch?" is not self-determination. *Journal of Vocational Rehabilitation*, 33(2), pp. 77–88.

Akyüz, E., *et al.* (2021) Elucidating the potential side effects of current anti-seizure drugs for epilepsy. *Current Neuropharmacology*, 19(11), pp. 1865–1883.

Antonsson, H., *et al.* (2008) Caregivers' reflections on their interactions with adult people with learning disabilities. *Journal of Microscopy*, 15(6), pp. 484–491.

Araten-Bergman, T. and Bigby, C. (2020) Forming and supporting circles of support for people with intellectual disabilities – a comparative case analysis. *Journal of Intellectual and Developmental Disability*, 47(2), pp. 1–13.

Ayer, S. (1998) Use of multi-sensory rooms for children with profound and multiple intellectual disabilities. *Journal of Intellectual Disabilities for Nursing, Health and Social Care*, 2(2), pp. 89–97.

Aylott, J. (2001) The new intellectual disabilities white paper: Did it forget something? *British Journal of Intellectual Disabilities*, 10(8), p. 512.

Barden, O., *et al.* (2022) Antonia's story: Bringing the past into the future. *British Journal of Learning Disabilities*, 50(2), pp. 258–269.

Barnes, C.M. and Drake, C.L. (2015) Prioritizing sleep health: Public health policy recommendations. *Perspectives on Psychological Science*, 10(6), pp. 733–737.

Barrow, M. (2012) NHS gives 'second-rate care' to mentally disabled patients. *The Times (London)*, 27 January.

Bates, C., Terry, L. and Popple, K. (2017) The importance of romantic love to people with learning disabilities. *British Journal of Learning Disabilities*, 45(1), pp. 64–72.

Bauer, M., *et al.* (2014) Supporting residents' expression of sexuality: The initial construction of a sexuality assessment tool for residential aged care facilities. *BMC Geriatrics*, 14(1), pp. 82–82.

Bawden, A. and Campbell, D. (2012) NHS accused over deaths of disabled patients: Mencap inquiry finds institutional discrimination against people with learning disabilities led to at least 74 deaths. *The Guardian (Manchester)*, 3 January.

Beadle-Brown, J., Hutchinson, A. and Whelton, B. (2012) Person-centred active support – increasing choice, promoting independence and reducing challenging behaviour. *Journal of Applied Research in Intellectual Disabilities*, 25(4), pp. 291–307.

Beadle-Brown, J., *et al.* (2016) Quality of life and quality of support for people with severe intellectual disability and complex needs. *Journal of Applied Research in Intellectual Disabilities*, 29(5), pp. 409–421.

Beghi, E. (2020) The epidemiology of epilepsy. *Neuroepidemiology*, 54(2), pp. 185–191.

Belifore, P.J. and Toro-Zambrana, W. (1994) *Recognising choices in community settings by people with significant disabilities*. Washington, DC: American Association on Mental Retardation.

Bellamy, G., *et al.* (2010) A study to define: Profound and multiple learning disabilities (PMLD). *Journal of Intellectual Disabilities*, 14(3), p. 221.

Box, M. and Shaw, J. (2014) The experiences of adults with learning disabilities attending a sexuality and relationship group: "I want to get married and have kids". *Journal of Family Planning and Reproductive Health Care*, 40(2), pp. 82–88.

Brison, S.J. (2021) Valuing the lives of people with profound intellectual disabilities. *Philosophical Topics*, 49(1), pp. 99–122.

Brown, I. and Brown, R.I. (2009) Choice as an aspect of quality of life for people with intellectual disabilities. *Journal of Policy and Practice in Intellectual Disabilities,* 6(1), pp. 11–18.

Brown, M., Hoyle, L. and Karatzias, T. (2016) The experiences of family carers in the delivery of invasive clinical interventions for young people with complex intellectual disabilities: Policy disconnect or policy opportunity? *Journal of Clinical Nursing,* 25(3–4), pp. 534–542.

Caldwell, P. (1997) Getting in touch' with people with severe learning disabilities. *British Journal of Nursing,* 6(13), pp. 751–756.

Calveley, J. (2017) Gaining the power of initiation through intensive interaction. *Learning Disability Practice,* 20(1), pp. 19–23.

Cambridge, P. and Carnaby, S. (2000a) A personal touch: Managing the risks of abuse during intimate and personal care. *The Journal of Adult Protection,* 2(4), pp. 4–16.

Cambridge, P. and Carnaby, S. (2000b) *Making it personal: Providing intimate and personal care for people with intellectual disabilities.* Brighton: Pavilion.

Cameron, A., *et al.* (2020) Making sense of multi-sensory environments: A scoping review. *International Journal of Disability, Development, and Education,* 67(6), pp. 630–656.

Cannella-Malone, H.I. and Sabielny, L.M. (2020) Preference assessments, choice, and quality of life for people with significant disabilities. In Stancliffe, R., Wehmeyer, M., Shogren, K. and Abery, B. (Eds.), *Choice, preference, and disability: Positive psychology and disability series.* New York: Springer.

Carnaby, S. (2001) Editorial. *Tizard Intellectual Disability Review,* 6(2), pp. 2–5.

Carter, M. and Stephenson, J. (2011) The use of multi-sensory environments in schools servicing children with severe disabilities. *Journal of Developmental and Physical Disabilities,* 24(1), pp. 95–109.

Casey, C., *et al.* (2021) *Annual report of the National Ability Supports System (NASS) 2021.* Dublin: Health Research Board.

Chadwick, D., Buell, S. and Goldbart, J. (2019) Approaches to communication assessment with children and adults with profound intellectual and multiple disabilities. *Journal of Applied Research in Intellectual Disabilities,* 32(2), pp. 336–358.

Clegg, J.A. (2020) Dedifferentiation in context. *Journal of Intellectual & Developmental Disability,* 45(4), pp. 305–308.

Cocquyt, C. (2018) Development of a multidisciplinary care pathway for people with profound and multiple learning disabilities. *Learning Disability Practice,* 21(6), pp. 15–19.

Collins, J. and Murphy, G.H. (2021) Detection and prevention of abuse of adults with intellectual and other developmental disabilities in residential services: A systematic review. *Journal of Applied Research in Intellectual Disabilities,* 35(2), pp. 338–373.

Cooper, V. and Ward, C. (2011) Valuing people now and people with complex needs. *Tizard Learning Disability Review,* 16(2), pp. 39–43.

Courtenay, K. and Cooper, V. (2021) Covid 19: People with learning disabilities are highly vulnerable. *British Medical Journal,* 374(n1701). doi:10.1136/bmj.n1701.

Davies, D. and Evans, L. (2001) Assessing pain in people with profound intellectual disabilities. *British Journal of Nursing,* 10(8), pp. 513–516.

De Haas, C. and Ryan, R. (2016) Family centred care in a health care setting. In Runin, I.L., Merrick, J., Greddanus, D.E. and Patel, D.R. (Eds.), *Health care for people with intellectual and developmental disabilities across the lifespan* (3rd edition). Switzerland: Springer, pp. 49–58.

DH (2001) *Valuing people: A new strategy for intellectual disability for the 21st century.* London: The Stationary Office.

DH (2009) *Valuing people now.* Leeds: Department of Health.

DH (2012) *Compassion in practice, nursing, midwifery and care staff: Our vision and strategy.* Leeds: Department of Health.

Devinsky, O., Friedman, D. and Besag, F.M. (2018) Nocturnal monitoring in epilepsy: Evidence mounts. *Neurology,* 91(16), pp. 731–732.

Doody, O. and Bailey, M.E. (2019) Interventions in pain management for persons with an intellectual disability. *Journal of Intellectual Disabilities,* 23(1), pp. 132–144.

Doukas, T., *et al.* (2017) *Supporting people with profound and multiple learning disabilities: Core and essential service standards.* Available at: www.pmldlink.org.uk/wp-content/uploads/2017/11/Standards-PMLD-h-web.pdf (Accessed 28 July 2022).

Education Scotland (2021) *Communication passports.* Available at: https://education.gov.scot/improvement/practice-exemplars/communication-passports/ (Accessed 28 July 2022).

Emerson, E. (2009) *Estimating future numbers of adults with profound multiple learning disabilities in England.* Lancaster: Centre for Disability Research.

Emly, M., Wilson, L. and Darby, J. (2001) Abdominal massage for adults with learning disabilities. *Nursing Times,* 97(30), pp. 61–62.

Engel, G.L. (1981) The clinical application of the biopsychosocial model. *The Journal of Medicine and Philosophy: A Forum for Bioethics and Philosophy of Medicine,* 6(2), pp. 101–124.

Entzeridou, E., Markopoulou, E. and Mollaki, V. (2018) Public and physician's expectations and ethical concerns about electronic health record: Benefits outweigh risks except for information security. *International Journal of Medical Informatics,* 110, pp. 98–107.

Esteban, L., *et al.* (2021) Community living, intellectual disability and extensive support needs: A rights-based approach to assessment and intervention. *International Journal of Environmental Research and Public Health,* 18(6), p. 3175.

Finlay, K.A., Peacock, S. and Elander, J. (2018) Developing successful social support: An interpretative phenomenological analysis of mechanisms and processes in a chronic pain support group. *Psychology & Health,* 33(7), pp. 846–871.

Flick, U. (2017) Challenges for a new critical qualitative inquiry. *Qualitative Inquiry,* 23(1), pp. 3–7.

Flynn, M. (2012) *Winterbourne view hospital: A serious case review.* Gloucester: Gloucestershire Safeguarding Adults Board.

Flynn, S., *et al.* (2017) Measurement tools for mental health problems and mental well-being in people with severe or profound intellectual disabilities: A systematic review. *Clinical Psychology Review,* 57, pp. 32–44.

Foreman, P., *et al.* (2004) Evaluating the educational experiences of students with profound and multiple disabilities in inclusive and segregated classroom settings: An Australian perspective. *Research and Practice for Persons with Severe Disabilities,* 29(3), pp. 183–193.

Forster, S. (2020) Approaching a person with profound intellectual and multiple disabilities: What do you think, what do you do? In Nind, M. and Strnadova, I. (Eds.), *Belonging for people with profound intellectual and multiple disabilities.* London: Routledge, pp. 133–158.

Fyson, R. and Patterson, A. (2020) Staff understandings of abuse and poor practice in residential settings for adults with intellectual disabilities. *Journal of Applied Research in Intellectual Disabilities,* 33(3), pp. 354–363.

Gale, E. and Hegarty, J.R. (2000) The use of touch in caring for people with learning disability. *The British Journal of Developmental Disabilities,* 46(91), pp. 97–108.

Garrard, B., Lambe, L. and Hogg, J. (2010) *Invasive procedures: Minimising risks and maximising rights: Improving practice in the delivery of invasive procedures for people with profound and multiple learning disabilities*. Dundee: PAMIS and White Top Research Unit.

Gates, B. and Atherton, H. (2001) The challenge of evidence-based practice for learning disability professionals in health and social care. *British Journal of Nursing*, 10(8), pp. 173–178.

Gates, B. and Wray, J. (2000) The problematic nature of evidence. In Gates, B., Gear, J. and Wray, J. (Eds.), *Behavioural distress: Concepts and strategies*. London: Bailliere Tindall.

Ghogomu, E., *et al.* (2017) *Implementation of care planning in long term care: A Bruyère rapid review*. Ottawa: Bruyère Research Institute.

Gjermestad, A., Skarsaune, S.N. and Bartlett, R.L. (2022) Advancing inclusive research with people with profound and multiple learning disabilities through a sensory-dialogical approach. *Journal of Intellectual Disabilities*. doi:10.1177/17446295211062390.

Glover, G. and Ayub, M. (2010) *How people with learning disabilities die*. Durham: Improving Health and Lives Learning Disabilities Observatory.

Gooding, L. (2004) Valuing people has yet to make a real impact. *Learning Disability Practice*, 7(3), p. 6.

Guerin, S., *et al.* (2021) Bereavement, grief reactions and end of life. In Prasher, V.P., Davidson, P.W. and Santos, F.H. (Eds.), *Mental health, intellectual and developmental disabilities and the ageing process*. New York: Springer.

Halladay, P.M. and Harrington, C. (2015) Scandals of abuse: Policy responses in intellectual disabilities. *International Journal of Sociology and Social Policy*, 35(1–2), pp. 107–124.

Harding, C. and Wright, J. (2010) Dysphagia the challenge of managing eating and drinking difficulties in children and adults who have learning disabilities. *Tizard Learning Disability Review*, 15(1), pp. 4–13.

Haslam, S.A., *et al.* (2021) Rethinking the nature of the person at the heart of the biopsychosocial model: Exploring social changeways not just personal pathways. *Social Science and Medicine*, 272(113566). doi:10.1016/j.socscimed.2020.113566.

Hatton, C., *et al.* (2004) *Religious expression, a fundamental human right: The report of an action research project on meeting the needs of people with learning disabilities*. London: The Mental Health Foundation.

Hendry, A., Snowden, A. and Brown, M. (2018) When holistic care is not holistic enough: The role of sexual health in mental health settings. *Journal of Clinical Nursing*, 27(5–6), pp. 1015–1027.

Heslop, P., *et al.* (2013) *Confidential inquiry into premature deaths of people with learning disabilities, final report*. Bristol: Norah Fry Research Centre.

Hewett, D. (2012) *Intensive interaction: Theoretical perspectives*. London: Sage.

Hewett, D., *et al.* (2012) *The intensive interaction handbook*. London: Sage.

Ho, A. (2004) To be labelled, or not to be labelled: That is the question. *British Journal of Learning Disabilities*, 32(2), pp. 86–92. https://doi.org/10.1111/j.1468-3156.2004.00284.x

Hollins, S. and Esterhuyzen, A. (1997) Bereavement and grief in adults with learning disabilities. *British Journal of Psychiatry*, 170, pp. 497–501.

Hollins, S., *et al.* (1998) Mortality in people with learning disability: Risks, causes and death certification findings in London. *Developmental Medicine and Child Neurology*, 40(1), pp. 50–56.

Human rights act 1998. London: HMSO.

Humber, L.A. (2016) The impact of neoliberal market relations of the production of care on the quantity and quality of support for people with learning disabilities. *Critical and Radical Social Work*, 4(2), pp. 149–167.

Jacobs, P., *et al.* (2021) Relationships matter! – Utilising ethics of care to understand transitions in the lives of adults with severe intellectual disabilities. *British Journal of Learning Disabilities*, 49(3), pp. 329–340.

Javaid, A., Nakata, V. and Michael, D. (2019) Diagnostic overshadowing in learning disability: Think beyond the disability. *Progress in Neurology and Psychiatry*, 23(2), pp. 8–10.

Kersten, M.C., *et al.* (2022) Contextual factors related to the execution of knowledge strategies in intellectual disabilities organizations. *Knowledge and Process Management*. doi:10.1002/kpm.1700.

Klotz, J. (2004) Sociocultural study of intellectual disability: Moving beyond labeling and social constructionist perspectives. *British Journal of Learning Disabilities*, 32(2), pp. 93–94.

Krogh, K., Chiarioni, G. and Whitehead, W. (2017) Management of chronic constipation in adults. *United European Gastroenterology Journal*, 5(4), pp. 465–472.

Lacey, P. and Ouvry, C. (Eds.). (1998) *People with profound and multiple intellectual disabilities: A collaborative approach to meeting complex needs*. London: David Foulton.

Ladha, M., Wagg, A. and Dytoc, M. (2017) An approach to urinary incontinence for dermatologists. *Journal of Cutaneous Medicine and Surgery*, 21(1), pp. 15–22.

Legere, T. (1984) A spirituality for today. *Studies in Formative Spirituality*, 5(3), pp. 375–385.

Maes, B., *et al.* (2021) Looking back, looking forward: Methodological challenges and future directions in research on persons with profound and multiple learning disabilities. *Journal of Applied Research in Intellectual Disabilities*, 34(1), pp. 250–262.

Male, D. (1996) Who goes to SLD schools? *Journal of Applied Research in Intellectual Disabilities*, 9(4), pp. 307–323.

Mansell, J. (2010) *Raising our sights: Services for adults with profound intellectual and multiple disabilities*. Kent: Tizard Centre.

Marsland, D., Oakes, P. and Bright, N. (2015) It can still happen here: Systemic risk factors that may contribute to the continued abuse of people with intellectual disabilities. *Tizard Learning Disability Review*, 20(3), pp. 34–146.

Martin, A.M., *et al.* (2022) Reconciling communication repertoires: Navigating interactions involving persons with severe/profound intellectual disability, a classic grounded theory study. *Journal of Intellectual Disability Research*, 66(4), pp. 332–352.

Martinello, E. (2015) Reviewing risks factors of individuals with intellectual disabilities as perpetrators of sexually abusive behaviors. *Sexuality and Disability*, 33(2), pp. 269–278.

Mathew, R., *et al.* (2021) A primary care approach to constipation in adults with intellectual and developmental disabilities. *Advances in Medicine*. doi:10.1155/2021/3248052.

Mattousova-Done, S. and Gates, B. (2006) The nature of care planning and delivery in intellectual disability nursing. In Gates, B. (Ed.), *Care planning and delivery in intellectual disability nursing*. Oxford: Blackwell, pp. 1–20.

McNally, S. (2004) Plus change? Progress achieved in services for people with an intellectual disability in England since the publication of valuing people. *Journal of Learning Disabilities*, 8(4), pp. 323–329.

Medina-Rico, M., López-Ramos, H. and Quiñonez, A. (2017) Sexuality in people with intellectual disability: Review of literature. *Sexuality and Disability*, 36(3), pp. 231–248.

Mencap (2001) *No ordinary life: the support needs of families caring for children and adults with profound and multiple intellectual disabilities*. London: Mencap.

Mencap (2004) *Treat me right! Better healthcare for people with a learning disability*. London: Mencap.

Mencap (2007) *Death by indifference: Following the treat me right! Report*. London: Mencap.

Mencap and PMLD Network (2022) *About profound and multiple learning disabilities*. Available at: https://www.mencap.org.uk/sites/default/files/2016-11/PMLD%20 factsheet%20about%20profound%20and%20multiple%20learning%20disabil- ities.pdf (Accessed 26 November 2022).

Michael, J. (2008) *Healthcare for all: A report of the independent inquiry into access to healthcare for people with learning disabilities*. London: HMSO.

Morrison, J., Bradshaw, J. and Murphy, G. (2021) Reported communication chal- lenges for adults with intellectual disabilities giving evidence in court. *Journal of Applied Research in Intellectual Disabilities*, 34(5), p. 86.

Moulster, G., Ames, S. and Griffiths, T. (2012) Implementation of a new framework for practice. *Learning Disability Practice*, 15(7), pp. 21–26.

Moulster, G., *et al.* (2019) *The Moulster and Griffiths learning disability nursing model: A framework for practice*. London: Jessica Kingsley.

Muñoz-Neira, C., *et al.* (2012) The technology – activities of daily living question- naire: A version with a technology-related subscale. *Dementia and Geriatric Cogni- tive Disorders*, 33(6), pp. 361–371.

Narayanasamy, A., Gates, B. and Swinton, J. (2002) Spirituality and intellectual dis- abilities: A qualitative study. *British Journal of Nursing*, 11(14), pp. 948–957.

Nieuwenhuijse, A.M., *et al.* (2019) Quality of life of persons with profound intellec- tual and multiple disabilities: A narrative literature review of concepts, assessment methods and assessors. *Journal of Intellectual and Developmental Disability*, 44(3), pp. 261–271.

Nind, M. and Hewett, D. (2004) *A practical guide to intensive interaction*. Kiddermin- ster: BILD Publications.

Nind, M. and Strnadová, I. (2020) *Belonging for people with profound and multiple learning disabilities: Pushing the boundaries of inclusion*. Oxford: Routledge.

NMBI (2016) *Nurse registration programmes standards and requirements* (4th edition). Dublin: Nursing and Midwifery Board of Ireland.

NMBI (2021) *Code of professional conduct and ethics for registered nurse and registered midwives*. Dublin: NMBI.

NMC (2018a) *Future nurse: Standards of proficiency for registered nurses*. London: NMC.

NMC (2018b) *The code: Professional standards of practice and behaviour for nurses, mid- wives and nursing associates*. London: NMC.

Northway, R., *et al.* (2013) Researching policy and practice to safeguard people with intellectual disabilities from abuse: Some methodological challenges. *Journal of Policy and Practice in Intellectual Disabilities*, 10(3), pp. 188–195.

Northway, R., *et al.* (2017) Hospital passports, patient safety and person-centred care: A review of documents currently used for people with intellectual disabilities in the UK. *Journal of Clinical Nursing*, 26(23–24), pp. 5160–5168.

O'Shea, A., *et al.* (2020) Experiences of LGBTIQA+ people with disability in health- care and community services: Towards embracing multiple identities. *International Journal of Environmental Research and Public Health*, 17(21), p. 8080. doi:10.3390/ ijerph17218080.

Oswin, M. (1991) *Am I allowed to cry? A study of bereavement amongst people who have learning difficulties*. London: Human Horizons.

Oxford English Dictionary (2002) 10th ed. Revised. Oxford: Oxford University Press.

Palmer, C. and Walmsley, J. (2020) Are people with profound and multiple learn- ing disabilities and their families welcome in the wider learning disability community? In Nind, M. and Strnadova, I. (Eds.), *Belonging for people with profound intellectual and multiple disabilities*. London: Routledge, pp. 129–132.

PAMIS (2022) *Digital passports supporting inclusive communication*. Available at: https://pamis.org.uk/services/digital-passports/#:~:text=Family%20carers%20worked%20with%20PAMIS,build%20positive%20interaction%20and%20truly (Accessed 28 July 2022).

Pedrazza, M., *et al.* (2018) Variables of individual difference and the experience of touch in nursing. *Western Journal of Nursing Research*, 40(11), pp. 1614–1637.

Phillips, C. (2016) Wales' safeguarding policy and practice: A critical analysis. *The Journal of Adult Protection*, 18(1), pp. 14–27.

PMLD Network (2001) *No ordinary life: The support needs of families caring for children and adults with profound and multiple learning disabilities*. London: Mencap.

PMLD Network (2002) *Valuing people with profound and multiple intellectual disabilities (PMLD)*. London: Mencap.

PMLD Network (2013) *About profound and multiple learning disabilities*. Available at: www.mencap.org.uk/about-learning-disability/information-professionals/pmld/about-pmld (Accessed 31 May 2022).

Public Health England (2016) *Dysphagia in people with learning difficulties: Reasonable adjustments guidance*. Avail able at: www.gov.uk/government/publications/dysphagia-and-people-with-learning-disabilities/dysphagia-in-people-with-learning-difficulties-reasonable-adjustments-guidance#:~:text=More%20recent%20studies%20have%20shown,disability%20services%20will%20have%20dysphagia (Accessed 28 July 2022).

RCSLT (2015) *Dysphagia – guidance*. Available at: www.rcslt.org/members/clinical-guidance/dysphagia/dysphagia-guidance/ (Accessed 22 July 2022).

Richards, M. (2020) Whorlton Hall, Winterbourne . . . person-centred care is long dead for people with learning disabilities and autism. *Disability and Society*, 35(3), pp. 500–505.

Robertson, J., *et al.* (2015) Prevalence of epilepsy among people with intellectual disabilities: A systematic review. *Seizure*, 29, pp. 46–62.

Robertson, J., *et al.* (2018) Postural care for people with intellectual disabilities and severely impaired motor function: A scoping review. *Journal of Applied Research in Intellectual Disabilities*, 31(S1), pp. 11–28.

Rodgers, J. and Lipscombe, J. (2005) The nature and extent of help given to women with intellectual disabilities to manage menstruation. *Journal of Intellectual and Developmental Disability*, 30(1), pp. 45–52.

Royal College of Nursing (2013) *Meeting the health needs of people with learning disabilities: RCN guidance for nursing staff*. London: RCN.

Rukasha, T., Woolley, S.I. and Collins, T. (2020) Wearable epilepsy seizure monitor user interface evaluation: An evaluation of the empatica 'embrace' interface. *Adjunct Proceedings of the 2020 ACM International Joint Conference on Pervasive and Ubiquitous Computing and Proceedings of the 2020 ACM International Symposium on Wearable Computers*, pp. 110–114. doi:10.1145/3410530.3414382.

Sanderson, K.A., Bumble, J.L. and Kuntz, E.M. (2020) Meeting the daily needs of adults with IDD: The importance of informal supports. *International Review of Research in Developmental Disabilities*, 58, pp. 51–105.

Sawhney, I., *et al.* (2020) Awareness of bone health risks in people with epilepsy and intellectual disability. *British Journal of Learning Disabilities*, 48(3), pp. 224–231.

Schalock, R.L., Luckasson, R. and Tassé, M.J. (2021) *Intellectual disability: Definition, classification, and systems of supports* (12th edition). Silver Spring, MD: American Association on Intellectual and Developmental Disabilities.

Simmons, B. (2021) From living to lived and being-with: Exploring the interaction styles of children and staff towards a child with profound and multiple learning disabilities. *International Journal of Inclusive Education*, 25(6), pp. 657–670.

Son, Y.G., Shin, J. and Ryu, H.G. (2017) Pneumonitis and pneumonia after aspiration. *Journal of Dental Anesthesia and Pain Medicine*, 17(1), pp. 1–12.

Spassiani, N.A., *et al.* (2022) 'Now that I am connected this isn't social isolation, this is engaging with people': Staying connected during the COVID-19 pandemic. *British Journal of Learning Disabilities*. doi:10.1111/bld.12478.

Stancliffe, R.J. (2020) Choice availability and people with intellectual disability. In Stancliffe, R., Wehmeyer, M., Shogren, K. and Abery, B. (Eds.), *Choice, preference, and disability. Positive psychology and disability series*. New York: Springer.

Standley, D. (2016) Respiratory care in people with PMLD and complex physical disability. *PMLD Link*, 28(3), pp. 23–28.

Stannard, D. (2019) A practical definition of evidence-based practice for nursing. *Journal of PeriAnesthesia Nursing*, 34(5), pp. 1080–1084.

Strnadová, I., Johnson, K. and Walmsley, J. (2018) ". . . but if you're afraid of things, how are you meant to belong?" What belonging means to people with intellectual disabilities? *Journal of Applied Research in Intellectual Disabilities*, 31(6), pp. 1091–1102.

Sun, J.J., *et al.* (2020) Seizure and sudden unexpected death in epilepsy (SUDEP) characteristics in an urban UK intellectual disability service. *Seizure*, 80, pp. 18–23.

Talman, L., *et al.* (2019) Staff members and managers' views of the conditions for the participation of adults with profound intellectual and multiple disabilities. *Journal of Applied Research in Intellectual Disabilities*, 32(1), pp. 143–151.

Tbaily, C., *et al.* (2022) SPLASH study: Exploring caregiver perspectives of adults with severe or profound and multiple learning disabilities accessing sedentary hydrotherapy. *Physiotherapy*, 114, pp. e230–e23. doi:10.1016/j.physio.2021.12.219.

Thurman, S., Jones, J. and Tarleton, B. (2005) Without words meaningful information for people with high individual communication needs. *British Journal of Learning Disabilities*, 33(2), pp. 83–89.

Tittensor, P., *et al.* (2021) UK framework for basic epilepsy training and oromucosal midazolam administration. *Epilepsy Behavior*, 122, p. 108180. doi:10.1016/j.yebeh.2021.108180.

Tracy, J., Grover, S. and Macgibbon, S. (2016) Menstrual issues for women with intellectual disability. *Australian Prescriber*, 39(2), pp. 54–57.

Truesdale, M. and Brown, M. (2017) *People with learning disabilities in Scotland: 2017 health needs assessment update report*. Edinburgh: NHS Health Scotland.

U.K. Chief Nursing Officers (2012) *Strengthening the commitment: The report of the UK modernising learning disabilities nursing review*. Edinburgh: Scottish Government.

Van de Wouw, E., Evenhuis, H. and Echteld, M. (2012) Prevalence, associated factors and treatment of sleep problems in adults with intellectual disability: A systematic review. *Research in Developmental Disabilities*, 33(4), pp. 1310–1332.

Voegeli, D. (2018) Incontinence-associated dermatitis: Management. *Nursing and Residential Care*, 20(10), pp. 506–512.

Voegeli, D. and Hillery, S. (2021) Prevention and management of moisture-associated skin damage. *British Journal of Nursing*, 30(15), pp. S40–S46.

Walsh, N., *et al.* (2022) Peripheral bone density measurement: An interdisciplinary initiative for improving health outcomes for people with learning disabilities. *Journal of Intellectual Disabilities*, 26(1), pp. 18–28.

Whittle, C. and Butler, C. (2018) Sexuality in the lives of people with intellectual disabilities: A meta-ethnographic synthesis of qualitative studies. *Research in Developmental Disabilities*, 75, pp. 68–81.

Wolverson, M. (2003) Challenging behaviour. In Gates, B. (Ed.), *Learning disabilities: Toward inclusion*. London: Churchill Livingstone.

Yi, Y.G., *et al.* (2019) Dysphagia-related quality of life in adults with cerebral palsy on full oral diet without enteral nutrition. *Dysphagia*, 34(2), pp. 201–209.

Yoost, B.L. and Crawford, L.R. (2020) *Fundamentals of nursing* (2nd edition). London: Elsevier.

Yu, P. and Qian, S. (2018) Developing a theoretical model and questionnaire survey instrument to measure the success of electronic health records in residential aged care. *PloS One*, 13(1), p. e0190749. doi:10.1371/journal.pone.0190749.

Further Reading

Nind, M. and Strnadova, I. (Eds.). (2020) *Belonging for people with profound intellectual and multiple disabilities*. London: Routledge.

Useful Resources

Cerebral palsy: www.scope.org.uk/advice-and-support/cerebral-palsy-introduction/

Eating and swallowing difficulties: www.rcslt.org/speech-and-language-therapy/clinical-information/dy sphagia/

www.ndti.org.uk/assets/files/Dysphagia_RA_report_FINAL.pdf

Epilepsy: www.epilepsy.org.uk/

General information: www.learningdisabilities.org.uk/

Intensive interaction: www.intensiveinteraction.org/

PAMIS: https://pamis.org.uk/

PMLD: www.pmldlink.org.uk/resources/

Resource Buddy: www.resourcebuddy.co.uk/

Well-being: www.nacwellbeing.org/

Active Support: https://arcuk.org.uk/activesupport/files/2015/05/CAOL-Project-Publication.pdf

Postur al Care: www.nes.scot.nhs.uk/media/dzwncusg/postural_care_learning_byte.pdf

CHAPTER 7

Paul McAleer and Pepsi Takawira

Intellectual disability nursing in forensic settings

Introduction

This chapter explores key competencies, skills, and the knowledge base required for intellectual disability nurses working in a range of forensic settings. Explicit links will be made to the Nursing and Midwifery Council (NMC) (2018a) *Future Nurse: Standards of Proficiency For Registered Nurses*, and the Nursing and Midwifery Board of Ireland (NMBI) (2016) domains of competences for entry to the professional register for nurses that demonstrate how these prepare nurses to care for people with forensic health and social care needs. Forensic is an adjective, which, when used with other terms, has come to mean an activity that is linked to courts and criminal investigation. In relation to intellectual disabilities the term forensic is usually applied, although not always, to people who have offended and been dealt with by the courts. In relation to those who have not offended, the term forensic is often applied to people with intellectual disabilities who present a significant risk to others and who *may* commit an offence. Additionally, they may also present a significant risk to themselves through self-injurious behaviour, although this is not always the case.

It therefore follows that forensic nursing involves assessing and planning the care of people who have usually offended and have had contact with the criminal justice system. Forensic health and social care services for people with intellectual disabilities are now well established in many parts of the UK and Ireland, and contemporary provision has been aligned with national policies on service planning and development (NHS England, 2015). Providing intellectual disability nursing to people with forensic needs is a highly complex area of practice that involves balancing the tensions between offering person-centred and therapeutic care within contemporary rights-based cultures, and the need to manage and reduce risk within a legally authorised framework of restrictive practices or environments.

DOI: 10.4324/9781003296461-7

Box 7.1 This chapter will focus on the following issues:

- Case study
- Epidemiology/prevalence
- Service development and configuration
- Sexually harmful behaviour
  - Assessment
  - Formulation
  - Treatment
- Arson
  - Causation
  - Assessment
  - Interventions
- Risk assessment and risk management
- The Mental Health Act
  - Section 17: Supervised community treatment – compulsory treatment orders (CTOs)
  - Section 37: Hospital order
  - The Mental Capacity Act (MCA) 2005 Deprivation of Liberty Safeguards (DOLS)
- De-escalation, physical intervention and restrictive practice

People with intellectual disabilities and forensic presentations have a diverse range of complex needs. Their behaviours constitute a risk, and often result in offending, and include physical aggression or violence, sexually harmful behaviour, arson, destruction of property, substance misuse, and self-injurious behaviours. The causation of these behaviours is often extremely complex with a multifactorial range of contributory factors, including a dual diagnosis of mental disorder and intellectual disabilities, the presence of Autistic Spectrum Disorder, acquired brain injury, and psychosocial disorders, such as complex post-traumatic stress disorders which arise from adverse life experiences such as abuse, and institutionalisation. People with intellectual disabilities and a forensic history will often have had involvement with a wide range of clinical professionals and agencies, including psychiatry, psychology, education, the police, and criminal justice system.

It is evident that this complex area of practice requires intellectual disability nurses who specialise in this area to acquire an evidence-based body of knowledge, and the requisite skills and competencies to deliver effective nursing care within a multidisciplinary and multiagency context. Whilst there has been a lack of clarity in relation to the core nursing competencies expected of the forensic intellectual disability nurse, evidence suggests that competencies should reflect the ever-expanding knowledge base that supports the move away from hospital-centred care, and towards community models which support trauma-informed approaches to care (Lovell and Skellern, 2020).

This chapter explores this core knowledge base and the core competencies by specifically focusing on sexually harmful behaviour, arson, managing risk, and the Mental Health Act 1983. The case illustration provided by 'Jason' will be used to illustrate key points throughout.

Box 7.2 Competences

Nursing and Midwifery Council (2018a) Proficiencies

Platform 1: Being an accountable professional – 1.1, 1.2, 1.8, 1.9, 1.14, 1.18

Platform 2: Promoting health and preventing ill health – 2.1, 2.2, 2.3, 2.4, 2.5, 2.6, 2.7, 2.8, 2.11

Platform 3: Assessing needs and planning care – 3.1, 3.3, 3.4, 3.5, 3.6, 3.9, 3.13, 3.16

Platform 4: Providing and evaluating care – 4.8, 4.11

Platform 5: Leading and managing nursing care and working in teams – 5.4, 6.5

Nursing and Midwifery Board of Ireland (2016) Competences

Domain 2: Nursing practice and clinical decision-making competences – 2.1, 2.2, 2.3, 2.4, 2.5

BOX 7.3 CASE STUDY 7.1

Jason is 19 years of age and is currently detained under section 37/41 of the Mental Health Act 1983 in a medium-secure unit operated by a private company. He is accommodated in a 12-bedded unit within a large forensic hospital campus, which has six other units that provide treatment for specific groups of people requiring treatment in a forensic setting. The campus, which is eight miles from the town centre and 130 miles from Jason's hometown, is on the site of a pre-existing psychiatric hospital and some of the older buildings have been retained and modernised. The specific purpose of Jason's unit (which is referred to as a ward) is to assess and treat men with intellectual disabilities who have offended in law. It is predominantly staffed by intellectual disability nurses and unqualified support staff, although there are two registered mental nurses and one registered general nurse. The hospital also employs an extensive multidisciplinary team, including two psychiatrists, psychologists, occupational therapists, and psychotherapists.

Jason has a long history of sexually harmful and offending behaviours, which first came to the attention of services when he was 12. At this age, teachers at his school for people with special educational needs expressed concerns about both sexually harmful behaviour and fire setting. Jason would regularly expose his genitals and attempt to touch the genitals of both male and female pupils. He would also set fire to waste bins and the school bags of other pupils, and the police arrested him for setting fire to a large haystack. At this stage he was referred to both the children's community intellectual disability team and the Child and Adolescent Mental Health Service (CAMHS). Both teams assessed Jason, and some services where offered. These included respite care and structured care plans that required family involvement. At this stage, intellectual disability nurses and other members of the multidisciplinary team gathered important information that could explain some of the reasons why Jason displayed these behaviours of concern.

Jason lived in an overcrowded house, provided by social housing on a deprived estate. He has six siblings who have three different fathers. It became evident that Jason, and all his siblings, had been sexually, physically, and psychologically abused by his father and by the fathers of his siblings. It was noted that Jason's mother colluded with the abuse and attempted to justify it by blaming her children for it. Currently, Jason's father is serving a prison sentence for abuse and there was no contact with the fathers of his siblings. Because of this, it was recommended that Jason should remain in the family home as the risk of abuse had been considerably reduced.

Jason had regular contact with intellectual disability nurses from this stage. Jason's sexually harmful behaviour was assessed and treated by members of the community intellectual disability team and CAHMS. His behaviours did remain concerning but were assessed as becoming less dangerous and more manageable. Jason's dangerous behaviour suddenly escalated when he was 18.

At this stage, Jason's father was due to be released from prison and Jason was just about to leave school. He was arrested by the police because he had set fire to two large waste bins outside a leisure centre, and he was seen by members of the public to try to 'grab' passing children while threatening to throw them into the burning bins. When he was interviewed by the police, an intellectual disability nurse who knew Jason was present as an appropriate adult. She was also the diversion from custody officer who was present in court where she advised that Jason would benefit from assessment and treatment in a specialist forensic unit.

Box 7.4
Learning Activity 7.1

In the case study, Jason has been detained under the Mental Health Act in a medium-secure unit in which he has his own room. He has access to communal areas, involvement from the multidisciplinary team, and escorted trips into the community as part of his care plan. Consider what could be done to ensure that Jason is treated in as person-centred a way as is possible within this predominantly controlled environment. Make a list of your ideas and then go to Learning Activity 7.2.

> **Box 7.5**
> **Learning Activity 7.2**
>
> Learning Activity 7.1 requested that you consider and make a list of things that could be done so that Jason could be treated in person-centred ways. You should now think about the 'barriers' within forensic settings that could prevent you from implementing your ideas. Make a list of these barriers and then think of ways in which you can overcome them.

Epidemiology/prevalence

Hayes (2018) has suggested that due to a combination of inter-linking factors, the prevalence and epidemiology of offending in intellectual disability remains extremely difficult to accurately define. It is a fact that historically, and particularly in the first half of the twentieth century, there was a widespread belief that people with intellectual disabilities had a higher propensity to offend than did the general public. Johnston (2005) contends that this belief was to some extent the result of misconception, prejudice, and the stigmatisation of people with intellectual disabilities in general.

From approximately 1950, and particularly within the last 30 years, attempts have been made through research studies to ascertain the proportion of people more accurately with intellectual disabilities who offend within the population of people with intellectual disabilities and compare this with that of the general public. Talbot (2009) has reported that there is an overrepresentation of people with intellectual disabilities in criminal justice settings with a prevalence of 7% in UK prisons (people with intellectual disabilities represent approx. 2% of the overall population). Hayes (2018) reports that a combination of variable factors can lead to a degree of inaccuracy in identifying people with intellectual disabilities in the criminal justice system and suggests that only evidence derived from whole population samples, and which use reliable diagnostic instruments will provide an accurate estimate. Variable factors and limited knowledge of intellectual disabilities within the criminal justice system may lead to an individual with intellectual disabilities receiving admission to prison rather than person-centred, specialist support (Talbot, 2011). These variables include applying the arbitrary IQ of 70 to include and exclude those studied, which can result in those with 'mild or borderline' intellectual disabilities with a forensic history being dealt with inappropriately. Other variables include the belief that people with intellectual disabilities who commit crimes are less likely to be able to conceal their offences than can people in the general public and lack insight into their offending behaviour and its outcomes. They can be suggestible and therefore manipulated by others to commit offences, and an eagerness to please may make them more likely to confess to offences.

Harding, Deeley and Robertson (2010) have attempted to summarise the evidence base in relation to the epidemiology of offending behaviour and people with intellectual disabilities. They suggest that there is some degree of correlation between intellectual disabilities and offending with people with mild intellectual disabilities being more likely than the general public to commit offences, and those with moderate or severe intellectual disabilities less likely to offend. Hayes (2018) reports that the overrepresentation of people with intellectual disabilities in the criminal justice system may be explained through psychosocial factors such as cognitive impairment and limitations in moral reasoning, emotional dysregulation, memory difficulties, lack of knowledge about the law and legal system, and communication barriers. Socio-economic factors such as poverty, limited access to adapted health services (for example, substance misuse programmes), prosocial community supports, adequate housing, and educational and employment opportunities may also play a significant role. It should be noted that Hodgins (1992) has reported that a birth cohort study indicated that women with intellectual disabilities are four times more likely to offend than women with an average IQ, and that the likelihood of committing a violent offence is 25 times greater. These figures are very different from those relating to the general public, as men are responsible for 90% of violent crimes.

Johnston (2005) has commented that there is a lack of clarity as to whether the personal characteristics of offenders who have intellectual disabilities are the same as those of the general public. It does seem to be the case that there are some comorbid factors associated with intellectual disabilities that predispose a propensity to offend, but also that many predisposing psychosocial factors are the same as those of the general public. Intellectual disability nurses working in forensic settings need to be aware of the factors that influence epidemiology so that they can effectively assess and plan care. A comprehensive knowledge of comorbid factors and broad psychosocial issues is therefore a requirement of forensic intellectual disability nursing.

Service development and configuration

Beacock (2005) and Mason, Phipps and Melling (2010) have outlined the development of forensic intellectual disability services from historical and political perspectives. The overarching political and philosophical agenda of the closure of the large institutions to be replaced by care in the community has resulted in the contemporary provision of forensic intellectual disability services. This process can be tracked back in a timeline commencing with the publication in 1971 of *Better Services for the Mentally Handicapped*, followed by a plethora of subsequent key policy documents such as the Reed Report (DH, 1992), the *NHS and Community Care Act* (DH, 1990), *Valuing People* (DH, 2001), *Valuing People Now* (DH, 2009a), The Bradley Report (DH, 2009b), NICE guidelines for challenging behaviour (2015), and NICE guidelines for mental health and intellectual disabilities (2016). This chapter cannot focus in any depth on the specific detail of each of these reports and other similar documents. They have been mentioned to demonstrate that government policy and clinical practice agendas have resulted in the development of the current provision of forensic intellectual disability services and that this to a large extent dictates the way that health and social care is delivered to people with intellectual disabilities, across a range of forensic care settings. It should be noted that some of this policy guidance can be interpreted as being, at best, contradictory, and, at worst, difficult to implement within forensic settings. For example, a person with intellectual disabilities who has offended and is detained under a section of the Mental Health Act 1983 could be excluded from all four key principles from *Valuing People* (rights, independence, choice, and inclusion) as a result of their detention.

Mason and Phipps (2010) have suggested that the development of forensic intellectual disability service provision that resulted from the de-institutionalisation of intellectual disability services and gathered pace in the 1980s lacked coordination and strategic planning. Whilst this initially resulted in a range of forensic intellectual disability service provision that varied in scope and function depending on locality and the historical development of local services, regional models of care have now been developed to provide consistency in composition and delivery of forensic health and social care services (Kennedy, 2022). The spectrum of forensic services that has developed includes high-, medium-, and low-secure units for inpatients and services that are part of the functions of the following

- Community intellectual disability teams
- Specialist community forensic intellectual disability teams
- Generic mental health services
- Youth offending teams
- Forensic child and adolescent mental health (CAMHS) teams
- Specialist mental health teams for people with intellectual disabilities
- Local multiagency networks involving police, probation, courts and diversion from custody schemes

Mason, Phipps and Melling (2010) have commented that these differing service models can create internal tensions between clinicians as a result of differing assumptions about the primary functions and purposes of forensic services. Forensic services can be seen to be influenced by the law, the biopsychosocial model, politics, protection of the public, and therapeutic treatment. Irrespective of these sometimes-contradictory factors, the primary purpose of forensic services and of intellectual disability nurses in forensic settings is to assess and treat people in therapeutic ways. Whereas this is the stated intention of forensic intellectual disability services, the Department of Health (2007) has reported that in many instances inpatient units can become controlling mini-institutions that do not provide a therapeutic environment and often intensify mental distress. The most egregious example of this is provided by the recent gratuitous abuse of people at Winterbourne View (DH, 2012). It is evident that forensic intellectual disability nurses need to operate from an ethical value base and attempt to offer personalised care within systems that by their very nature can be extremely controlling.

So far, this chapter has begun to outline some of the complexities involved with delivering nursing care to people with intellectual disabilities with forensic needs, in a range of secure or community settings. It would seem self-evident that there should be consensus in relation to the core competencies, requisite skills, and role expectations of intellectual disability nurses working in forensic settings; however, there is limited evidence to support this. Lovell *et al.* (2014) contend that nurses perceive knowledge assimilation, personal attributes, effective team working, communication, and decision-making skills as being the competencies most critical to high quality forensic nursing care. Whilst Mason, Phipps and Melling (2010) have previously expressed concern about the preparation that intellectual disability nurses receive during their pre-registration nurse training, the NMC (2018a) have developed new guidelines for undergraduate nursing that standardise a range of core competencies which can be applied to forensic nursing within existing fields of practice. Thus, it can be argued that the core competencies required for intellectual disability nursing in forensic settings are introduced at the earliest point in the nurse's career and developed in practice settings to reflect the diverse and complex needs of the people being treated within them. A research study by Mason and Phipps (2010) has attempted to ascertain what practising intellectual disability and mental health nurses working in intellectual disability forensic settings considered to be the 10 most required core competencies for their role. In summary the skills and competencies identified were the following

1. Risk assessment and risk management
2. Multidisciplinary (and multiagency) working
3. De-escalation
4. Identification of triggers
5. Management of aggression
6. Interventions to manage specific offences
7. Communication
8. Physical intervention and restrictive practices
9. Early interventions
10. Clear boundaries

Whilst Lovell and Bailey (2016) contend that the competencies required for forensic nursing in intellectual disability health and social care are in a state of continuous evolution to meet the ever-changing needs of people intellectual disabilities, it is clear that some of these areas, such as multidisciplinary working and communication continue to be linked directly to the generic domains of competence within the NMC (2018a) *Future nurse: Standards of proficiency for registered nurses*, and the Nursing and Midwifery Board of Ireland (2016) standards. It is also evident that others, such as risk assessment and risk management, are linked to field-specific competencies. However, it should be noted that important issues such as interventions to manage specific offences are unlikely to be explicitly incorporated into NMC field-specific competencies. Because of this, intellectual disability nurses working within forensic settings should develop knowledge and skills relating to areas not covered by field-specific competencies through preceptorship and continuous professional development. The most common behaviours associated with people with intellectual disabilities in forensic settings, and which are unlikely to be incorporated in depth into field competencies, are destruction of property, self-injurious behaviour, arson, and sexually harmful behaviour. The chapter will now offer an exploration of sexual offending and arson, which are the two areas of offending behaviour associated with intellectual disabilities that result in the involvement of forensic services.

Sexually harmful behaviour

Riding (2005) has commented that, although on balance research findings can be equivocal, people with intellectual disabilities are more likely to enter the criminal justice system as a result of sexual offending than the general public. One significant factor to consider is the increased prevalence of childhood and lifetime adversity that is experienced by people with intellectual disabilities. A study by Reavis (2013) found that sexual abuse lay alongside disproportionately higher rates of adverse childhood experiences (ACEs), experienced by people convicted of sexual offences. Furthermore, people with intellectual disabilities are acknowledged to be at higher risk of becoming exposed to ACEs and to experience sexual abuse (Byrne, 2018).

The assessment and treatment of people with intellectual disabilities who exhibit sexually harmful behaviour presents some extremely difficult and complex challenges to nurses working within forensic environments. Taylor (2021) has stressed the necessity of using a trauma-informed approach to delivering person-centred and holistic care planning in relation to people with intellectual disabilities who display sexually harmful behaviours. Person-centred and holistic care planning using the nursing process (assessment, planning, implementation, and evaluation) is explicitly covered both within competencies detailed within the NMC (2018a) *Future nurse: Standards of proficiency for registered nurses*, and the Nursing and Midwifery Board of Ireland (2016) standards. Intellectual disability nurses working within forensic settings will therefore be expected to be able to engage in trauma-sensitive, holistic, person-centred care planning. Because there are some specific skills and areas of knowledge that relate to care planning and sexually harmful behaviour, nurses working in forensic settings will, at post-qualification, be required to expand their knowledge and skills base to effectively assess and treat people with intellectual disabilities who display sexually harmful behaviour.

Sexually harmful and offending behaviour encompasses a wide range of manifestations. Riding (2005) has explained that sexual offences can be divided into three areas as follows

- Behaviour that involves another person or people regardless of whether there has been physical contact
- Behaviour where there are issues of consent
- The illegality or unacceptable deviance of a behaviour, irrespective of whether this has resulted in a conviction

Within these categories specific examples of sexual offending include rape (vaginally, orally, and anally), touching of body parts, paedophilia, bestiality, voyeurism, exhibitionism, and the downloading of obscene images from the Internet. This list of offending behaviours serves to illustrate not only the diverse nature of offending behaviour but also the serious nature of these offences and how these often elicit moral revulsion from members of the public and nurses.

The generic domains within the NMC (2018a) *Future nurse: Standards of proficiency for registered nurses*, and the Nursing and Midwifery Board of Ireland (2016) *Nurse registration programme standards and requirements* reinforce the necessity of treating clients in non-judgemental and therapeutic ways, and these competencies often need to be reinforced when working with people who have committed sexual offences such as paedophilia.

The causation and development of sexually harmful and offending behaviours displayed by people with intellectual disabilities can be highly complex and multifactorial. Hepworth and Wolverson (2006) have emphasised the necessity of using global and robust assessment processes to ascertain the cause(s) of an individual's sexually harmful behaviour. Effective formulations and appropriate interventions can only be arrived at and implemented when based on thorough and accurate assessment. Bennet and Henry (2010) have pointed out that the reasons why people with intellectual disabilities commit sexual offences can be similar or the same as those that apply to the general public, but there are some specific factors relating to people with intellectual disabilities that increase the propensity to commit sexual offences.

When considering the factors which lead to the perpetration of sexually harmful behaviour by an individual with intellectual disabilities, it is important to think about 'mens rea' or in other words the intentionality of the individual's actions. Behaviours which could constitute a sexual offence can be categorised into two ways which are dependent on an individual's cognitive capacity and degree of insight. People with severe or moderate intellectual disabilities who engage in sexually harmful behaviour, for example, may not have the capacity to understand the risks or potential consequences of the behaviour for themselves or others. In these instances, the behaviours may be considered as behaviours that challenge. Offending behaviours, on the other hand, are those which are intentionally perpetrated by an individual who has 'mens rea', that is, the capacity to understand that the behaviour would constitute legal wrongdoing (Hounsome, Newton and Banks, 2018). These individuals may have deviant ideas about sexuality and have some understanding that these are socially unacceptable or illegal. Bennet and Henry (2010) explain how various models can be applied to understand this type of offending. Finklehor's model, which was originally proposed in relation to sexual offences against children, has been adapted so that it can be used with people who have intellectual disabilities. The model has four components as follows

1. The motivation to sexually abuse, or the 'thinking stage', which includes having a strong sexual attraction to children and fantasising about sexual activity with them.
2. Overcoming moral restraint: This involves 'rationalising' sexual offences by providing cognitive distortions or 'excuses', such as the victim 'enjoyed' the sexual contact or 'deserved' it due to their provocative behaviour.

3. Overcoming external barriers or creating the opportunity for sexual assault: This involves overcoming the victim's resistance and planning where the offence will take place.
4. Overcoming the victim's resistance: This can include grooming, threats, or force (Finklehor, 1986).

Wolf (1988) has proposed a similar model, which is often applied to people with intellectual disabilities who commit sexual offences. This model explains sexual offending as a 'vicious cycle' that leads to repetitive offending. The cycle begins with an individual experiencing a negative self-concept and low self-esteem, which leads to social isolation and the expectation of sexual rejection. To manage these negative emotions, and in the absence of appropriate coping strategies, the individual engages in deviant escapist fantasies, which will eventually lead to stages 2, 3, and 4 of the Finklehor model. Riding (2005) has suggested that having a physical disability alongside intellectual disabilities may compound associated factors that lead to low self-esteem and therefore entrench the 'vicious cycle' outlined within Wolf's model.

Some other causative factors of sexual offending apply equally to the general public and people with intellectual disabilities. It is widely recognised that a dysfunctional family upbringing can lead to sexual offending, particularly where sexually harmful behaviour is accepted (McBrien, Newton and Banks, 2010). Other causative theories are the following:

- emotional dysregulation
- impulsivity
- the self-perception that the individual does not conform to stereotypical views of masculinity.

Offences that are perpetrated by people who do not understand that their behaviours are illegal or unacceptable are sometimes collectively as referred to as 'counterfeit deviance' (Griffiths *et al.*, 2013), and some specific aspects of this are:

- Lack of opportunity to develop appropriate sexual relationships.
- Poor sex education.
- Limited interpersonal and social skills.
- Sexual naivety.
- Lack of appropriate role models or lack of encouragement to adopt appropriate behaviour.
- Relating to pedophilia: It has been suggested that the psychosexual developmental age of the offender is congruent with the age of those that they commit offences against.
- Sexually harmful behaviour lacks a sexual motive and serves a communicative function: This is particularly so for people with poor verbal skills, who may use sexually harmful behaviour to draw attention to abuse, 'escape' from uncomfortable situations, or to gain attention.

Most research findings relating to sexual offending in intellectual disabilities focuses on psychosocial causative factors. Although this is the case, it should be noted that there are some potential organic causations, which are listed in Box 7.1. In the case of Jason, a thorough assessment indicated that there was no apparent organic causation; it did reveal a combination of psychosocial causations relating to his intellectual disability and history of abuse. Jason did have some awareness that his offending behaviour was illegal; however, his intellectual disability also contributed to his offending as a result of some aspects on counterfeit deviance, particularly his limited interpersonal skills, lack of appropriate role models, and lack of opportunity to form appropriate sexual relationships.

Box 7.6 The potential organic causations of sexually harmful behaviours

- Damage to the frontal lobe of the brain
- Side effects of medication
- Neurological abnormalities
- Klinefelter's syndrome
- Temporal lobe epilepsy
- Acquired brain injury

Assessment

The discussion of the causative factors that can lead to an individual with a intellectual disability committing a sexual offence indicates the complex and diverse nature of this behaviour. To reflect this complexity and to plan targeted interventions it is therefore imperative that intellectual disability nurses working in forensic settings have the necessary competencies to be involved in the assessment of individuals who have committed sexual offences. Lofthouse *et al.,* (2013) state that historical assessments on risk of sexual harm have attempted to predict recidivism by focusing on static factors, that is, factors that are unlikely to change over time. More recent research has demonstrated that risk assessments which include dynamic assessment of stable and acute factors alongside static factors, are a more reliable method of proactively identifying and managing risk factors associated with sexual offending in people with intellectual disabilities (Lofthouse *et al.,* 2013). One such assessment tool, the Armidilo-S (Boer *et al.,* 2013) provides an assessment of risk factors, and protective factors, which may predict future risk of sexually offending in people with intellectual disabilities with a medium to large degree of accuracy (Lindsay *et al.,* 2018). The assessment approach itself supports the nurse to assess a range of dynamic factors that relate to both the individual and to the environments they are in. It also supports the assessment of protective factors, that is, effective treatment or interventions which positively reduce risk (Lindsay *et al.*, 2018).

When assessing the risk of sexual offending by a person with intellectual disabilities it is essential that the nurse uses a standardised and evidence-based risk assessment model, has accredited training in the use of the model, and conducts the assessment as part of a multidisciplinary or multiagency approach. The wider assessment may be informed by thorough history taking using a biopsychosocial assessment, an assessment of the individual's capacity or cognitive functioning, an assessment of the individual's sexual knowledge or an assessment of the individual's social functioning and domestic circumstances. The accuracy of these assessments will be reliant on contributions of other professions such as psychiatry, psychology, speech and language therapy, occupational therapy, and/or the social worker. It is also essential to facilitate authentic involvement of the individual, his or her advocate and/or their carers or family.

Formulation

Formulation is the process of drawing together all the information gathered from assessments and reports so that hypotheses can be made that explain why an individual engages in offending behaviour and which treatments might be the most effective to implement (McMurran, Sturmey and Wiley, 2017). Formulation can be interpreted as a form of applied functional analysis, and some methods of doing this use the S.T.A.R. approach, which involves organising assessment information into setting conditions, triggers, action, and results. Formulation can be used to form hypotheses relating to both long-term setting conditions and fixed functions, as well as more immediate situations (see Box 7.2 for an example).

In the case of Jason, the S.T.A.R. approach enabled staff to develop a formulation in relation to the complex causation and functions of his sexually harmful

Setting – The environment/social context (both long term and immediate).	Triggers.	Action – Give a detailed description of the incident.	Responses – What happened after the incident, what impact did the responses have on the individual and others within the setting.
History of dysfunctional family dynamics and sexual abuse. Limited interpersonal skills and lack of appropriate role models. Difficulties with the transition after leaving school.	Father's imminent release from prison.	Setting fire to two large waste bins outside of a leisure centre. Attempting to grab passing children while threatening to throw them into the burning bins.	Arrested by the police and sectioned under the Mental Health Act. Detention in a medium-secure unit.

Source: Zarkowska, E. (2018) *Problem Behaviour and People with Severe Intellectual Disabilities; the S.T.A.R Approach.* London: Routledge.

Table 7.1 The S.T.A.R. approach to formulation

behaviour (see Box 7.2). A range of hypotheses were drawn from the information collected in the S.T.A.R. chart with a consensus emerging that Jason's dysfunctional family background and exposure to sexual abuse, alongside his intellectual disability, were clearly causative factors in the development of his sexually harmful behaviour. Formulation also led to an understanding that his sexually harmful behaviour served a variety of functions, including an expression of emotional distress, poor anger management, displaced aggression, and desperate attempts to 'escape' from his current situation.

Formulation is a recognised tool that structures clinical decision-making of intellectual disability nurses working in forensic settings, and as such it has clear links to the NMC (2018a) *Future nurse: Standards of proficiency for registered nurses*, and the Nursing and Midwifery Board of Ireland (2016) *Nurse registration programme standards and requirements*.

Treatment

Riding (2005) has suggested that until the early 1980s treatment options were limited to close supervision, use of libido-lowering medications, and elimination of deviant sexual arousal. From the early 1980s onwards, a spectrum of largely psychosocial treatments has been developed and tested in forensic intellectual disability services (Newton *et al.*, 2011). This spectrum includes the following

- Developing appropriate interpersonal skills
- Changing offence-related attitudes through prosocial role-modelling
- Self-monitoring and regulation techniques
- Developing victim empathy
- Strategies for relapse prevention
- Cognitive restructuring and problem solving
- Increasing sexual knowledge and competence
- Addressing sexual preoccupation
- Psychological therapies (Jones and Chaplin, 2017; Morrissey and Ingamells, 2011)
- Applied service models for example, The Good Lives Model/Positive Behaviour Support

Many of the fundamental aspects of the causation and maintenance of sexually harmful behaviour, and the assessment and treatment of it also apply to other manifestations of offending behaviour such as arson, which will now be discussed.

Arson

As is the case for offending in general and in relation to sexual offences, there has been an historical belief that there was a correlation between intellectual disabilities and fire setting. It was also thought that women, and particularly pubescent girls with intellectual disabilities and psychosocial difficulties, were more likely to deliberately set fires than men with intellectual disabilities and members of the general public (Chaplin, 2010). Alexander *et al.* (2015) report that there is a plethora of research studies that suggest that people with intellectual disabilities are more likely to commit arson than other groups of people, however, they also contend that accurate numbers and comparisons are difficult to ascertain. Generalising the data from these studies is beset by difficulties as each study varies widely in terms of definition of intellectual disabilities, study samples, methodological approach, and results (Alexander *et al.*, 2015). What is clear is that arson, alongside sexual offending, is one of the two most common offences that lead to admission to forensic intellectual disability services (Hall *et al.*, 2005).

Arson is a complex phenomenon that may arise due to a combination of psychosocial causative factors, and it may serve a variety of functions for the perpetrator. As such, different terms may be used to describe phenomena, for example, arson or fire-setting. Whilst terminology is generally used interchangeably, arson refers to the criminal conviction one may receive for deliberately starting a fire with the intention of causing harm. Fire-setting refers to the behavioural act of setting fires. The assessment, treatment, and management of arson demands a skilled nursing approach from intellectual disability nurses working in forensic settings. Some of the NMC (2018a) *Future nurse: Standards of proficiency for registered nurses,* and the Nursing and Midwifery Board of Ireland (2016) will help prepare intellectual disability nurses to practise safely and offer effective and appropriate care planning skills in relation to arson.

Causation

The causation of arson is multifactorial, and Chaplin (2010) has explained that there are two typologies of arsonist who have different motivations for committing the offence. They are the following

1. *Non-pathological arson:* This is often a single offence, with the motivation of deliberately using arson as method for achieving an outcome. Examples of this include concealment of another crime, to claim insurance, to make a political statement, or for revenge.
2. *Pathological arson:* This often involves a repeated pattern of fire setting, with high rates of recidivism. It can be associated with mental ill health, personality disorder and psychosocial issues associated with intellectual disabilities.

The likelihood is that intellectual disability nurses working in forensic settings will be involved in the assessment and treatment of people who are diagnosed as 'pathological arsonists'. It is worth noting that the terms non-pathological and pathological arson is the terminology of choice in the United States, and that 'pyromania' is a diagnosis in the DSM V (TR) (American Psychiatric Association, 2022) and the ICD-11 (World Health Organisation, 2019). In the DSM V (TR), pyromania is categorised as a disruptive, impulse control, and conduct disorder.

Although the term pyromania is rarely used in practice, it illustrates that there is a belief that arson can be strongly linked to mental disorder and mental illness, and this can add to the complexity of care planning.

Alexander *et al.* (2015) and Hall *et al.* (2005) have all outlined a range of psychosocial factors that can lead to an individual with intellectual disabilities committing arson. Intellectual disability nurses working in forensic settings will be involved in the assessment of psychosocial factors that predispose an individual to commit arson and the subsequent functional analysis of this behaviour. Kelly *et al.* (2009) suggests that arson can be viewed as a maladaptive attempt to cope with intolerable situations or emotions. A study by Devapriam *et al.* (2007) found that 60% of people with intellectual disabilities who engaged in fire-setting behaviours also had a diagnosis of Emotionally Unstable Personality Disorder.

Some other suggested psychological motivations for arson include the following

■ Seeking sensational impacts from fire setting and fantasising about being involved in firefighting.
■ Seeking sexual release and pleasure from fire setting.
■ Exerting power.
■ Displaced aggression: The individual can display aggression without direct contact with other people.

Other personal and social characteristics that can predispose an individual to commit arson are social isolation/deprivation and an inability to communicate effectively. It can also be the case that an individual with intellectual disabilities may not fully understand the potentially devastating consequences of arson and may not intend to cause harm as a result of fire setting. The case study provided by Jason demonstrates how a combination of personal and social characteristics, particularly low self-esteem, poor regulation of emotions, and displaced aggression can explain his propensity to commit arson.

Assessment

There are some specific assessment tools that can be used as part of a global assessment process. There is the Fire Assessment Schedule (Murphy and Clare, 1996), which is a structured interview divided into two sections that help to assess an individual's pre- and post-fire setting thought processes. Whilst this assessment schedule remains one of the only tools specifically designed for people with intellectual disabilities, a lack of evidence about its validity, reliability and application in practice may affect confidence in its use (Collins, Langdon and Barnoux, 2022). A broader global multidisciplinary/agency range of assessments will also be necessary. In essence, these should incorporate the components already outlined earlier in this chapter in relation to sexual offending with some added assessment criteria to reflect some arson-specific issues. These criteria are that people with intellectual disabilities are the following:

- More likely than other people with intellectual disabilities to commit other offences.
- Extremely likely to re-offend if convicted for arson for a second time, and
- Often have a history of long-term behavioural problems that are most likely to be related to the destruction of property rather than direct aggression toward people.

As with the discussion of sexual offending, findings from the assessment process should be amalgamated into a formulation to help explain the development of fire-setting behaviour so that appropriate treatment can take place. This can be based on a broad behavioural functional analysis incorporating a timeline of events as outlined in the S.T.A.R. approach (see Table 7.1). Box 7.7 outlines the components of behavioural analysis in relation to fire setting.

Box 7.7 The components of behavioural analysis

Antecedents: Assessment of the psychosocial setting and circumstances, such as family background, and history of behavioural difficulties and fire setting. The presence of a mental disorder. Peer pressures, coping strategies, and impulsivity. Immediate triggers.

Behaviour: How was the offence committed? What did the individual do during the fire? Were accelerants used, and did the individual commit the offence alone?

Consequences: What did the individual gain from the fire setting, and how did he or she feel?

Interventions

Some of the treatments and interventions, particularly those based on cognitive behavioural approaches and victim empathy, are very similar to those already outlined in the discussion of sexual offending and can be applied to people who have committed arson. Specifically, components for the treatment of arson include the following:

- Helping individuals to understand the link between emotions and fire setting and to develop alternative and appropriate ways of coping with emotions, reducing impulsivity and problem solving, and
- Treating any underlying mental disorder.

It is most important to note that people with intellectual disabilities who commit arson are perceived to be dangerous and that they constitute a significant risk to the public. Although this is the case, they often present as being passive within forensic settings (Hall, Clayton and Johnson, 2005). Because of this, intellectual disability nurses working in forensic settings will need to be able to assess and manage risk. The next section of this chapter discusses risk management in forensic settings in a general way; however, it should be noted that the risk presented by people who commit arson is managed by some practical measures within forensic settings. These involve policies and procedures that apply to patients, staff, and all visitors for removing and searching for any inflammable materials.

Risk assessment and risk management

Assessing and managing risk is an essential part of practice for all intellectual disability nurses practicing in forensic settings. The discussion around offending behaviour in people with intellectual disabilities has necessitated that intellectual disability nurses working in forensic settings must be aware of and have the necessary knowledge and skills to assess and manage risk specific to forensic settings. Some of the NMC (2018a) *Future nurse: Standards of proficiency for registered nurses*, and the Nursing and Midwifery Board of Ireland (2016) *Nurse registration programme standards and requirements* will help intellectual disability nurses to effectively assess and manage risk in forensic settings. These standards and competencies relate, to some extent, to the general management of risk and being accountable for this.

The most usual and simplest definition of risk is that risk is the combination of the chance that something may occur and the harm that this could cause (Fisher and Scott, 2013). Alaszewski and Alaszewski (2011) have argued that there is a range of more complex and culturally specific definitions of risk including that of balancing person-centred positive risk taking within risk-averse services, such as forensic settings. This is key as intellectual disability nurses may be working in forensic settings that place more emphasis on the minimisation of the risks presented by patients than on person-centred therapeutic risk taking. The National Patient Safety Agency (2007) has explained that risk assessment is a sequential process based on the following five steps:

1. Identify the risk, e.g., aggression.
2. Decide who might be harmed and how, e.g., the patient, other patients, physical or emotional harm.
3. Evaluate the risk and decide on precaution(s), e.g., how significant is it, how often does it occur.
4. Record findings and implement them, including monitoring of existing risk, change in patterns of behaviour, and emergent risks.
5. Regularly review the assessment and revise as required.

Risk assessment should involve the gathering together, from as many relevant and appropriate sources as possible, of as much information as possible that relates to the level of dangerousness or risk that individual poses. Some assessment tools such as the Sainsbury Centre Risk Management Tool are particularly comprehensive in collecting important information enabling robust and effective risk assessment and planning. Keller (2016) has discussed the components of effective risk assessment, and these can be seen in Box 7.4.

These general components should underpin risk assessment and risk management in forensic settings, and they can form part of a global risk strategy alongside specific assessments for specific behaviours. Another useful assessment tool, which Lindsay *et al.* (2004) have reported to be reliable, is the Dynamic Risk Assessment and Management System (DRAMS). DRAMS predicts risk in relation to psychotic symptoms, mood, self-regulation, and compliance with routines.

As well as individual risk assessments, intellectual disability nurses working in forensic settings will also need to be aware of, and be accountable for, some aspects of managing environmental risk. Examples of this might relate to managing access to items that might heighten the level of risk posed by an individual. These procedures can apply both within forensic inpatient environments and when service-users are on escorted leave. Other examples can be seen in Box 7.5. It is important to note that these examples may constitute a deprivation of the individual's liberties, and any actions that are taken must be supported by relevant legislation, and clearly outlined in the individual's care plan. To promote accountability, any restrictions on a person's liberty should be regularly reviewed by the multidisciplinary team to ensure that they are utilised for the least amount of time necessary (NICE, 2015).

Box 7.8 The components of robust risk assessment

- The collecting together of as much personal history as possible
- A multidisciplinary approach with named professionals being given responsibility for key tasks
- Clear identification and prioritisation of behaviour(s) most likely to constitute a risk to self and others
- Identification of immediate, acute, and long-term risk
- Patient involvement whenever possible
- Relational security
- Identification of factors that could increase or decrease future risk
- Identification of factors that are likely to trigger dangerous behaviour
- Contingency options
- Arrangements for regular evaluation and revision of risk management plan

Source: Keller, J. (2016) Improving Practices of risk assessment and intervention planning for persons with intellectual disabilities who sexually offend. *Journal of Policy and Practice in Intellectual Disabilities*, 13(1), pp. 75–85.

Box 7.9 Practical precautions for managing risk in forensic inpatient settings

- Observing levels and ratio of staff to clients.
- Using safety alarms.
- Monitoring and preventing where required access to vulnerable groups such as children.
- Ensuring, if necessary, that the client is always in sight or that 'sight lines' within forensic units are kept clear.
- Minimising control or preventing access to materials that could cause harm to the client or others, such as CD cases, batteries, aerosols, and cutlery.
- Monitoring or preventing access to materials that could be used for deviant arousal, e.g., magazines containing images of children or photographs of children.

Intellectual disability nurses working in forensic settings are likely to take a lead role in assessing and managing risk, and they may have some responsibility for delegating tasks in relation to this. The NMC seven platforms of proficiency (2018a) underpin the skills necessary for practice. Both the proficiencies and other NMC future nurse standards can also support intellectual disability nurses in their involvement as named care coordinators or when providing therapeutic interventions or activities which are designed to help the individual to mitigate against risk. The role of the care coordinator has evolved from the Care Programme Approach (CPA) which was the standard framework for provision of care in secondary mental health and intellectual disabilities services in England. Approaches and frameworks for providing secondary intellectual disability services will be slightly direct in each of the home nations Wales, Scotland and Northern Ireland, and in Ireland.

The CPA Framework was a comprehensive, person-centred, systematic, and integrated approach to multiagency care planning that also involves the management of risk. CPA was introduced originally in 1991 as a result of public concerns relating to the perceived lack of supervision of people who were known to mental health services and who had been previously sectioned under the Mental Health Act 1983. A main component of the original CPA was that the supervision of CPA care plans would be the responsibility of named care coordinators. The role of the care coordinator is mostly undertaken by nurses, however, in some services it could be a social worker or Occupational Therapist.

The CPA was superseded in 2019 by the Community Mental Health Framework for Adults and Older Adults, a policy designed to place greater focus on delivering care to people within their own communities (NHS England, 2019). Whilst the Community Framework retains some of the high-quality functions of the CPA approach, it aims to provide a flexible, responsive, and personalised approach to comprehensive risk assessment and management which places emphasis on

- The complexity of an individual's needs.
- Providing greater choice for the individual.
- Attention to the views of carers and family members.
- Positive risk management.
- Professional judgement (NHS England, 2021).

The framework is well can be aligned with established support models currently utilised in forensic intellectual disability health and social care services, such as the Good Lives Model. The Good Lives model is a human rights-based approach to assessment, treatment and management which seeks to focus on and understand the reasons or needs that ground the actions of offenders. At its core, the Good Lives Model views offending behaviour as a socially unacceptable attempt to pursue a primary need; that is, the problem is not with the need itself but the ways in which the individual attempts to meet those needs (Barnao, Ward and Robertson, 2016).

This chapter has discussed that the criteria outlined previously are often characteristics associated with people with intellectual disabilities who are involved with forensic services. Because of this, intellectual disability nurses working in forensic settings will need to develop the requisite skills and use their competencies to coordinate and deliver care for these individuals. Further practice-based experience will usually be required to develop competence in this role.

Mental health legislation

Each of the home nations England, Wales, Scotland, and Northern Ireland have their own local mental health legislation. The broad purpose of the Mental Health Act is to compel people with a mental disorder to be assessed and treated for that disorder. The Mental Health Act 1983 as amended in 2007 is the most important and influential piece of legislation relating to intellectual disability nursing within forensic settings. It dictates fundamental aspects of how people detained under the Act must be treated. It also instructs and guides the operational function of nurses treating people who are detained under the Act. When working in forensic settings nurses should develop their knowledge of the most relevant sections of the Act that relate to the people in their care and ensure that they operate within the legal parameters set out in the Act.

In respect of the Mental Health Act for England, before 2007 the scope of the intellectual disability nurse to act autonomously within the Act was limited to being able to detain people for six hours under Section 5.4 (see Box 7.6 for details of this) and to involvement with CPA as a provision of Section 117 (as outlined in the previous section). After much political debate the Mental Health Act 1983 was amended in 2007. The amendments to the Mental Health Act 1983 (amended 2007), most of which went into effect in November 2008, have provided some new opportunities and challenges for intellectual disability nurses working in forensic settings. The amendments to the Act were intended to limit the impact of mental disorder on the individual and society, including safeguards against the abuse of process and access to independent review. The amendments that impact most on intellectual disability nursing within forensic settings will be explained, in turn, beginning with the change of definitions used within the Act.

Box 7.10 Section 5.4: Nurses' Holding Powers

This section of the Mental Health Act authorises registered mental health nurses and registered intellectual disability nurses to prevent a person from leaving an inpatient setting if it is in the best interests of the individual or others. This holding power can last for six hours. Nurses who intend to use Section 5.4 should base the decision to do so on the following:

- Likelihood of the patient harming themselves or others.
- Patient's expressed intentions.
- Evidence of disordered thinking.
- Recent disturbances on the ward.
- Likelihood of the individual being violent.
- Whether the individual has received any disturbing news from relatives or friends.
- Changes in usual patterns of behaviour.
- Relevant involvement with other patients.
- History of impulsivity or unpredictability.
- Formal risk assessments that have been conducted and other relevant information from the multidisciplinary team.

One fundamental amendment to the Act relates to the definitions used to apply to people who could be treated under the Act. Before the 2007 amendments, the Act attempted to define the types of mental disorder that might require an individual assessed as having that disorder to be treated under the Act (see Box 7.7 for these definitions). The two definitions most pertinent to intellectual disabilities were 'severe mental impairment' and 'mental impairment'. These definitions alone were not a reason for detention under the Act unless they were 'associated with abnormally aggressive or seriously irresponsible conduct of the person concerned'. However, it should be noted that no other specific client group was specifically identified within the 1983 Act, and this was perceived to be potentially stigmatising for people with mental impairments/ intellectual disabilities. Mental impairment and severe mental impairment are no longer definitions within the amended Act, and there is now only one definition of mental disorder. Mental disorder is now defined as 'any mental disorder of the mind'. It should be noted that, whereas this definition includes autism spectrum conditions, intellectual disabilities alone is no longer categorised as a mental disorder. This amendment therefore excludes people with intellectual disabilities from treatment or guardianship orders unless an individual's intellectual disability is 'associated with seriously irresponsible or abnormally aggressive conduct'.

A further amendment that directly applies to intellectual disability nurses is the changes to professional roles. Before the amended Act, intellectual disability nurses could only autonomously detain a person under Section 5.4 of the Act and other than this had very limited involvement with the decision to detain an individual under the Act. Prior to the amendments to the Act, the Responsible Medical Officer (RMO) and Approved Social Worker (ASW) were responsible for making applications and recommendations for detention under the Act and for making reports to Mental Health Act Tribunals. The amended Act broadens the scope of professionals who can apply and train to become an Approved Mental Health Professional (AMHP).

Box 7.11 Definitions within the Mental Health Act 1983

Mental disorder: This included mental illness, arrested or incomplete development of mind, psychopathic disorder, or disability of mind.

The Act then offers three subcategories of mental disorder as follows:

1. *Severe mental impairment:* A state of arrested or incomplete development of mind, which includes severe impairment of intelligence and social functioning, and is associated with abnormally aggressive or seriously irresponsible conduct on the part of the person concerned.
2. *Mental impairment:* A state of arrested or incomplete development of mind (not amounting to severe impairment), which includes severe impairment of intelligence and social functioning, and is associated with abnormally aggressive or seriously irresponsible conduct on the part of the person concerned.
3. *Psychopathic disorder:* A persistent disorder or disability of mind (whether or not including significant impairment of intelligence), which results in abnormally aggressive or seriously irresponsible conduct on the part of the person concerned.

Box 7.12 The role and function of the Approved Mental Health Professional

A core responsibility of the Approved Mental Health Professional (AHMP) is to conduct an independent assessment about whether to make an application to have a person compulsorily admitted to hospital. Unlike doctors, it is not the responsibility of the AHMP to diagnose a mental disorder rather they must decide whether the use of compulsory powers is the only way a person can receive the treatment and care required. The AHMP should make an application for someone to be detained under the Act only if the AHMP is satisfied that detention in hospital is the most appropriate way of providing treatment. Other duties include the following:

■ Formal engagement with a person's nearest relative.

■ Taking or arranging for a person to be taken to hospital when an application has been made.

■ Returning a person who has been absent without leave.

■ Interviewing someone detained under Section 136 by the police.

■ Involvement in deciding whether to continue or end a Community Treatment Order.

The AMHP can now take on some of the functions previously limited to the RMO and ASW. The professional groups that can apply to become AMHPs are social workers, occupational therapists, chartered psychologists, mental health nurses, and intellectual disability nurses. The role and functions of AMHPs are like those undertaken by the ASW before the amendments to the Act (see Box 7.8 for an outline of the role and function of the AMHP) with some added responsibilities relating to Section 17, Supervised community treatment (see later).

Registered medical practitioners (doctors) and the professional groups that can apply to become AMHPs can also apply to become 'approved clinicians' (ACs). An AC has the authorisation to conduct specific duties under the Act that cannot be carried out by anyone else, such as writing court reports on some patients and being responsible for certain treatments. An AC who is given overall responsibility for an individual's case becomes a responsible clinician (RC), and the functions of this role replace those of the RMO in the amended Act. To become an approved clinician/responsible clinician, it is necessary to undertake post-registration training, and to demonstrate key competencies. The competencies for approved clinicians include the following:

■ Assessment skills, such as being able to identify and evaluate the severity of mental disorder and to determine whether this requires compulsory treatment.

■ Ability to assess risk.

- Ability to include biological, psychosocial, and cultural factors within the assessment process.
- Ability to consider different treatment options.
- Demonstration of a high level of skills in determining capacity to consent.
- Ability to effectively work within a multidisciplinary context.
- Ability to make decisions without supervision in complex cases.
- Report writing and presenting evidence to courts and tribunals.

Clearly the functions of the role of the AMHP and approved clinician/responsible clinician are demanding and complex and require post-qualification training. However, it is important to note that many of the NMC generic and field-specific standards of competence can underpin the competencies required to become an AC/RC as outlined previously. These new roles require post-qualifying experiences and a lengthy training course before they can be applied for, and it is therefore unlikely that many intellectual disability nurses are currently fulfilling these roles. However, it should be noted that intellectual disability nurses are the only professional group with a specific qualification that equips them to work with people with intellectual disabilities. Because of this, the competencies gained as part of their nurse training provide a good level of underpinning skills that make them ideally suited to develop into the new roles. This is acknowledged within the Mental Health Act Code of Practice (DH, 2015), which states:

> If possible, either a consultant psychiatrist in intellectual disabilities or an AMHP with knowledge and experience of working with people with intellectual disabilities should be available to make the assessment where it appears that the detained person has an intellectual disability.

(Department of Health, 2015, p. 148)

Section 17: Supervised community treatment – Compulsory Treatment Orders (CTOs)

Another major change to the Mental Health Act 1983 was the introduction of compulsory treatment orders (CTOs). CTOs allow for people with a mental disorder to be compulsorily treated outside of hospital. An intention of this was to prevent the multiple readmissions to and discharges from hospital of 'revolving door' patients. A CTO imposes 'conditions' on the individual who is to be compulsorily treated outside of hospital. Two conditions are obligatory and are that the individual must make themselves available for medical examination

- If consideration is needed to extend the CTO.
- By second opinion doctor if required.

People who are compulsorily treated under a CTO can be recalled to hospital if there is a risk to the health and safety of the individual or a risk to other people. The clinical decision-making skills of the AHMP and the AC/RC are vital to the CTO process. It is the RC who has the responsibility for making the order to discharge an individual onto a CTO, and the AHMP must agree that it is appropriate. The RC with agreement from the AHMP can also set additional conditions other than the two obligatory ones so that the individual receives treatment for his or her mental disorder or to prevent harm to him or her or other people. The RC can recall an individual to hospital by serving notice in writing. If the individual requires more than 72 hours to be in hospital for treatment the RC should consider revoking the CTO and the AHMP must agree to this.

Section 37: Hospital order

If an individual is convicted of an offence punishable by a prison sentence, a court can authorise detention in hospital under section 37 of the MHA 1983, if it is satisfied that the offender has a mental disorder, and this includes intellectual disabilities (mental impairment). Before the 2007 amendments, this mental impairment must have been associated with seriously irresponsible or abnormally aggressive conduct, which was likely to alleviate or prevent deterioration in the individual's condition. This became known as the 'treatability test', and it has caused a degree of controversy, as it was seen to exclude some individuals from treatment.

The 2007 amendments replaced the 'treatability test' with an 'appropriate treatment test'. This requires that 'appropriate treatment' must be available in a hospital before an individual can be detained under section 37. The definition of 'appropriate treatment' is very wide and considers psychosocial factors relating to the individual such as gender, ethnicity, and culture. Intellectual disability nurses working in forensic settings have many of the requisite skills to respond to the demands of the diverse, person-centred, and holistic treatments that fall within the 'appropriate treatment' test.

The Mental Capacity Act (MCA) 2005 Deprivation of Liberty Safeguards (DOLs)

The Mental Capacity Act Deprivation of Liberty Safeguards, which came into effect in April 2009, do not apply to people who are under a section of the Mental Health Act. The MCA DOLS provide legal protection from harm for individuals who lack capacity to give informed consent for their care or treatment, and who might be deprived of their liberty in hospitals or care homes. Further elements of the MCA DOLS are that people are cared for in the least restrictive ways, and that it must be in their best interests if they are deprived of their liberty. When a care home or hospital identifies a person as being at risk of being deprived of his or her liberty, then that entity must apply to a supervisory body for authorisation of the deprivation of liberty. For care homes, the supervisory body is the local authority and for hospitals, it is the health authority. For authorisation to be granted, the supervisory body must obtain six assessments, which are conducted by assessors. Nurses are one of the professional groups identified as being suitable assessors for this purpose. One key assessment is in relation to best interests, and intellectual disability nurses working in forensic settings will need to demonstrate well-developed decision-making skills based on often competing ideas about what constitutes an individual's best interests.

Transforming care: care and treatment reviews

Following the public enquiry into the criminal abuse of people with intellectual disabilities and autism detained at Winterbourne view the department of health in England established Transforming care as a public response to the criminal abuse at Winterbourne. This response established the beginning of Care and Treatment Reviews (CTRs). CTRs were developed to improve the care of those people with intellectual disabilities, autism, or both; the aim being to reduce the admissions and unnecessary lengthy stays in hospitals including forensic settings DH, (2012). Individuals with intellectual disabilities and or autism have a right to CTRs if they are in hospital for behaviour that challenges services, mental health problems or are diverted from the criminal justice system. They are also entitled to a CTR if they are at risk of being admitted into hospital. The CTR panel is independent, however, it is chaired by a commissioner or a private chair (NHS England, 2017).

De-escalation, physical intervention and restrictive practice

Intellectual disability nurses working in forensic settings are likely to be involved in the management of threatening, hostile, and, at times, aggressive behaviour. All clinical guidance at the national and local level demands that the management of aggressive behaviour be managed in the least restrictive ways possible, and that physical restraint must be the last option. De-escalation involves responding to changes in an individual's emotional arousal level before he or she becomes physically aggressive, thus avoiding physical restraint. Kaplan and Wheeler (1983) have linked de-escalation to what they termed the 'assault cycle'. The assault cycle involves changes in physiology, such as the increased production of adrenaline, which results in heightened levels of emotional arousal and can result in overt aggression. De-escalation is a proactive response that involves observing and identifying changes in an individual's usual or 'baseline' behaviour (Pickard, Henry and Yates, 2010). Some common changes to baseline behaviour include the following

- Changes in usual communication such as raised volume, muttering, making verbal threats
- Changes in physical presentation and activity such as dilated pupils, pallor, rapid breathing, pacing, and increasing agitation
- Changes in levels of interaction such as increased demands and invading personal body space.

Intellectual disability nurses in forensic settings can use a range of communication skills to respond to these changes in arousal. Egan and Reese (2018) have developed the SOLER model of body language that can be used as a basis for how to approach an individual with increased levels of emotional arousal. The definition of SOLER follows

S – Face the individual squarely but at a slight angle
O – Adopt an open posture with arms unfolded
L – Lean slightly forward toward the individual
E – Maintain eye contact but do so intermittently as constant eye contact can be threatening
R – Model relaxed, calm, and non-threatening body language

Broader de-escalation techniques related to communication involve understanding that some individuals may have communication and comprehension difficulties and responding to these differences in ways that ensure individuals feel listened to. One practical consideration is that if several members of staff are present, then one member of staff should take the lead in communicating with an aroused individual and use short, simple, and comprehensible words and language. Chapter 26 of the Mental Health Act Code of Practice (DH, 2015) offers guidance on best practice in relation to restrictive practices

> Restrictive interventions should be used in a way that minimises any risk to the patient's health and safety and that causes the minimum interference to their autonomy, privacy and dignity, while being sufficient to protect the patient and other people. The patient's freedom should be contained or limited for no longer than is necessary. Unless there are cogent reasons for doing so, staff must not cause deliberate pain to a patient in an attempt to force compliance with their instructions (for example, to mitigate an immediate risk to life).

(DH, 2015, p. 289)

Intellectual disability nurses working in forensic settings will need the required skills and knowledge to implement physical restraint, seclusion, and rapid tranquilisation. Rapid tranquilisation involves the administration of PRN medication. The NMC Future nurse standards and the NMBI domains will have, to some extent, prepared nurses for these tasks. However, additional specific training and regular refresher training maybe required. NMC-approved nursing courses within the United Kingdom and Ireland have a mandatory requirement that nursing students cover verbal de-escalation. Competent medications management, including the use of PRN medication, is also a requirement for entry to nursing registers. Specific NICE guidelines for 2015 state that only suitably trained staff can implement these procedures. These required skills and competencies can be developed further as part of preceptorship and in-house training in forensic settings.

Conclusion

This chapter has explored the evolving role and contemporary practice of intellectual disability nursing for people with intellectual disabilities in their contact with forensic services. The implications of legislation and how this can lead to tensions between managing risk and maintaining a secure environment and person-centred approaches have been discussed.

This chapter has made evident that intellectual disability nursing in forensic settings is an increasingly specialised role that requires the development of a specifically focused knowledge base and the mastery of nursing competencies. It has been discussed that people with intellectual disabilities in forensic settings are a stigmatised, marginalised, and often vulnerable client group. Further, it has been argued that intellectual disability nurses are the only specifically trained professionals with the requisite skills and knowledge that can advocate on behalf of this stigmatised client group and offer some degree of person-centredness within forensic environments.

References

Alaszewski, A. and Alaszewski, H. (2011) Positive risk taking. In Atherton, H. and Crickmore, D. (Eds.), *Intellectual disabilities: Toward inclusion* (6th edition). London: Churchill Livingstone, pp. 179–195.

Alexander, R.T., *et al.* (2015) Arson or fire setting in offenders with intellectual disability: Clinical characteristics, forensic histories, and treatment outcomes. *Journal of Intellectual and Developmental Disability*, 40(2), pp. 189–197.

American Psychiatric Association (2022) *Diagnostic and statistical manual of mental disorders DSM – V* (text revision). Washington, DC: American Psychiatric Association.

Barnao, M., Ward, T. and Robertson, P. (2016) The good lives model: A new paradigm for forensic mental health. *Psychiatry, Psychology and Law*, 23(2), pp. 288–301.

Beacock, C. (2005) The policy context. In Riding, T., Swann, C. and Swann, B. (Eds.), *The handbook of forensic intellectual disabilities*. Padstow: Radcliffe Publishing, pp. 1–14.

Bennett, C. and Henry, J. (2010) Working with sexual offenders with intellectual disabilities. In Chaplin, E., Henry, J. and Hardy, S. (Eds.), *Working with people with intellectual disabilities and offending behaviour: A handbook*. Brighton: Pavilion Publishing, pp. 97–108.

Boer, D., *et al.* (2013) *ARMIDILO: The assessment of risk and manageability of individuals with developmental and intellectual limitations who offend*. Available at: www.armidilo.net/ (Accessed 20 June 2022).

Byrne, G. (2018) Prevalence and psychological sequelae of sexual abuse among individuals with an intellectual disability: A review of the recent literature. *Journal of Intellectual Disabilities*, 22(3), pp. 294–310.

Chaplin, E. (2010) Working with fire setters with intellectual disabilities. In Chaplin, E., Henry, J. and Hardy, S. (Eds.), *Working with people with intellectual disabilities and offending behaviour: A handbook*. Brighton: Pavilion Publishing, pp. 109–120.

Collins, J., Langdon, P.E. and Barnoux, M. (2022) The adapted fire setting assessment scale: Reliability and validity. *Journal of Intellectual Disability Research*, 66(7), pp. 642–654.

DH (1990) *The NHS and community care act. London:* HMSO.

DH (1992) *Reed report: Review of mental health and social services for mentally disordered offenders and others requiring similar services: Vol. 1 final summary report.* London: HMSO.

DH (2001) *Valuing people: A strategy for intellectual disability for the 21st century.* London: TSO.

DH (2007) *Services for people with intellectual disabilities and challenging behaviour or mental health needs.* London: TSO.

DH (2009a) *Valuing people now: A new strategy for people with intellectual disabilities.* London: TSO.

DH (2009b) *The Bradley report: Lord Bradley's review of people with mental health problems or intellectual disabilities in the criminal justice system.* London: Department of Health.

DH (2012) *Transforming care: A national response to winterbourne view hospital: Department of health review: Final report.* London: Department of Health.

DH (2015) *Mental health act 1983: Code of practice (amended 2015).* London: The Stationery Office.

Devapriam, J., *et al.* (2007) Arson: Characteristics and predisposing factors in offenders with intellectual disabilities. *The British Journal of Forensic Practice,* 9(4), pp. 23–27.

Egan, G. and Reese, R.J. (2018) *The skilled helper: A problem-management and opportunity-development approach to helping* (11th edition). Boston, MA: Cengage.

Finklehor, D. (1986) *A source on child sexual abuse.* Beverley Hills, CA: Sage.

Griffiths, D., *et al.* (2013) 'Counterfeit deviance' revisited. *Journal of Applied Research in Intellectual Disabilities,* 26, pp. 471–480.

Hall, I., Clayton, P. and Johnson, P. (2005) Arson and intellectual disability. In Riding, T., Swann, C. and Swann, B. (Eds.), *The handbook of forensic intellectual disabilities.* Padstow: Radcliffe Publishing, pp. 51–72.

Harding, D., Deeley, Q. and Robertson, D. (2010) History, epidemiology and offending. In Chaplin, E., Henry, J. and Hardy, S. (Eds.), *Working with people with intellectual disabilities and offending behaviour: A handbook.* Brighton: Pavilion Publishing, pp. 13–20.

Hayes, S. (2018) Criminal behavior and intellectual and developmental disabilities: An epidemiological perspective. In Lindsay, W. and Taylor, J.L. (Eds.), *Handbook on offenders with intellectual developmental disabilities: Research, training, practice.* Chichester: Wiley.

Hepworth, K. and Wolverson, M. (2006) Care planning and delivery in forensic settings for people with intellectual disabilities. In Gates, B. (Ed.), *Care planning and delivery in intellectual disability nursing.* Oxford: Blackwell Publishing, pp. 125–157.

Hodgins, S. (1992) Mental disorder, intellectual deficiency, and crime: Evidence from a birth cohort. *Archives of General Psychiatry,* 6, pp. 476–483.

Hounsome, J., *et al.* (2018) The structured assessment of violence risk in adults with intellectual disability: A systematic review. *Journal of Applied Research in Intellectual Disabilities,* 31(1), pp. e1–e17. doi:10.1111/jar.12295.

Johnston, S. (2005) Epidemiology of offending in intellectual disability. In Riding, T., Swann, C. and Swann, B. (Eds.), *The handbook of forensic intellectual disabilities.* Padstow: Radcliffe Publishing, pp. 15–30.

Jones, E. and Chaplin, E. (2017) A systematic review of the effectiveness of psychological approaches in the treatment of sex offenders with intellectual disabilities. *Journal of Applied Research in Intellectual Disabilities,* 33(1), pp. 79–100.

Kaplan, S.G. and Wheeler, E.G. (1983) Survival skills for working with potentially violent clients. *Social Case Work: The Journal of Contemporary Social Work,* 64(6), pp. 339–346.

Keller, J. (2016) Improving practices of risk assessment and intervention planning for persons with intellectual disabilities who sexually offend. *Journal of Policy and Practice in Intellectual Disabilities*, 13(1), pp. 75–85.

Kelly, J., *et al.* (2009) A retrospective study of historical risk factors for pathological arson in adults with mild intellectual disabilities. *British Journal of Forensic Practice*, 11(2), pp. 17–23.

Kennedy, H.G. (2022) Models of care in forensic psychiatry. *British Journal of Pyschiatric Advances*, 28(1), pp. 46–59.

Lindsay, W.R., *et al.* (2004) The dynamic risk assessment and management system: An assessment of immediate risk of violence for individuals with offending and challenging behaviour. *Journal of Applied Research in Intellectual Disabilities*, 17, pp. 267–274.

Lindsay, W.R., *et al.* (2018) The protective scale of the Armidilo-S: The importance of forensic and clinical outcomes. *Journal of Applied Research in Intellectual Disabilities*, 33(4), pp. 654–661.

Lofthouse, R.E., *et al.* (2013) Prospective dynamic assessment of risk of sexual reoffending in individuals with an intellectual disability and a history of sexual offending behaviour. *Journal of Applied Research in Intellectual Disabilities*, 26(5), pp. 394–403.

Lovell, A. and Bailey, J. (2016) Nurses' perceptions of personal attributes required when working with people with a intellectual disability and an offending background: A qualitative study. *Journal of Psychiatric and Mental Health Nursing*, 24(1), pp. 4–14.

Lovell, A. and Skellern, J. (2020) Making sense of complexity: A qualitative investigation into forensic intellectual disability nurses' interpretation of the contribution of personal history to offending behaviour. *British Journal of Intellectual Disabilities*, 48, pp. 242–250.

Lovell, A., *et al.* (2014) Working with people with intellectual disabilities in varying degrees of security: Nurses' perceptions of competencies. *Journal of Advanced Nursing*, 70(9), pp. 2041–2050.

Mason, T. and Phipps, D. (2010) Forensic intellectual disability nursing skills and competencies: A study of forensic and non-forensic nurses. *Issues in Mental Health Nursing*, 31, pp. 708–715.

Mason, T., Phipps, D. and Melling, K. (2010) Forensic intellectual disability nursing role analysis. *British Journal of Intellectual Disabilities*, 39, pp. 121–129.

McBrien, J., Newton, L. and Banks, J. (2010) The development of a sex offender assessment and treatment service within a community intellectual disability team (the SHEALD project): Mapping and assessing risk. *Tizard Intellectual Disability Review*, 15(1), pp. 31–43.

McMurran, M., Sturmey, P. and Wiley, J. (2017) *Forensic case formulation*. Chichester: Wiley-Blackwell.

Mental Capacity Act (2005) *Deprivation of liberty safeguards: Code of practice to supplement the main mental capacity act 2005 code of practice*. London: TSO.

Mental Health Act (2007) *New roles: Guidance for approving authorities and employers on approved mental health professionals and approved clinicians 2008*. National Institute for Mental Health in England. London: TSO.

Morrissey, C. and Ingamells, B. (2011) Adapted dialectical behaviour therapy for male offenders with intellectual disability in a high secure environment: Six years on. *Journal of Intellectual Disabilities and Offending Behaviour*, 2(1), pp. 10–17.

Murphy, G.H. and Clare, I.C.H. (1996) Analysis of motivation in people with mild intellectual disabilities (mental handicap) who set fires. *Psychology Crime and Law*, 2, pp. 153–164.

National Patient Safety Agency (2007) *Healthcare risk assessment made easy*. London: National Patient Safety Executive.

NHS England (2015) *Supporting people with a intellectual disability and/or autism who display behaviour that challenges, including those with a mental health condition; Service model for commissioners of health and social care services*. London: NHS England.

NHS England (2017) *Care and treatment reviews*. Available at: www.england.nhs.uk/intellectual-disabilities/care/ctr/ (Accessed 15 June 2022).

NHS England (2019) *The community mental health framework for adults and older adults*. Available at: www.england.nhs.uk/wp-content/uploads/2019/09/community-mental-health-framework-for-adults-and-older-adults.pdf (Accessed 15 June 2022).

NHS England (2021) *Care programme approach: NHS England and NHS improvement position statement Ref: PAR526*. Available at: www.england.nhs.uk/wp-content/uploads/2021/07/Care-Programme-Approach-Position-Statement_FINAL_2021.pdf (Accessed 15 June 2022).

NICE (2015) *Challenging behaviour and intellectual disabilities: Prevention and interventions for people with intellectual disabilities whose behaviour challenges*. Available at: www.nice.org.uk/guidance/ng11/resources/challenging-behaviour-and-intellectual-disabilities-prevention-and-interventions-for-people-with-intellectual-disabilities-whose-behaviour-challenges-pdf-1837266392005 (Accessed 15 June 2022).

NICE (2016) *Mental health problems in people with intellectual disabilities: Prevention, assessment and management*. Available at: www.nice.org.uk/guidance/ng54/resources/mental-health-problems-in-people-with-intellectual-disabilities-prevention-assessment-and-management-pdf-1837513295557 (Accessed 15 June 2022).

Newton, L., *et al.* (2011) The development of a sex offender assessment and treatment service within a community intellectual disability team (the SHEALD Project): Part 2. *Tizard Intellectual Disability Review*, 16(3), pp. 6–16.

Nursing and Midwifery Board of Ireland (2016) *Nurse registration programmes standards and requirements*. Dublin: NMBI.

Nursing and Midwifery Council (2018a) *Future nurse: Standards of proficiency for registered nurses*. London: NMC.

Nursing and Midwifery Council (2018b) *Standards framework for nursing and midwifery education*. London: NMC.

Pickard, M., Henry, J. and Yates, D. (2010) Working with violent offenders with intellectual disabilities. In Chaplin, E., Henry, J. and Hardy, S. (Eds.), *Working with people with intellectual disabilities and offending behaviour: A handbook*. Brighton: Pavilion Publishing, pp. 121–132.

Reavis, J. (2013) Adverse childhood experiences and adult criminality: How long must we live before we possess our own lives? *The Permanente Journal*, 17(2), pp. 44–48.

Riding, T. (2005) Sexual offending in people with intellectual disabilities. In Riding, T., Swann, C. and Swann, B. (Eds.), *The handbook of forensic intellectual disabilities*. Padstow: Radcliffe Publishing, pp. 31–50.

Talbot, J. (2009) No one knows: Offenders with intellectual disabilities and intellectual difficulties. *International Journal of Prisoner Health*, 5(3), pp. 141–152.

Talbot, J. (2011) Working with offenders. In Atherton, H. and Crickmore, D. (Eds.), *Intellectual disabilities: Toward inclusion* (6th edition). London: Churchill Livingstone Elsevier, pp. 339–356.

Taylor, J. (2021) Compassion in custody: Developing a trauma sensitive intervention for men with developmental disabilities who have convictions for sexual offending. *Advances in Mental Health and Intellectual Disabilities*, 15(5), pp. 185–200.

Wolf, S.C. (1988) A model of sexual aggression/addiction (Special issues: The sexually unusual guide to understanding and helping). *Journal of Social Work and Human Sexuality*, 7, pp. 131–148.

World Health Organisation (2019) *ICD – 11 classifications of mental and behavioural disorder: Clinical descriptions and diagnostic guidelines*. Geneva: World Health Organisation.

Zarkowska, E. (2018) *Problem behaviour and people with severe intellectual disabilities the S.T.A.R approach*. London: Routledge.

Further Reading

Bennett, C. and Henry, J. (2010) Working with sexual offenders with intellectual disabilities. In Chaplin, E., Henry, J. and Hardy, S. (Eds.), *Working with people with intellectual disabilities and offending behaviour: A handbook*. Brighton: Pavilion Publishing, pp. 97–108.

Chaplin, E., Henry, J. and Hardy, S. (Eds.) (2010) *Working with people with intellectual disabilities and offending behaviour: A handbook*. Brighton: Pavilion Publishing.

Craig, L.A., Lindsay, W.R. and Browne, K.D. (Eds.) (2010) *Assessment and treatment of sexual offenders with intellectual disabilities: A handbook*. Chichester: Wiley-Blackwell.

Department of Health and Social Care (2010) *Positive practice outcomes: A handbook for professionals in the criminal justice system working with offenders with intellectual disabilities*. Available at: www.gov.uk/government/publications/positive-practice-positive-outcomes-a-handbook-for-professionals-in-the-criminal-justice-system-working-with-offenders-with-a-learning-disability (Accessed 28 July 2022).

Fisher, M. and Scott, M. (2013) *Patient safety and managing risk in nursing*. London: Sage.

McMurran, M., Sturmey, P. and Wiley, J. (2017) *Forensic case formulation*. Chichester: Wiley-Blackwell.

Swann, C. and Swann, B. (Eds.). (2005) *The handbook of forensic intellectual disabilities*. Padstow: Radcliffe Publishing.

Useful Resources/Addresses

ARMIDILO (The Assessment of Risk and Manageability of Individuals with Developmental and Intellectual Limitations who Offend): www.armidilo.net/

Sainsbury Centre for Menta l Health: https://mentalhealthpartnerships.com/publisher/sainsbury-centre-for-mental-health/

British Institute of Intellectual Disa bilities: www.bild.org.uk

Tizar d Centre: www.kent.ac.uk/tizard/

The Ann Cra ft Trust: www.anncrafttrust.org/?gclid=Cj0KCQjwio6XBhCMARIsA C0u9aHCflqTXMTGCk2yzDyyFv_Euj-UCLFxAtTcNvDdbhIqTLh2sQELoB0 aAlxKEALw_wcB

CHAPTER 8

Linda Hume, Jo Delrée and Ailish McMeel

Challenging and distressed behaviour in people with intellectual disabilities: the role of intellectual disability nursing

Introduction

The support of people with intellectual disabilities who present with challenging or distressed behaviour by intellectual disability nurses has never been so important. This chapter promotes the unique contribution that intellectual disability nursing can provide in promoting holistic support, whilst drawing from a strong value and professional base. This chapter discusses the role of the intellectual disability nurse in leading change and improving the quality of services and supports for people with intellectual disabilities who display distressed and challenging behaviour.

The abuse of people with intellectual disabilities who have challenging behaviours and/or mental health needs in care settings has, sadly, been reported numerous times over the past few decades, but most recently at Whorlton Hall, Ely hospital and Winterbourne View in England, and at Muckamore Abbey Hospital in Northern Ireland as recently as 2020. These have led to Government commissioned investigations and reports, and changes to policy and good practice guidance (DH, 2012; Bubb, 2014; Lenehan, 2017; Willis, 2020). Targets were set in these documents for reductions in hospital care for people with intellectual disabilities who also have mental health needs or complex challenging behaviours. In England, reports have shown that targets have been repeatedly missed, and that standards of care and support are still below that which this group of people deserve.

The registered intellectual disability nurse has a key role to play in changing this situation. They also have an important safeguarding role, being alert to the signs and symptoms of abuse, and taking appropriate action to prevent and address abusive situations. The knowledge and skills of the intellectual disability nurse are crucial in assessing the needs of individuals with complex needs and challenging behaviours, and in developing appropriate supports, alongside the multidisciplinary team to ensure that people with intellectual disabilities can be supported in their communities, rather than in institutional care. Later sections in this chapter will provide an overview of the background and philosophy of Positive Behavioural Supports, a key philosophy and strategy for supporting individuals with challenging behaviour, and other interventions that intellectual disability nurses, along with colleagues from other disciplines, can implement to avoid the need for institutional care.

DOI: 10.4324/9781003296461-8

Box 8.1 This chapter will focus on the following issues:

- Definitions and terminology
- Prevalence of challenging behaviour
- Understanding behaviour
  - Behavioural Phenotypes
  - Physical illness, Pain and Distress
  - Mental illness and challenging behaviour
  - Trauma-informed practice
- Supporting challenging behaviour
  - Applied Behavioural Analysis
  - Positive Behaviour Support
  - Assessment
  - Social construct of behaviour
  - Ecological systems theory
  - Functional behaviour assessment
  - Formulation and functions of behaviour
- Positive Behaviour Support plans
  - Ecological Strategies
  - New Skills and Opportunities
  - Prevention (Focused Support) Strategies
  - Reactive Strategies
- Restrictive Practices
  - Implementation
  - Evaluation
- Other evidence-based approaches
  - Person-Centred Active Support
  - Communication

The content of this chapter is contextualised within the Nursing and Midwifery Council (NMC, 2018) of the United Kingdom and Nursing and Midwifery Board of Ireland (2016) standards and requirements for competence.

Box 8.2 Competences

Nursing and Midwifery Council (2018) Proficiencies

Platform 1: Being an accountable professional - 1.1, 1.9, 1.11, 1.12, 1.13, 1.14, 1.15, 1.18, 1.20

Platform 2: Promoting health and preventing ill health - 2.1, 2.2, 2.3, 2.4, 2.5, 2.6, 2.7, 2.8, 2.9, 2.10, 2.11, 2.12

Platform 3: Assessing needs and planning care - 3.1, 3.2, 3.3, 3.4, 3.5, 3.6, 3.7 3.8, 3.9 3.10 3.11, 3.12, 3.13, 3.14, 3.15, 3.16,

Platform 4: Providing and evaluating care - 4.1, 4.6, 4.8, 4.10, 4.13, 4.14, 4.15, 4.18

Platform 5: Leading and managing nursing care and working in teams - 5.2, 5.12

Platform 6: Improving safety and quality of care - 6.1, 6.3, 6.5, 6.6

Platform 7: Coordinating care - 7.1, 7.2, 7.3, 7.4, 7.5

Nursing and Midwifery Board of Ireland (2016) Competences

Domain 2: Nursing practice and clinical decision-making competences - 2.1, 2.2, 2.3, 2.4, 2.5

Domain 3: Knowledge and cognitive competences - 3.1, 3.2

Domain 4: Communication and interpersonal competences - 4.1, 4.2

Domain 6: Leadership potential and professional scholarship competences - 6.1

Definitions and terminologies

Firstly, however, we will establish some basic principles and terminologies relating to challenging behaviour in people with intellectual disabilities. There has been some debate in recent years over what terminologies are most appropriate. The authors of this chapter believe that if it is understood and applied correctly, *'challenging behaviour'* is acceptable. There is a need for a widely understood, functionally useful term that opens doors for people and allows them access to appropriate services and supports. It should not be used as a label but as a key.

It is important to note that the 'challenge' is to the people and/or services around the individual. It is inaccurate and unhelpful to think of a person as 'challenging'; evidence shows us that most challenging behaviours have a communicative function, and there is always a reason for the behaviour (Emerson and Enfield, 2011; NICE, 2015).

Probably the most widely used definitions of challenging behaviour are from Emerson (2001) and Royal College of Psychiatrists, British Psychological Society and Royal College of Speech and Language Therapists (2007). These are as follows:

Culturally abnormal behaviour(s) of such an intensity, frequency, or duration that the physical safety of the person or others is likely to be placed in serious jeopardy, or behaviour which is likely to seriously limit use of, or result in the person being denied access to, ordinary community facilities.

(Emerson, 2001)

Behaviour can be described as challenging when it is of such an intensity, frequency, or duration as to threaten the quality of life and/or the physical safety of the individual or others and it is likely to lead to responses that are restrictive, aversive or result in exclusion.

(Royal College of Psychiatrists, British Psychological Society and Royal College of Speech and Language Therapists, 2007)

From these definitions, we can see that there is a quantitative element, i.e., in understanding challenging behaviour – how long does the behaviour occur for, and how often. But also, there are qualitative and subjective elements to deciding whether a behaviour is perceived as 'challenging'. We need to look not just at the behaviour, but at the impact of this behaviour. Essentially, we are asking, 'does this behaviour harm the individual displaying it, or the people around them in any way?'. Sometimes the answer to this will be clear-cut. If someone is using physically aggressive behaviour, and this has led to a broken bone in their hand and physical injury to a carer, then we can say that yes, that behaviour is causing harm to them and to others. But what about a person who is verbally aggressive, or makes loud vocalisations? Is that 'challenging behaviour'? This leads us back to the question of impact. Although neither of these behaviours would cause immediate or obvious physical harm to the individual, if those behaviours were intense and/or frequent enough they could have a significant impact on the emotional well-being of those around them, and lead to the individual not being able to access community facilities. This is the qualitative element of challenging behaviour mentioned earlier. If the vocalisations are loud enough to cause discomfort, and occur every 30 seconds, a trip to a café, cinema, or library would be very uncomfortable, and the emotional well-being of the individual and their carers could be significantly impacted. If they were not very loud, or very infrequent, this would be a different picture. Then there is the issue of subjectivity. Some people are more sensitive to loud noise than others, so the impact would be greater for them. Let us also consider verbal aggression in the form of swearing. The impact of this would depend again on the intensity (what words are being used and at what volume) the frequency (every minute or a couple of times each day?) subjectivity (how offensive you find swearing), but also the culturally typical behaviour in any given location, that is, the context – when and where such behaviour occurs. Swearing loudly and aggressively at a football match, or in a pub at 10 pm is not likely to have much of an impact, at least in most cases. It might be considered culturally typical. However, in a playground, on a bus, in a café, library or cinema it most likely would be a different matter. This really brings home the point that the 'challenge' lies outside of the individual, and is subjective, and contextual, being deeply dependent on social norms in various situations, and upon personal values and beliefs. The impact, however, can most certainly felt by the individual, in terms of exclusion and limited life opportunities. Place the person in the right environment, with the right people, and the perceived challenge can be reduced. Although these are simplified examples, and challenging behaviour can be anything but simple, it does bring home why it is so important to understand what the term 'challenging behaviour' really means, and to establish, and perhaps challenge, ways of thinking about these behaviours and the individuals that display them.

At times, challenging behaviour has been used almost as a diagnosis – 'George has challenging behaviour' in the same way that 'Ahmed has diabetes'. We need to remember that the challenge is to services, the person themself is not 'challenging' – they are communicating, possibly distressed, reacting to circumstances that are overwhelming to them, or just trying to cope with what is happening in the moment with what skills that they have. 'Challenging behaviour' is not a diagnosis rather it is a description of a person's actions in particular circumstances. There is a temptation to think that challenging behaviour only applies to people with intellectual disabilities, or perhaps those who live with mental illness; this of course is not true. Any person, in the right (or wrong, as the case may be) circumstances, can demonstrate challenging behaviours. Think of a time when you yourself really lost your temper or were so stressed about something you wanted to run away. How did you behave? How would that look on paper, in a file about your behaviour?

On that occasion, what were the reasons for your behaviour? Were you frustrated at not being listened to, or being misunderstood? Were you feeling threatened? Was it something small that triggered the incident, but your frustration and anger had been building for some time? Whatever the reason, the important thing to note is that there *was* a reason. And, of course, that is the same for people with intellectual disabilities. *Nobody does anything without reason!*

It is important to recognise that behaviours that we as professionals label as challenging aren't only displayed by people with intellectual disabilities; they are displayed by all sorts of people. They are a human response to situations that we find frustrating, overwhelming, or threatening. Unfortunately, people with intellectual disabilities can find themselves in these types of situations more often than others.

Box 8.3
Learning Activity 8.1

Think of a time when you were really upset or angry and lost your temper.

What led up to it? Make a list of all the factors and triggers – were you tired, hungry, in pain, unwell, misunderstood, treated unfairly, ignored . . .

When you are angry, what makes it worse? Make a list of all the things that people can do exacerbate the situation, e.g., being talked over, being told to calm down, being patronised or told what to do, people getting too close to you, being ignored . . .

What makes it better? How can you help yourself to calm down and what can others do? Make a list of all the things that help, e.g., being left alone, being allowed to talk, or cry, listening to music, going for a walk, having a glass of wine . . .

Ask another person to do the same and discuss your answers. Everyone will be slightly different in what helps and what doesn't but there will be some common themes – what are they?

Now think of an example from your experience where a person with intellectual disabilities in a residential setting who is as upset and angry as you were. Did they receive the help to calm down and resolve this situation that most of us need (the common themes that you have just identified), or did others respond in a way that made it worse? What could have been done differently to help the person?

Why might it be difficult for people with intellectual disabilities to get the help they need to feel better when they are upset or angry? What barriers are there?

Prevalence of challenging behaviour

Reported prevalence rates of challenging behaviour for people with intellectual disabilities vary. Studies may focus on specific aspects of challenging behaviour such as self-injury or on a particular group of people, such as people with profound and multiple intellectual disabilities; other research has focused on population-based studies. Population-based studies, also known as epidemiology studies, consider the characteristics of specific parts of the population. These studies have consistently reported a prevalence rate of challenging behaviour for people with intellectual disabilities between 18–22% (Bowring, Painter and Hastings, 2019; Jones *et al.*, 2008; Lunqvist, 2013).

Other research has focused on topographies of challenging behaviour; in the UK reported prevalence rates for aggressive behaviour have been as high as 51.7% (Crocker *et al.*, 2006), self-injurious behaviour at 35%, and destructive behaviour at 32% (Lowe *et al.*, 2007). Such statistics demonstrate that challenging behaviour is a concern for many people with intellectual disabilities and will continue to be so for many over their lifespan.

Understanding challenging behaviour

As we have already discussed, challenging behaviour is complex and with many contributing factors. The next sections of this chapter introduce some of these factors.

Behavioural phenotypes

Behavioural phenotypes are patterns of behaviour linked to specific syndromes that are caused by genetic atypicalities. These syndromes may also be associated with intellectual disabilities.

Understanding behavioural phenotypes can help us to understand the individual, how they interact with their environment, and what adaptations to that environment may support their needs (Waite *et al.*, 2014). It should be noted that the severity of any syndrome-associated behaviour can vary, and each person remains very much an individual regardless of any particular syndrome and condition. As such any supports should still be personalised.

The following is by no means an exhaustive list, nor is it intended to provide a detailed description of these conditions and syndromes. The aim here is simply to highlight some of the more common syndromes associated with challenging behaviour, in order to better help practitioners, and support the people who live with them.

Lesch-Nyhan syndrome

This genetic syndrome is linked with serious self-injurious behaviour, notably biting hands, fingers, lips, and cheeks, leading to serious damage to those areas (Jathar *et al.*, 2016). These behaviours are thought to be physiologically and neurologically driven, and a range of interventions including medications, prosthetics (for example, mouth shields) and behavioural interventions to promote quality of life and reduce anxiety are generally used in combination to support the individual. Although these interventions can help reduce the harm caused by the behaviours, it is extremely unlikely that the behaviours will be eliminated completely.

Cornelia de lange syndrome

Cornelia de Lange Syndrome is associated with autistic-type behaviours that includes social anxiety, and self-injurious behaviours, most notably self-biting, headbanging and skin picking (Giani *et al.*, 2022; Kline *et al.*, 2018). Mood disorders, and repetitive behaviours are also common, as are sensory processing problems. People with Cornelia de Lange Syndrome also experience a range of physical conditions, such as gastroesophageal reflux, requiring medical treatment, and which may cause pain, so this must be considered before any behavioural intervention. Multi-element interventions are often required to support people with Cornelia de Lange Syndrome, including medical, pharmaceutical, and behavioural interventions.

Cri du chat syndrome

Cri du Chat Syndrome is also associated with self-injurious behaviour, as well as self-stimulatory/repetitive behaviours, aggression, hyperactivity, poor concentration/distractibility, and impulsivity (Cochran et al., 2019). These factors need to be considered when planning any behavioural supports – the individual's sensory needs should be particularly considered, as should their attention span, but again this must be in the context of the individual, and their needs and preferences. There are some physical features of this condition which should also be considered, and as always pain, psychological and medical issues must be addressed simultaneously.

Smith-Magenis syndrome

This syndrome is also associated with self-injurious behaviour, including skin picking, self-biting and self-hitting. Self-stimulatory behaviours such as flapping and hand licking are also noted, along with distractibility, impulsivity and anxiety. Additionally, reduced sensitivity to pain and temperature is a feature of the syndrome, as is chronic sleep disturbance (Smith et al., 1998). Again, knowing this should help understand the individuals needs and what situations pose risks or challenges when planning and individualising behavioural supports.

Prader-Willi syndrome

Prader-Willi syndrome is typified by problems in the mechanism for satiation of appetite, meaning that individuals with this condition feel compelled to eat very frequently (hyperphagia). This leads to complicated behaviours around food and eating, which require sensitive and skilled handling to meet the individual's needs. Compulsions, issues with impulse control and compulsive skin picking are also common (Butler, Miller and Forster, 2019).

There are also musculoskeletal and endocrine issues which will need consideration and medical intervention.

Fragile X syndrome

Individuals with Fragile X syndrome can show impulsive behaviours, as well as hand flapping or biting. Fragile X is associated with autism, with about one in three people with the condition also being autistic. As such, behaviours are often linked to anxiety, changing from one activity to another, or sensory processing issues, such as feeling overwhelmed by noise, or any other sensory stimuli (Hardiman and McGill, 2018).

Autism

Autism is a condition believed to be caused by a range of neurological differences, and resulting in difficulties with social interaction and communication, as well as restricted and repetitive behaviours. Communication difficulties can lead to unmet needs and frustration, which, in the absence of the right support, can lead to challenging behaviours (Matson and Kozlowski, 2011). People with autism often live with anxiety (Spain *et al.*, 2018), which exacerbates this, and should also be considered when thinking of any supports or interventions. Autistic people also have sensory processing issues, which can lead to over-stimulation and behaviours designed to avoid this, or under stimulation, in which case the person's behaviour can have a self-stimulatory function (Fernandez-Prieto *et al.*, 2021). Challenging behaviour is more prevalent in people with autism for this reason, however, once more it must be remembered that it is not the person who is challenging. They simply find themselves in challenging situations more frequently than other people, and without the skills or support to negotiate these, they may use behaviour that we find challenging in order to attempt to meet their needs.

It should also be considered that people with autism are more likely to live with some mental health conditions such as anxiety disorders, depression, and schizophrenia (Hollocks *et al.*, 2019; Lai *et al.*, 2019) which will also impact on behaviour.

Physical illness, pain, and distress

There is surprisingly scant research which addresses the link between ill health, pain, and challenging behaviour. Physical health, and in particular pain, are recognised as being expressed through behaviour and contributing to challenging behaviours (de Winter, Jansen and Evenhuis, 2011; de Knegt *et al.*, 2013). In this instance, the term distressed behaviour can be applied – the behaviour that we see is the externalisation of distress caused by poor health and or pain.

There is inherent danger when an expression of discomfort or pain, due to ill health or injury, is assumed to be a function of the person's intellectual disabilities. This is termed 'diagnostic overshadowing' and has been acknowledged as a contributory factor in health inequality and the avoidable premature deaths of some people with intellectual disabilities, and this has been known for some years (Doody and Bailey, 2017; Mencap, 2007, 2012).

It is important therefore that changes in behaviour are potential indicators of pain or illness (Doody and Bailey, 2017; Breau and Camfield, 2011; Findlay *et al.*, 2015), and a full physical health assessment should be carried out to rule out any physical causes for behaviour change, or exacerbation of an existing behaviour.

This is a key skill for the registered intellectual disability nurse; firstly, to acknowledge that behaviour change can have an underlying physical reason, and then to use their clinical skills to carry out a health assessment to identify any potential physical health conditions that may need intervention or further investigation.

Mental illness and challenging behaviour

Evidence suggests that mental illnesses are more common in people with intellectual disabilities, with some studies suggesting that it is twice as prevalent (Cooper *et al.*, 2015; Emerson and Hatton, 2007; Hatton *et al.*, 2017). Symptoms of mental ill health can sometimes be difficult to identify in people with intellectual disabilities, and those with autism, especially where people do not use speech, or there are communication issues. It is easy for mental illness to be overlooked, or for diagnostic overshadowing to conflate diagnosis. For this reason, mental health checking should be integral to overall health checks and should also be considered as part of the plan to support individuals with challenging behaviour, particularly if there has been behaviour change.

Trauma-informed practice

The next sections of this chapter explore strategies to support people who present challenging behaviour. Whatever approaches are used, these should be trauma-informed. This means that they should be underpinned by an understanding of the traumatic experiences that an individual may have gone through, and the impact that this trauma has had on their behaviour and all aspects of their health and well-being.

Enduring, safe, and empowering relationships are a fundamental human need. This need for human connection is innate to all individuals, yet for people with intellectual disabilities, it is often an area fraught with disappointment, threat, and trauma (Beail, Frankish and Skelly, 2021; Crates *et al.*, 2013).

Historically the need for connection and relationship has been largely ignored or not seen as a priority by intellectual disability services. Institutionalised models of care have sometimes resulted in exclusion, and a lack of love and friendships, and oppression which are dehumanising for all people (Rogers, 2016).

Beail, Frankish and Skelly (2021) have identified that everyone has a key role in in recognising, preventing, and responding to the trauma experienced by people with intellectual disabilities. The Learning Disability Professional Senate (2019) have identified that people with intellectual disabilities are most at risk of trauma, and provide '10 top tips' for Trauma-Informed Care. For registered nurses this includes being trauma-aware and understanding the skills needed in preventing people being traumatised and supporting people who may be traumatised.

There is now wide acknowledgment of the trauma experienced by people with intellectual disabilities and the need for more trauma-informed services. However, the trauma experienced by families trying to navigate the systems which should support them is largely unrecognised. A family survey carried out by The Challenging Behaviour Foundation (2020) identified the risk factors families associated with an increased likelihood of trauma. The survey shows that the trauma of family carers of children and adults with intellectual disabilities and autism is multi-layered and complex. Many families experience a wide range of trauma and receive little to no support for this. Families also experience an additional burden by needing to search for their support independently.

The role of the registered intellectual disability nurse is to mediate and support families to navigate systems in order to access support their family needs and consider how their practice can identify and mitigate the impact of trauma for families.

Understanding and supporting challenging behaviour

Applied behavioural analysis

Evidence-based approaches to understanding behaviour are a relatively new phenomenon and are evolving. One of the early applications of this understanding was Applied Behaviour Analysis. Applied Behaviour Analysis (ABA) has been defined as:

> *A scientific approach for discovering environmental variables that reliably influence socially significant behaviour and for developing a technology of behaviour change that takes practical advantage of those characteristics.*

> (Cooper *et al.*, 2007, p. 3)

ABA is evidence-based, but there are concerns regarding some of its applications. For example, autism and neurodiversity rights groups express concerns about the use of ABA to 'treat' autism, and some historical literature, which includes the use of punishment or other aversive approaches such as electric shock, are unacceptable in current practice (Leaf *et al.*, 2021). However, an evidence-based approach to understanding behaviour requires intellectual disability nurses and other members of the multidisciplinary team to undertake detailed and, at times, comprehensive assessment of individuals, their environment, and the contexts where their behaviour occurs. Such assessments provide an evidence-based understanding of why behaviour occurs and what variables support behaviour change. These principles of ABA are a foundation of several approaches, and that includes Positive Behaviour Support.

Positive behaviour support

Positive Behaviour Support (PBS) is an evidence-based approach with the primary goal of increasing a person's quality of life and a secondary goal of decreasing the frequency and severity of challenging behaviour (LaVigna and Willis, 2012; Gore *et al.*, 2013; Hardiman and McGill, 2018).

Gore *et al.* (2013) have described PBS as a multi-component framework which includes those important to the person to develop an understanding of the challenging behaviour. This involves an assessment of the social and physical environments and broader context within which the behaviour occurs. Using this assessment, it is possible to develop, implement, and evaluate the effectiveness of a personalised system of support that enhances the quality of life outcomes for the person and their stakeholders (Gore *et al.*, 2013).

Assessment

Research demonstrates that challenging behaviour is socially constructed (see Figure 8.1); it is the product of individual and environmental factors interacting together (Emerson and Enfield, 2011; Bowring, Painter and Hastings, 2019).

Individual factors are characteristics unique to the individual, for example, the severity of their intellectual disabilities, the presence of additional sensory needs, along with communication or their personal history of relationships and experiences. Understanding what the person does is one of the first steps in understanding the function of a behaviour. Firstly, there is a need to state what the behaviour looks like by describing precisely; what the person does, i.e., the topography of behaviour. This is usually described in terms of intensity, duration, and frequency (Emerson and Enfield, 2011).

Environmental factors can include characteristics of services, numbers of staff, training experience of staff, how they work with people and with each other, quality of the support that staff or family members receive, and the quality of the environment and the opportunities this presents (The Royal College of Psychiatrists and the British Psychological Society, 2016; Bowring, Painter and Hastings, 2019). The principles of assessment, planning, implementing, and evaluating behaviour support plans are based on a systematic, problem-solving, and a strengths-based approach and can be understood using Bronfenbrenner's (1992) ecological systems theory (see Figure 8.2).

This framework should guide registered intellectual disability nurses to consider the variables and interactions of each environment where challenging behaviour occurs and what supports are required. Assessments by nurses should adopt a holistic, non-linear approach by looking more broadly than antecedents and consequences of behaviour, considering the contexts and systems that influence behaviour. This approach is known as non-linear functional

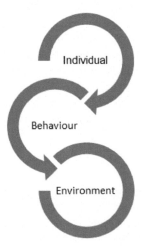

Figure 8.1

Social construct of behaviour.

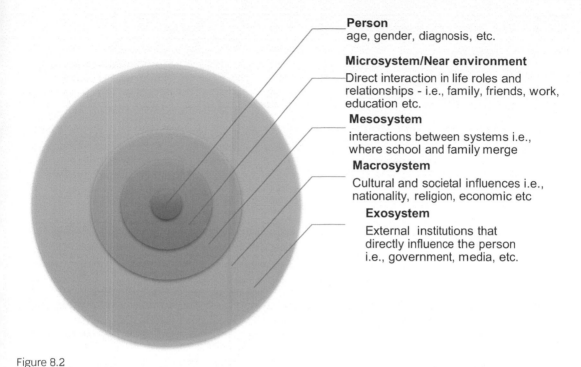

Figure 8.2

Approaches to systematic assessment.

behaviour assessment. It is a method of assessment that identifies the events and contexts in which the behaviour occurs. Functional behaviour assessment commonly involves:

- Identifying and defining behaviour in a way that is measurable and can be observed.
- Collecting information about the behaviour, considering the person, their history, and all components of the ecological system.
- Presenting a hypothesis about the function of the behaviour.
- Developing a plan which identifies the functional support needed to optimise quality of life.

Functional behavioural assessment is supported by several tools, the choice of which may be determined by the behaviour presented and the type of assessment required.

Formulation

Following assessment of a person's needs and environment, this information can be used to develop a formulation to understand why the behaviour may be happening and provide some context. This formulation should provide

Tools to support systematic assessment	Description
Physical/mental health – Nursing assessment, pain assessments, dementia screening, Bristol stool charts, dental health, medication reviews (Emerson and Enfield, 2011; NICE, 2015)	Internal factors such as physical or mental health should be considered as a function of the challenging behaviour. These internal factors require comprehensive nursing assessment, for potential underlying conditions and to gather baseline information to monitor for deterioration as described previously in behavioural phenotypes.
Observations – ABCs, Incident reports, other observation forms (Emerson and Enfield, 2011)	Direct observation in natural situations and the interplay of the immediate environment on other environments (ecological systems theory); this helps to objectively verify the contexts of why behaviours could be happening rather than biased assumptions.
Rating Scales – Behaviour Problem Inventory Short (Rojahn *et al.*, 2012) Motivation Assessment Scale (Durand and Crimmins, 1992)	Rating scales can provide a structured approach to analyse behaviour presentation as well as showing changes in topography over time. Rating scales can suggest the potential function of the behaviour, but it is not recommended these are used in isolation.
Checklists – Aberrant Behaviour Checklist (Aman and Singh, 1985; Aman, 2012) Mini PASADD & PAS-ADD (Moss *et al.*, 1998)	A rating scale that measures the severity of symptoms and behaviour presentation for people with intellectual disabilities. Tools to help recognise the presence of a mental health need so further referrals/investigations can occur.
Interviews/Questionnaires – (O'Neil *et al.*, 2015; Cooper, Heren and Heward, 2007)	A systematic approach using verbal or written reports of behaviour in natural situations and formal checklist and observations to aid development of an intervention plan.
Functional analysis – (Cooper *et al.*, 2007)	Examination of the functional nature of the behaviour, whether this is sensory, escape, social interaction or tangible, and considering the internal and external factors that reinforce the behaviour and the impact of the context in which the behaviour occurs.
Active Support Measure – (Mansell, Elliot and Beadle-Brown, 2005)	Can be used as a measure for quality of engagement and staff support.
Quality of life measures – Family Quality of Life Scale (FQLS) (Hoffman *et al.*, 2006) Guernsey Community Participation and Leisure Assessment (GCPLA) (Baker, Taylor-Roberts and Jones, 2021) Health of the Nation Outcome Scales – Learning Disability (HONOS-LD) (Roy *et al.*, 2002) The Maslow Assessment of Needs Scales – Learning and intellectual disabilities (MANS-LD) (Skirrow and Perry, 2009)	Can be used pre- and post-intervention to assess changes in quality of life.

Table 8.1   Methods of assessment

information about the potential function(s) of the behaviour, which are commonly referred to as:

■ Escape: The need to avoid a situation or interaction.
■ Tangible: The need to have access to something.

- Sensory: The need to remove or add a sensation.
- Social Attention: The need to connect or interact with someone.
- Pain/Health: The need to have a healthcare need met.

It is important to note that these are categories, not diagnostic labels, and a summary of the function of behaviour should always consider why this may be happening. Following this formulation, a behaviour support plan may be developed. The plan should summarise the supports the person and their carers, staff, and family need to make and these should be seen as positive changes to address unmet needs. It should include strategies for improving the quality of life through systems change, development of skills, and environmental redesign; these are known as proactive strategies.

Positive behaviour support plans

A positive behaviour support plan is a detailed plan with strategies to improve the person's quality of life by outlining supports to meet their needs better and uphold their human rights. It is acknowledged that there are a variety of formats for plans, given the individual nature of their content, however, they generally include the elements outlined as follows. This example is based upon the multi-element behaviour support plan outlined by LaVigna and Willis (2005) and LaVigna *et al.* (2022).

Ecological strategies

Ecological strategies can include changing factors such as staff attributions (through providing training), supporting the family, or physical factors such as altering noise/stimulation levels or ensuring increased choices and development of positive relationships with the individual (LaVigna and Willis, 2012). Individual's sensory needs should be considered when planning ecological strategies.

New skills and opportunities

Strategies can include:

- supporting the person to experience success and personal satisfaction across a variety of settings, such as work, social, community, educational and family settings.
- developing more functional ways to communicate their needs.
- developing skills that meet potential gaps in being able to engage in meaningful activities.
- enhancing the knowledge and skills of people who support the person so they can implement effective environmental and systems change (Hardiman and McGill, 2018).

■ accessing other psychological approaches such as Cognitive Behavioural Therapy, Dyadic Developmental Psychotherapy (Beail, Frankish and Skelly, 2021).

Prevention (focused support) strategies

Prevention strategies aim to prevent the need for reactive strategies by preventing challenging behaviour occurring or escalating. This can be achieved by managing antecedents; removing the 'triggers' known to escalate a situation or cause further distress. For example, if making a request is likely to escalate the situation, then a strategy could be not to make that request. Another example could be introducing something or someone to the situation (a preferred person, activity, or object) in the knowledge this will likely prevent escalation resulting in the avoidance of reactive strategies.

Reactive strategies

These are strategies that aim to gain rapid and safe control over a situation, resolving the issue as quickly and as safely as possible (LaVigna *et al.*, 2022), and must be included in a behavioural support plan. Reactive strategies are not intended to impact the future occurrence of the behaviour, that is to teach or provide consequences in the hope that the behaviour will not occur again in the future.

Interventions can include strategies such as active listening, changing something in the environment, redirecting to a preferred activity. Emerging evidence shows that such non-aversive reactive strategies may be more effective to bring resolution and reduce the severity of challenging behaviours than more restrictive practices (LaVigna and Willis, 2016; Royal College of Psychiatrists and the British Psychological Society, 2016; Spicer and Crates, 2016).

Ecological strategies	New skills and opportunities	Prevention (focused support) strategies	Reactive strategies
Physical environment • Predictable • Sensory needs • Interpersonal environment • Considers attachment • Relationships • Staff rapport and support style • Programmatic environment • Stimulating with interesting people and activities	Fun Skills • What the person wants or likes to do/learn • General skills • Better meeting own needs • Functional skills • Meet the same functional needs as behaviour of concern • Replacement skills • Better way to exert choice and control • Coping skills • Ensure resilience and ways to cope when things change or go wrong	Managing antecedents • Increasing preferred events (including people) • Differential schedules of reinforcement	Non-Functionally based • Increase preferred event • Ask them to help you • Relaxation • Remove what you know is causing the problem • Functionally-based • Give the person what they want/need • Active listening • Comfort • Remove demands

Table 8.2   Multi-element behaviour support plan (Adapted from LaVigna and Willis, 2005; LaVigna *et al.*, 2022; Crates *et al.*, 2013)

Box 8.4 Learning Activity 8.2: Case study

Susan is 19 years old with a diagnosis of intellectual disabilities and autism. She lives with her family, two parents, and one younger sibling in a town location. Susan attends a local college with other young adults with intellectual disabilities, where she enjoys access to computer courses, art, and other social activities. Susan enjoys listening to her iPod, swimming, walking, and attending craft fairs. Susan is full of curiosity and adventure and is always smiling. Susan has good physical health, is allergic to pollen, cats, and dairy products, and presents with breathing difficulties and skin irritations needing treatment with oral antihistamine and topical creams. Susan has never had an anaphylactic reaction because of allergies. Susan communicates verbally using single words or short, learned phrases and uses symbols, gestures, and objects to augment her communication.

Recently, Susan has presented with the following behaviour:

> Susan will undress from the waist up, then wrap herself in a blanket. She rolls onto her back and bangs her head off the floor, saying, 'hot'. If people approach, she will hit them with her fist or kick them. This episode can last for an hour and happen three times per day at college and once a month at home.

Susan can cause bruising to herself and others while doing this. College staff report that she has appeared dizzy on one occasion after a particularly forceful headbang. Family and staff report that Susan appears to be in pain, although she does not cry out.

Susan is showing less interest in previously enjoyed activities. Susan's family stated that at home, they offered Susan a cool bath with essential oils and her favourite music when she began to undress and rarely saw her banging her head on the floor.

Task:

- Define the challenging behaviour's frequency, duration, and severity.
- Consider any internal or external elements contributing to the challenging behaviour.
- Propose a function(s) of this behaviour.
- Identify strategies to form a positive behaviour support plan using the previous template.

Restrictive practices

Restrictive practices are defined as:

> *Interventions that restrict an individual's movement, liberty and/or freedom to act independently in order to: take immediate control of a dangerous situation: and end or reduce significantly the danger to the person or others; and contain or limit the patient's freedom for no longer than is necessary.*

(DH, 2014, p. 14)

Restrictive practices should only be used as a last resort; nurses must always choose the least restrictive option. An assessment of the person's capacity to make the decision about these restrictive practices must be undertaken in the context of relevant legislation and the individual's Human Rights. The use of restrictive practices should be used under extreme caution. It is known that their use can cause injury, psychological distress, and trauma (Royal College of Psychiatrists and the British Psychological Society, 2016; Spicer and Crates, 2016; Beail, Frankish and Skelly, 2021). Where restrictive practices are in place then a reduction plan must be in place with regular monitoring. Any restrictive practices must be based on the principles of data-informed practice, staff development, service user involvement and a commitment to post incident review all within a framework of effective leadership and restoration of the persons human rights (DH, 2014). Furthermore, the emotional impact of restraint on the service user and staff must also be considered (RCN, 2017).

Implementation

The implementation of a Behaviour Support Plan (BSP) requires collaboration with all services involved in supporting a person including the person, their families, carers and multi-disciplinary teams. It must be ensured that everyone fully understands their specific role in carrying out the strategies and has the necessary support or training is crucial. Support with implementation can involve direct mentoring and role modelling of the strategies, specific training and continued monitoring, and support to ensure evidence-based practice and efficacy of the plan (Beadle-Brown *et al.*, 2014, 2021; Horner, 1990; NICE, 2015).

Evaluation

BSPs should be regularly updated to reflect any changes in the presentation of behaviours. This may be as the risk reduces, or as strategies become less effective. The evaluation should seek to gather information on the effectiveness of the strategies and measure the outcomes of this on the quality of life for the person, as well as gathering data on the use of restrictive practices.

An audit of the service should also be undertaken to identify patterns or trends in restrictive practice use, frequency of incidents, the people involved in incidents, injuries sustained and any consequences of the challenging behaviour. There are several audit tools available for this, with the Periodic Service Review being a long-standing format (LaVigna *et al.*, 1994).

Some key questions for the registered nurse to consider are:

- Do people understand the plan?
- Do they have the skills and resources to implement the plan?
- How will you know if the plan is successful? What data or evidence do you need?
- Is the plan focused on quality of life, health and well-being and promotes rights?
- Are there improvements in the person's quality of life?
- How are these being measured/how will we know if this is the case?

Other evidence-based approaches

Person-Centred Active Support (PCAS)

PCAS is described a way to develop staff practices to support people in community settings. This approach recognises that for staff to support people with Intellectual disabilities to have a good quality of life and be meaningfully involved in activities and relationships, staff needed to be skilled in supporting this. Where this approach is used by staff, it helps them provide more individually tailored, reliable, and practical support to the people they support (Mansell *et al.*, 2005). There is continued evidence that the quality of staff support reflects the quality of life for people with intellectual disabilities, leading to increased engagement and participation and reductions in challenging behaviour (Bigby and Beadle-Brown, 2016; Hardiman and McGill, 2018; Hume, Khan and Reilly, 2020).

There are four essentials of PCAS, and registered intellectual disability nurses should work with staff teams and families to:

- Identify where the individual can be included in everyday activities: Every moment has potential.
- Engage people at their pace: Little and often.
- Provide just the right amount of support to engage in activities: Grading assistance.
- Provide the type of support the person wants and needs: Maximising choice and control.

Box 8.5
Learning Activity 8.3

Visit the person-centred active support YouTube channel to view recorded examples of each of the four essentials of PCAS.

Communication

Challenging behaviour is known to be connected to difficulties with communication (Matson and Kozlowski, 2011), and so communication strategies are central to supporting people presenting challenging behaviour. Communication skills are central to the role of the registered nurse, and are vital given that up to 90% of people with intellectual disabilities will require additional support with communication (Royal College of Speech and Language Therapists, 2016). The reason for such support is widely variable and very individual but can be because of:

■ Difficulties with understanding or expressing themselves.
■ Sensory needs associated with hearing or sight.
■ Limited literacy skills.
■ Lack of reasonable adjustments or opportunity to access communication supports.
■ Information is presented in a complicated or inaccessible way.

Without good communication support people with Intellectual disabilities are at risk of poor access to healthcare, low mood and anxiety, limited opportunities to develop relationships and are more at risk to abuse and hate crime, as well as challenging behaviours (Royal College of Speech and Language Therapists, 2016; Spicer and Crates, 2016; The Royal College of Psychiatrists and the British Psychological Society, 2016).

Good communication supports may require more specialist input for example from a Speech and Language Therapist, but many communications supports are easily available to those supporting individuals. Examples of communication supports include:

■ Objects of reference, photographs or symbols which represent the core 'message'.
■ Use of Makaton or other signing systems.
■ Communication or health passports.
■ The use of Talking Mats or Picture Exchange Communications System (PECS).
■ Rapport building approaches such as Intensive Interaction.

The *'five good communication standards'* for best practice (Royal College of Speech and Language Therapists, 2016) will assist nurses understand what good communication looks like as well as providing several resources to promote good communication. Some general principles about supporting communication are outlined in these standards.

These include:

■ Reduce the amount of information presented.
■ Simplify time concepts such as use of now and next.

■ Focus on the positive, for example, what you will do, not what you will not do.

■ Use the person's name at the beginning of the sentence.

Simple communication strategies such as these should underpin any supports for people whose behaviour can be challenging.

Conclusion

The intellectual disability nurse has a crucial role in supporting people who may at times show challenging behaviours. They may work directly with individuals who have complex and challenging needs in specialist support services. They may be involved in developing behavioural support plans, using their functional assessment skills. They may support families and carers in adopting communication strategies that support the individual and reduce the need for challenging behaviours. They may also undertake health assessments to rule out physical causes of pain and distress.

Some intellectual disability nurses specialise in working with people who display challenging behaviour, becoming behaviour specialist nurses. There are many master's level courses aimed at skilling professionals in undertaking behavioural assessments, with a view to developing positive behavioural support plans.

Whatever the role, the intellectual disability nurse is instrumental in supporting this group of people towards achieving a good quality of life and preventing the recurrence of such poor practice as was seen at Winterbourne View, Muckamore Abbey, and the other institutions that went before them and that were also reported as being unfit for purpose, and responsible for appalling abuses.

It is vital to remember that people with intellectual disabilities who have challenging behaviour need additional support to empower them to be supported in ways that promote their independence, autonomy, safety, and essentially, their human rights.

History bears witness as to what happens when this is not the case. As such, the role of the intellectual disability nurse in providing the range of supports described in this chapter cannot be underestimated.

There is a sound evidence base for the use of Positive Behavioural Supports, and this is now recognised as a key intervention to support individuals whose behaviour can challenge services. The theory is clear, and there is much guidance around its implementation.

Collectively we need to ensure that practice is supported to fully embrace the philosophy of PBS, focusing on improvements to quality of life for the individuals at its centre, so that we can see real improvements for this vulnerable group.

It is often said that the measure of any civilisation can be seen in how it treats is most vulnerable. At present there is still some way to go before we in the UK achieve this aim. What is clear, however, is that as intellectual disabilities nurses, we must use our specialist knowledge, skills, and value base to push boundaries towards improvements in the care and support of this group. We must continue to advocate for the rights of people with intellectual disabilities to live healthy, happy lives, free from abuse, and free to develop to their full potential. Arguably no other professional group has the unique knowledge, skills and value base nor is positioned to do this. Intellectual disability nurses must not lose sight of the privileged positions they hold in people's lives. They must continue to fight for the human rights and integrity of people with intellectual disabilities as citizens to be upheld, for equality, and ultimately their happiness.

References

Aman, M.G. (2012) Aberrant behavior checklist: Current identity and future developments. *Clinical & Experimental Pharmacology*, 2, p. e114. doi:10.4172/2161-1459.1000e114.

Aman, M.G. and Singh, N.N. (1985) *Aberrant behavior checklist manual*. East Aurora, NY: Slosson Educational Publications.

Baker, P., Taylor-Roberts, L. and Jones, F.W. (2021) Development of the Guernsey community participation and leisure assessment-revised (GCPLA-R). *Journal of Applied Research in Intellectual Disabilities*, 34(1), pp. 218–228.

Beadle-Brown, J., *et al.* (2014) Practice leadership and active support in residential services for people with intellectual disabilities: An exploratory study. *Journal of Intellectual Disability Research*, 58(9), pp. 838–850.

Beadle-Brown, J., *et al.* (2021) Outcomes and costs of skilled support for people with severe or profound intellectual disability and complex needs. *Journal of Applied Research in Intellectual Disabilities*, 34(1), pp. 42–54.

Beail, N., Frankish, P. and Skelly, A. (2021) *Trauma and intellectual disability*. Hove: Pavilion.

Bigby, C. and Beadle-Brown, J. (2016) Improving quality of life outcomes in supported accommodation for people with intellectual disability: What makes a difference? *Journal of Applied Research in Intellectual Disabilities*, 31(2), pp. e182–e200. doi:10.1111/jar.12291.

Bowring, D.L., Painter, J. and Hastings, R.P. (2019) Prevalence of challenging behaviour in adults with intellectual disabilities, correlates, and association with mental health. *Current Developmental Disorders Reports*, 6(4), pp. 173–181.

Breau, L.M. and Camfield, C.S. (2011) Pain disrupts sleep in children and youth with intellectual and developmental disabilities. *Research in Developmental Disabilities*, 32(6), pp. 2829–2840.

Bronfenbrenner, U. (1992) *Ecological systems theory*. London: Jessica Kingsley Publishers.

Bubb, S. (2014) *Winterbourne View-time for change: Transforming the commissioning of services for people with learning and intellectual disabilities and/or autism*. Transforming Care and Commissioning Steering Group. Available at: www.england.nhs.uk/wp-content/uploads/2014/11/transforming-commissioning-services.pdf (Accessed 9 August 2022).

Butler, M.G., Miller, J.L. and Forster, J.L. (2019) Prader-Willi syndrome-clinical genetics, diagnosis and treatment approaches: An update. *Current Pediatric Reviews*, 15(4), pp. 207–244.

Cochran, L., *et al.* (2019) Age-related behavioural change in Cornelia de Lange and Cri du Chat syndromes: A seven year follow-up study. *Journal of Autism and Developmental Disorders*, 49(6), pp. 2476–2487.

Cooper, J., Heren, E. and Heward, W. (2007) *Applied behavior analysis* (2nd edition). Saddle River, NJ: Pearson.

Cooper, S.A., *et al.* (2015) Multiple physical and mental health comorbidity in adults with intellectual disabilities: Population-based cross-sectional analysis. *BMC Family Practice*, 16, p. 110. doi:10.1186/s12875-015-0329-3.

Crates, N., *et al.* (2013) *Trauma informed support for people with disability: Australasian society for intellectual disability conference paper*. Available at: www.google.com.au/url?sa=t&rct=j&q=&esrc=s&source=web&cd=1&ved=0ahUKEwj6la Ge3cTOAhWDmJQKHeBzBtAQFggbMAA&url=https%3A%2F%2Fasid.asn.au%2F2Ffiles%2F219_24_n_crates_m_spicer.pdf&usg=AFQjCNGlyWFbUSUeij4M 2XJW4LzdfiLSeA&cad=rja (Accessed 28 July 2022).

Crocker, A.G., *et al.* (2006) Prevalence and types of aggressive behaviour among adults with intellectual disabilities. *Journal of Intellectual Disability Research*, 50(9), pp. 652–661.

de Knegt, N.C., *et al.* (2013) Behavioral pain indicators in people with intellectual disabilities: A systematic review. *The Journal of Pain*, 14(9), pp. 885–896.

de Winter, C.F., Jansen, A.A.C. and Evenhuis, H.M. (2011) Physical conditions and challenging behaviour in people with intellectual disability: A systematic review. *Journal of Intellectual Disability Research*, 55(7), pp. 675–698.

DH (2012) *Transforming care: A national response to Winterbourne View hospital.* Available at: www.gov.uk/government/publications/winterbourne-view-hospital-department-of-health-review-and-response (Accessed 28 July 2022).

DH (2014) *Positive and proactive care: Reducing the need for restrictive interventions.* Available at: Positive and Proactive Care: reducing the need for restrictive interventions (publishing.service.gov.uk) (Accessed 28 March 2022).

Doody, O. and Bailey, M.E. (2017) Pain and pain assessment in people with intellectual disability: Issues and challenges in practice. *British Journal of Learning Disabilities*, 45(3), pp. 157–165.

Durand, V.M. and Crimmins, D.B. (1992) *The motivation assessment scale (MAS) administration guide.* Topeka, KS: Monaco and Associates.

Emerson, E. (2001) *Analysis and intervention in people with severe intellectual disabilities* (2nd edition). Cambridge: Cambridge University Press.

Emerson, E. and Enfield, S. (2011) *Challenging behaviour* (3rd edition). Cambridge: Cambridge University Press.

Emerson, E. and Hatton, C. (2007) Mental health of children and adolescents with intellectual disabilities in Britain. *The British Journal of Psychiatry*, 191(6), pp. 493–499.

Fernandez-Prieto, M., *et al.* (2021) Executive functioning: A mediator between sensory processing and behaviour in autism spectrum disorder. *Journal of Autism and Developmental Disorder*s, 51(6), pp. 2091–2103.

Findlay, L., *et al.* (2015) Caregiver experiences of supporting adults with intellectual disabilities in pain. *Journal of Applied Research in Intellectual Disabilities*, 28(2), pp. 111–120.

Giani, L., *et al.* (2022) Behavioral markers of social anxiety in Cornelia de Lange syndrome: A brief systematic review. *Journal of Affective Disorders*, 299, pp. 636–643.

Gore, N.J., *et al.* (2013) Definition and scope for positive behavioural support. *International Journal of Positive Behavioural Support*, 3(2), pp. 14–23.

Hardiman, R.L. and McGill, P. (2018) How common are challenging behaviours amongst individuals with fragile X syndrome? A systematic review. *Research in Developmental Disabilitie*s, 76, pp. 99–109.

Hatton, C., *et al.* (2017) The mental health of british adults with intellectual impairments living in general households. *Journal of Applied Research in Intellectual Disabilitie*s, 30(1), pp. 188–197.

Hoffman, L., *et al.* (2006) Assessing family outcomes: Psychometric evaluation of the beach centre family quality of life scale. *Journal of Marriage and Family*, 68(4), pp. 1069–1083.

Hollocks, M.J., *et al.* (2019) Anxiety and depression in adults with autism spectrum disorder: A systematic review and meta-analysis. *Psychological Medicine*, 49(4), pp. 559–572.

Horner, R.H., *et al.* (1990) Towards a technology of 'nonaversive toward a technology of "nonaversive" behavioral support'. *Journal of the Association for Persons with Severe Handicaps*, 15(3), pp. 125–132.

Hume, L., Khan, N. and Reilly, M. (2020) Building capable environments using practice leadership. *Tizard Learning Disability Review*, 26(1), pp. 1–8.

Jathar, P., *et al.* (2016) Lesch-Nyhan syndrome: Disorder of self-mutilating behavior. *International Journal of Clinical Pediatric Dentistry*, 9(2), pp. 139–142.

Jones, S., *et al.* (2008) Prevalence of, and factors associated with, problem behaviors in adults with intellectual disabilities. *The Journal of Nervous and Mental Disease*, 196, pp. 678–686.

Kline, A.D., *et al.* (2018) Diagnosis and management of Cornelia de Lange syndrome: First international consensus statement. *Nature Reviews Genetics*, 19(10), pp. 649–666.

Lai, M.C., *et al.* (2019) Prevalence of co-occurring mental health diagnoses in the autism population: A systematic review and meta-analysis. *The Lancet Psychiatry*, 6(10), pp. 819–829.

LaVigna, G.W. and Willis, T.J. (2005) A positive behavioural support model for breaking the barriers to social and community inclusion. *Learning Disability Review*, 10(2), pp. 16–23.

LaVigna, G.W. and Willis, T.J. (2012) The efficacy of positive behavioural support with the most challenging behaviour: The evidence and its implications. *Journal of Intellectual and Developmental Disability*, 37(3), pp. 185–195.

LaVigna, G.W. and Willis, T.J. (2016) The alignment fallacy and how to avoid it. *International Journal of Positive Behavioural Support*, 6(1), pp. 6–13.

LaVigna, G.W., *et al.* (1994) *The periodic service review: Total quality assurance system for human services and education.* Baltimore, MD: Brookes Publishing.

LaVigna, G.W., *et al.* (2022) Needed independent and dependent variables in multi-element behavior support plans addressing severe behavior problems. *Perspectives on Behaviour Science*, 45(2), pp. 421–444.

Leaf, J.B., *et al.* (2021) Concerns about ABA-based intervention: An evaluation and recommendations. *Journal of Autism and Developmental Disorders*, 52(6), pp. 2838–2853.

Learning Disability Professional Senate (2019) *Top 10 tips: Trauma informed approaches for people who have ID*. Available at: www.google.com/url?sa=t&rct=j&q=&esrc=s&source=web&cd=&ved=2ahUKEwiWz5GRt8j3AhWJLMAKHWv6B2cQFnoEC AMQAQ&url=https%3A%2F%2Fwww.rcn.org.uk%2F-%2Fmedia%2Froyal-college-of-nursing%2Fdocuments%2Fclinical-topics%2Fsafeguarding%2Ftop-tips-for-trauma-infor (Accessed 28 July 2022).

Lenehan, C. (2017) *These are our children.* London: Department of Health.

Lowe, K., *et al.* (2007) Challenging behaviours: Prevalence and topographies. *Journal of Intellectual Disabilities*, 51(8), pp. 625–636.

Lunqvist, L. (2013) Prevalence and risk markers of behaviour problems among adults with intellectual disabilities: A total population study in Orebro County, Sweden. *Research in Developmental Disabilities*, 34, pp. 1346–1356.

Mansell, J., Elliot, T. and Beadle-Brown, J. (2005) *Active support measures* (revised edition). Canterbury: Tizard Centre.

Matson, J.L. and Kozlowski, A.M. (2011) The increasing prevalence of autism spectrum disorders. *Research in Autism Spectrum Disorders*, 5(1), pp. 418–425.

Mencap (2007) *Death by indifference.* London: Mencap.

Mencap (2012) *74 deaths and counting, a progress report 5 years on.* London: Mencap.

Moss, S., *et al.* (1998) Reliability and validity of the PAS-ADD checklist for detecting psychiatric disorders in adults with intellectual disability. *Journal of Intellectual Disability Research*, 42(2), pp. 173–183.

NICE (2015) *Challenging behaviour and learning and intellectual disabilities: Prevention and interventions for people with learning and intellectual disabilities whose behaviour challenges [NG11]*. Available at: www.nice.org.uk/guidance/ng11/resources/challenging-behaviour-and-learning-disabilities-prevention-and-inter ventions-for-people-with-learning-disabilities-whose-behaviour-challenges-pdf-1837266392005 (Accessed 28 March 2022).

Nursing and Midwifery Board of Ireland (2016) *Nurse registration programmes standards and requirements* (4th edition). Dublin: Nursing and Midwifery Board of Ireland.

Nursing and Midwifery Council (2018) *Future nurse: Standards of proficiency for registered nurses*. London: NMC.

O'Neill, R.E., *et al.* (2015) *Functional assessment and program development*. Boston, MA: Cengage Learning.

RCN (NI) (2017) *Three steps to positive practice: A rights-based approach when considering and reviewing the use of restrictive interventions*. Available at: www.rcn.org.uk/professional-development/publications/pub-006075 (Accessed 28 July 2022).

Rogers, C. (2016) *Intellectual disability and being human: A care ethics*. London: Routeledge.

Rojahn, J., *et al.* (2012) The behavior problems inventory-short form for individuals with intellectual disabilities: Part II: Reliability and validity. *Journal of Intellectual Disability Research*, 56(5), pp. 546–565.

Roy, A., *et al.* (2002) Health of the nation outcome scales for people with learning and intellectual disabilities (HoNOS-LD). *British Journal of Psychiatry*, 180(1), pp. 61–66.

Royal College of Psychiatrists and the British Psychological Society (2016) *Challenging behaviour: A unified approach*. Available at: www.bps.org.uk/sites/bps.org.uk/files/Policy/Policy-Files/Challenging behaviour-aunifiedapproach%28update%29.pdf (Accessed 28 July 2022).

Royal College of Psychiatrists, British Psychological Society and Royal College of Speech and Language Therapists (2007) *Challenging behaviour: A unified approach. Clinical and service guidelines for supporting people with learning disabilities who are at risk of receiving abusive or restrictive practices*. Available at: https://www.rcpsych.ac.uk/docs/default-source/improving-care/better-mh-policy/college-reports/college-report-cr144.pdf?sfvrsn=73e437e8_2 (Accessed 26 November 2022).

Royal College of Speech and Language Therapists (2016) *Five good communication standards*. Available at: www.rcslt.org/wp-content/uploads/media/Project/RCSLT/good-comm-standards.pdf (Accessed 28 July 2022).

Skirrow, P. and Perry, E. (2009) *The Maslow assessment of needs scales*. Available at: www.bps.org.uk/sites/www.bps.org.uk/files/Member%20Networks/Faculties/Intellectual%20Disabilities/MANS%20Manual.pdf (Accessed 28 July 2022).

Smith, A.C.M., Dykens, E. and Greenberg, F. (1998) Sleep disturbance in Smith-Magenis syndrome. *American Journal of Medicine and Genetics*, 8, pp. 186–191.

Spain, D., *et al.* (2018) Social anxiety in autism spectrum disorder: A systematic review. *Research in Autism Spectrum Disorders*, 52, pp. 51–68.

Spicer, M. and Crates, N. (2016) Non-aversive reactive strategies for reducing the episodic severity of aggression. *International Journal of Positive Behavioural Support*, 6(1), pp. 35–51.

The Challenging Behaviour Foundation (2020) *A family carer perspective*. Available at: www.challengingbehaviour.org.uk/wp-content/uploads/2021/03/brokencbffinalreportstrand1jan21.pdf (Accessed 28 July 2022).

Waite, J., *et al.* (2014) The importance of understanding the behavioural phenotypes of genetic syndromes associated with intellectual disability. *Paediatrics and Child Health*, 24(10), pp. 468–472.

Willis, D. (2020) Whorlton Hall, Winterbourne View and Ely Hospital: Learning from failures of care. *Learning Disability Practice*. doi:10.7748/ldp.2020.e2049.

Further Reading

Beail, N., Frankish, P. and Skelly, A. (2021) *Trauma and intellectual disability*. West Sussex: Pavilion.

Emerson, E. and Enfield, S. (2011) *Challenging behaviour* (3rd edition). Cambridge: Cambridge University Press.

Murphy, B., Bradshaw, J. and Beadle-Brown, J. (2017) *Person-centred active support self study guide* (2nd edition). Hove: Pavilion.

Useful Resources

Cerebra: https://cerebra.org.uk

Department of Health: Positive a nd Proactive Care: https://assets.publishing.service.gov.uk/government/uploads/system/uploads/attachment_data/file/300291/JRA_DoH_Guidance_on_RH_Summary_web_accessible.pdf

The Challenging Beh aviour Foundation: www.challengingbehaviour.org.uk

The Callan Institute: www.callaninstitute.org

The Institute of Applied Behavior Analysis: www.iaba.com

The Restraint Reduction Network: www.restraintreductionnetwork.org

CHAPTER 9

Rachel Morgan, Joanne Blair, Kirsty Henry and
Stacey Rees

Community intellectual disability nursing

Introduction

Community intellectual disability nurses work with a wide cross-section of people with intellectual disabilities and agencies. This chapter will explore current and changing roles of intellectual disability nurses working in the community. This will be contextualised within the Nursing and Midwifery Council for the United Kingdom (2018b) and Nursing and Midwifery Board of Ireland (NMBI) (2016) standards and requirements for competence.

Dependent upon the local configuration of services, community intellectual disability nurses often occupy several new and exciting roles across the lifespan. Many work as specialist practitioners, within multi-disciplinary teams and will work on time-limited interventions that can include epilepsy, ageing, personal and sexual relationships,

challenging behaviours, and supporting access to healthcare. This chapter will serve as a template for good care planning within the context of community intellectual disability teams, or where nurses are attached to local authorities or NHS providers.

Current health and social policy, for example, clinical commissioning, will inevitably make further demands on the development of the everyday practice of intellectual disability nurses working in the community. Seemingly the public health agenda is becoming central to the role of this group of healthcare workers. Implications for all fields of nursing and midwifery will be outlined with reference to the NMC (2018a, 2018b) and NMBI (2016) standards and requirements for competence.

DOI: 10.4324/9781003296461-9

Box 9.1 This chapter will focus on the following issues:

- Key concepts and policies
  - What is community nursing?
  - What is community intellectual disability nursing?
  - Community intellectual disability nursing roles in the United Kingdom
- A brief history of community intellectual disability nursing
  - Policy frameworks in the United Kingdom
- Community intellectual disability nursing practice
  - Models of community care

Box 9.2 Competences

Nursing and Midwifery Council (2018b) Proficiencies

Platform 1: Being an accountable professional – 1.2, 1.7, 1.8, 1.18

Platform 2: Promoting health and preventing ill health – 2.12

Platform 5: Leading and managing nursing care and working in teams – 5.1, 5.2, 5.3, 5.4, 5.5, 5.6, 5.7, 5.8, 5.9, 5.10, 5.11, 5.12

Platform 6: Improving safety and quality of care – 6.2, 6.4, 6.5, 6.6, 6.7

Platform 7: Coordinating care – 7.7, 7.8, 7.13

Nursing and Midwifery Board of Ireland (2016) Competences

Domain 2: Nursing practice and clinical decision-making competences – 2.1, 2.2, 2.3, 2.4, 2.5

Domain 3: Knowledge and cognitive competences – 3.2

Domain 5: Management and team competences – 5.1, 5.2

Domain 6: Leadership potential and professional scholarship competences – 6.1

Key concepts and policies

What is community nursing?

There is no universal definition of 'community nursing'. This is because the word community means different things to different people. To understand what 'community nursing' might mean, there is a need to understand the many definitions of what 'community' means. According to Laverack (2009), there are four main characteristics of a 'community', and these are the following:

1. Geographical location of a place
2. Shared identities or interests of groups of people
3. Social interactions that bond people together
4. Common needs

The dialogical and operational definition of community nursing has tended to incorporate some or all the four key characteristics (Chilton, 2012). What is important to note is the social construction of community nursing, which suggests that their roles may be defined and influenced by others (Kelly and Symonds, 2017).

What adds to the challenges of having a unified definition of community nursing is the range of specialties of community nursing practice. District nursing, health visiting, school nursing, community intellectual disability nursing, community mental health nursing, occupational health nursing, and practice nursing are all variations of community nursing (Buchan *et al.*, 2019). Within and between each of these nurses, there may be varied perceptions of their 'community nursing' roles.

What is community intellectual disability nursing?

Community intellectual disability nursing in the United Kingdom can be traced back to the 1970s. However, there is no legal or professional definition of community intellectual disability nursing. Furthermore, the four countries of the United Kingdom do not provide a working definition of community intellectual disability nursing.

The Royal College of Nursing has attempted to define community intellectual disability nursing (RCN, 1992). This definition has traditionally been accepted in practice, but it is constraining and no longer adequate. This is because the role of community intellectual disability nurses has evolved and continues to evolve in the practice setting (Boarder, 2002; Mobbs *et al.*, 2002; Barr, 2006; Rees, 2021; Mafuba *et al.*, 2021a, 2021b). Community intellectual disability teams have faced significant cuts since austerity began in 2010 in the United Kingdom (Aikaterini-Malli *et al.*, 2018). This has meant that the number of intellectual disability nurses working in these teams has reduced, services have been redesigned, nurses redeployed, and the activity of the community teams have changed their focus (RCN, 2021.) In 2004, the *NHS Knowledge and Skills Framework* outlined role expectations for community intellectual disability nurses in the United Kingdom (DH, 2004). In 2021, the Queens Nursing Institute (QNI) and Queen's Nursing Institute Scotland published a set of voluntary standards to support community intellectual disability nurse education and practice across all four countries of the UK. These standards are timely in terms of raising the profile of the community intellectual disability nurse, as all four countries of England's *Long-Term Plan* (NHS England, 2019; NHS Scotland, 2019; DH, 2016); the policy shift now focuses on promoting community based, integrated and inclusive health and social care in all UK countries with a specific focus on reducing the health inequalities that individuals with intellectual disabilities face.

The meaning of 'community intellectual disability nursing' is more likely to be influenced by the roles the nurse undertakes. These roles have evolved significantly in the recent past and will continue to evolve and increasingly focus on meeting the complex physical and healthcare needs of people with intellectual disabilities and their families (Barr, 2009; Mafuba, 2013; Mafuba *et al.*, 2021a, 2021b). In this book, 'community intellectual disability nurse' refers to a Nursing and Midwifery Council 'intellectual disability nurse' RN5 or RNLD registrant whose role involves provision of nursing care to people with intellectual disabilities in a wide range of community settings. In current practice, the 'community intellectual disability nurse' works in a multidisciplinary team, holds a caseload, and admits and discharges people with intellectual disabilities who have health needs.

Community intellectual disability nursing roles in the United Kingdom

The creation of community intellectual disability nursing roles was partly influenced by de-institutionalisation. Community intellectual disability nursing roles were first described in studies undertaken in the 1980s and 1990s (Mackay, 1989; Parahoo and Barr, 1994, 1996). Although these studies did not clearly describe community intellectual disability nursing roles at the time, they detailed the complex needs of people with intellectual disabilities who were supported in the community by the nurses. Broadly, these roles were focused on meeting the health and social care needs of people with intellectual disabilities living in the community.

Boarder (2002) in a study detailed the roles of community intellectual disability nurses as health maintenance; care planning; health promotion group work; team working; needs assessment; staff and carer training and support; advocacy; supporting community living; maintaining a place in the community; direct work with people with challenging behaviour, autism, mental illness, sensory, and communication difficulties; service development; working with play groups and schools; living skills development; personal relationship education and counseling; bereavement counseling; and research. In England, Mobbs *et al.* (2002) cites as the key roles of community intellectual disability nurses: needs assessment and health screening, provision of advice and support, health monitoring, provision of direct nursing care, counseling, ongoing health promotion, direct clinical procedures, crisis intervention, care reviews, health education and teaching, respite care provision, child protection work, supporting access to leisure and recreation, and other direct work with people with intellectual disabilities. In a study undertaken in Northern Ireland, Barr (2006) identified some of the key roles of community intellectual disability nurses as: health monitoring, provision of advice and support, direct clinical procedures, care reviews, needs assessment and health screening, education and training, care management/care coordination, health promotion, delivery of direct nursing case, counseling, respite care provision, child protection, and support with leisure and recreation. Mafuba and Gates (2013) and Mafuba *et al.* (2018, 2021a, 2021b) have detailed the public health role of community intellectual disability nurses.

BOX 9.3
CASE STUDY 9.1

Paul is a young man with a moderate intellectual disability living in a staffed residential home. Paul has diabetes for which he is on insulin. He also has epilepsy for which he takes 200 mg QDS sodium valproate and 200mg QDS carbamazepine.

He has been prescribed antibiotics for a urinary tract infection, but he has refused to take his medication and refused to discuss any issues with care staff. Whilst on duty one day, you hear one of the care staff trying to explain the importance of the antibiotics to Paul. You then hear this staff member say, '*You are not having your coffee until you take your medication*'. Paul then takes the medication.

Sometime later Paul is admitted to an acute medical ward in a general hospital to receive intravenous antibiotics and other treatments for his infection. He does not present any problems, but the busy nurses find it time-consuming to persuade him to take his medication. Paul tells the nurses that he would like to take his medication but needs constant reassurance. Subsequently, nurses crush his tablets and put them in his food without his knowledge.

a. Identify the roles of the community intellectual disability nurse in meeting Paul's health and healthcare needs.
b. Compare the roles you have identified with those that apply to your country in Table 8.1.
c. Identify relevant NMC/NMBI competencies that are applicable in this scenario.

What is clear from these studies (Boarder, 2002; Mobbs *et al.*, 2002; Barr, 2006; and Mafuba and Gates, 2013) is the increasing focus of the roles of community intellectual disability nurses in meeting the complex healthcare needs of people with intellectual disabilities. Brown *et al.* (2011), in a study of intellectual disability health liaison nurses, highlighted this increasing focus on meeting the continuing health and healthcare needs of people with intellectual disabilities. Furthermore, a study undertaken by Rees (2021) highlighted the significant role that community intellectual disability nurses have in supporting access to secondary care, at times working in partnership with the intellectual disability health liaison nurse.

These studies demonstrate significant developments in clarifying the roles and contributions to meet the often-complex health and healthcare needs of people with intellectual disabilities by community intellectual disability nurses.

However, several challenging issues need to be noted here. A study by Hames and Carlson (2006) have highlighted that local primary healthcare staff did not know about community intellectual disability teams. In addition, primary care staff lacked knowledge of the roles of local community intellectual disability teams, and there was confusion regarding the professionals within specialist community intellectual disability teams. Earlier research has discussed the importance of building the relationship between primary and secondary care (Powell, Murray and McKenzie, 2004), however, more recent research recognises the role of the community intellectual disability nurse in bridging any gap between primary and secondary healthcare and promoting a seamless pathway between primary and secondary healthcare (Rees, 2021). The issue of timely referrals and clear pathway between primary and secondary healthcare is fundamental, with Heslop et al. (2013) explaining that a key factor leading to the premature deaths of people with intellectual disabilities is a failure to undertake diagnostic investigations and necessary treatments in a timely manner. Lack of clarity of the health promotion and health facilitation roles of community intellectual disability nurses were also highlighted.

Agenda for Change (DH, 1999), *The NHS Knowledge and Skills Framework (NHS KSF)*, and *The Development Review Process* (DH, 2004) attempted to clarify the roles of community intellectual disability nurses in the United Kingdom. Mafuba (2013) noted a lack of consistency in role expectations for community intellectual disability nurses in the United Kingdom, suggesting that the evaluation of community intellectual disability nurses' roles through *Agenda for Change* had failed to adequately highlight the importance of these roles.

The changing nature of the role of the community intellectual disability nurse has been recognised for many years, with Boarder (2002), Mobbs *et al.* (2002) and Barr (2006) acknowledging such changes in their research. There may be two drivers; firstly, recognised that community intellectual disability nurses are strengthening their role through becoming increasingly more focused and selective in the work they are undertaking. Secondly, they are being proactive in meeting the identified needs of people with intellectual disabilities. Some evidence of this exists in the development of innovative health screening and health promotion tools, some of which date back over 20 years in Northern Ireland (Barr *et al.*, 1999). However, according to Mobbs (2002) evidence also exists that points to an alternative explanation namely that the role is fragmenting as other services (behaviour support, children's disability teams and epilepsy) increasingly work with individuals that would have previously been seen by community intellectual disability nurses. Consequently, Barr (2006) explains that the community intellectual disability nurse role is becoming much more about monitoring, coordinating and much less about individual client work.

In 2011 the Royal College of Nursing (RCN, 2012) reported that while overall community nursing statistics and those for certain specific areas of community nursing practice in the last decade show gradual increase in relation to the re-orientation of healthcare toward preventative care, community intellectual disability nursing numbers have been characterised by a gradual and consistent long-term decline (RCN, 2012) (see Figure 9.1). There are no recent reports on the numbers of community intellectual disabilities currently in practice in the UK. However, NHS Digital reports a continuing decline in the number of intellectual disabilities nurses practicing in the NHS in England (see Figure 9.2). This decline is more likely to reflect the current state of the community intellectual disability nursing population.

Although there are no clearly defined statutory roles, and limited studies regarding the roles of community intellectual disability nurses, important lessons emerge from literature. First, the complexity and increasingly specialised roles of the community intellectual disability nurses (Mobbs *et al.*, 2002) need to be understood by the nurses themselves, employers, and other health and social care professionals. Second, community intellectual disability nurses make an important contribution to meeting the health and healthcare needs of people

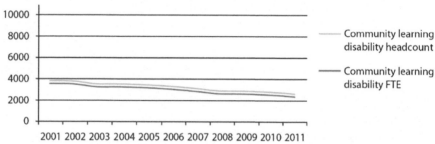

Figure 9.1   *Source:* From RCN (2012) *The Community Nursing Workforce in England.* London: Royal College of Nursing, p. 6

Community intellectual disability nurses in England.

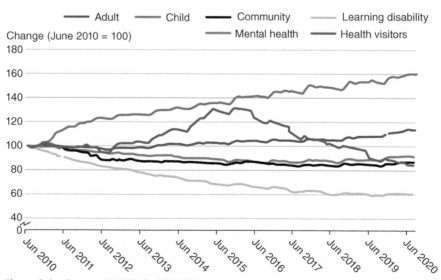

Figure 9.2   *Source:* NHS Digital (2020)

Change in registered nursing workforce (FTE) by work area – June 2010 to June 2020.

with intellectual disabilities in the community, primary care and secondary care (Bollard, 2002; Marshall and Moore, 2003; Barr *et al.*, 1999; Rees, 2021; Mafuba *et al.*, 2021a, 2021b). Third, primary and secondary care professionals have positive regard for community intellectual disability nurses' roles in meeting the health and healthcare needs of people with intellectual disabilities (Stewart and Todd, 2001, Rees, 2021). However, the lack of in-depth research to evaluate and validate the roles of community intellectual disability nurses need to be addressed to make clear their positive contributions to meeting the health and healthcare needs of people with intellectual disabilities in the community. What also needs to be addressed is the lack of clarity of community nursing roles among community intellectual disability nurses themselves, among other healthcare professionals, and among wider health and social care organisations (Boarder, 2002; Hames and Carlson, 2006; Mobbs *et al.*, 2002; Stewart and Todd, 2001; Mafuba, 2013). Making clear the roles of community intellectual disability nurses is important because a lack of role clarity may lead to confused and ambiguous expectations between healthcare professionals, resulting in reduced quality of care for people with intellectual disabilities in the community (Taylor, 1996; Mafuba, 2013).

A brief history of community intellectual disability nursing

The role of the community intellectual disability nurse in meeting the health needs of people with intellectual disabilities can be traced back to the 1960s (Jukes, 1994), influenced by the review of the Mental Health Act in 1959 and a movement lead by Enoch Powel (the Minister of Health at the time) towards community-based provision. Multidisciplinary community teams were first developed in the 1970s with the *Local Authorities Social Services Act 1970* and the first *White Paper* for people with an intellectual disability in England: *Better services for the Mentally Handicapped* (DHSS, 1971) called for the reduction of long stay hospital provision advocating a more integrated support within the community. The Jay report (1979) re-focused attention on the normalisation of community services for people with intellectual disabilities, the concept for which was defined by O'Brien and Tyne in 1981. Their Five Key Principles underpin community nursing practice today: Community Prescence, Choice, Competence, Respect and Community Participation (O'Brien and Tyne, 1981). In the 1980s, several attempts were made to identify and clarify the contribution of community intellectual disability nurses to health promotion (RCN, 1985). The Griffiths Report (Griffiths, 1988) and the NHS and Community Care Act (DH, 1990) emphasised the contribution of community intellectual disability nursing in meeting the health and healthcare needs of people with intellectual disabilities. However, there was a lack of clarity as to what this role entailed and how the role was supposed to be carried out in practice.

As a result, this role has evolved differently across the United Kingdom (Mobbs *et al.*, 2002; Boarder, 2002; Barr, 2006). Whilst Mansell and Harris

(1998) identified five key areas of practice – client-based interventions, coordination and planning of care, training, care management, and health promotion – healthcare and social care services across the United Kingdom had a differing understanding of the role and contribution of community intellectual disability nurses (McGarry and Arthur, 2001).

Policy frameworks in the United Kingdom

The policy agenda for the provision of healthcare for people with intellectual disabilities in the United Kingdom and the Republic of Ireland can be traced back to the beginning of the twentieth century (see Table 9.1). In England, the Mental Deficiency Act 1913 provided a distinct legal identity for people with intellectual disabilities.

Negative reports regarding segregated healthcare provision for people with intellectual disabilities (Department of Health and Social Security, 1969; Morris, 1969) led to a new policy direction through *Better Services for the Mentally Handicapped* (Department of Health and Social Security, 1971). This policy shift had two significant effects in relation to the roles of community intellectual disability nurses. The first effect was the shift of service provision from institutions to the community. The second effect was that intellectual disability nurses had to realign their roles with the new models of service provision based in the community. As de-institutionalisation gathered pace in the 1980s and 1990s, community intellectual disability nursing roles focusing on meeting the health needs of people with intellectual disabilities in the community began to emerge.

The *NHS and Community Care Act 1990* enabled people to stay in their own homes, and the *Health Services for People with Learning Disabilities (Mental Handicap)* (NHS Executive, 1992) highlighted the need for people with intellectual disabilities to access generic healthcare services. It could be argued that this position contributed to the development of some community intellectual disability nursing roles. *Signposts for Success* (NHS Executive, 1998) further outlined care pathways for people with intellectual disabilities in mainstream services, acknowledging that people with intellectual disabilities were experiencing poor access to services in the NHS. The document placed an emphasis on ensuring that the healthcare needs of people with intellectual disabilities were met through mainstream services, whilst recognising the need for continued specialist health and healthcare provision in areas such as mental health, epilepsy, and complex needs.

In 2001, *Valuing People: A New Strategy for Learning Disability for the 21st Century* (DH, 2001) highlighted the need to improve the health of people with intellectual disabilities in England and Wales (*The Same as You* in Scotland) (Scottish Executive, 2000). The complexity of the healthcare needs of people with intellectual disabilities are acknowledged, and the inadequacies of existing models of healthcare provision for people with intellectual disabilities in generic community healthcare settings highlighted. In Scotland, the *Health Needs Assessment Report: People with Learning Disabilities in Scotland* (NHS Health Scotland, 2004) highlighted the needs of people with intellectual disabilities and provided guidance to healthcare professionals on how these could be met.

Year	United Kingdom	Year	Republic of Ireland
1913	Mental Deficiency Act	1945	The Mental Treatment Act 1945
1957	Royal Commission on the Law Relating to Mental Illness and Mental Deficiency 1954–57	1947–2004	Government of Ireland – Health Acts 1947 to 2004
1963	Health and Welfare: The Development of Community Care (Ministry of Health)	1990	Needs and Abilities: A Policy for the Intellectually Disabled (Department of Health [DOH])
1969	Report of the Committee of Inquiry into Allegations of Ill-Treatment and Other Irregularities (Howe Report)		
1971	Better Services for the Mentally Handicapped (DHSS White Paper) Social Services Departments established (England and Wales) Social Work Departments established (Scotland)		
1979	Report of the Committee of Enquiry into Mental Handicap Nursing and Care (Jay Report)	2001	Quality and Fairness: A Health System for You (Department of Health and Children)
1981	Care in the Community (DHSS White Paper)		
1984	Registered Homes Act	2004	The Education of Persons with Special Educational Needs Act (Government of Ireland)
1989	Government Objectives for Community Care (DHSS White Paper)	2008	Government of Ireland – Mental Health Act 2008
1990	NHS and Community Care Act	2005	Disability Act (Government of Ireland)
		2007	Government of Ireland – Health Act 2007
2000	The Same as You (Scottish Executive)	2006	A Vision for Change (Ireland's national mental health policy framework) (Department of Health and Children)
2001	Valuing People (DH White Paper)	2009	Vision Statement for Intellectual Disability in Ireland for the 21st Century (National Federation of Voluntary Bodies)
2002	Review of Mental Health and Learning Disabilities (Northern Ireland) (Department of Health and Social Services)	2011	Time to Move on from Congregated Settings: A Strategy for Community Inclusion (Health Services Executive)
2003	Fulfilling the Promises (Welsh Assembly)	2012	Your Voice, Your Choice (National Disability Authority)
2008	Healthcare for all: report of the independent inquiry into access to healthcare for people with Learning disabilities (Department of Health)	2012	Value for Money and Policy Review of Disability Services in Ireland (Department of Health)
2012	Transforming Care: A national response to Winterbourne Hospital (England)	2013	National Standards for Residential Services for Children and Adults with Disabilities
2012	Health and Social Care Act (England)	2006–2015	Towards 2016: Ten-Year Framework Social Partnership Agreement 2006–2015 (Department of the Taoiseach)
2013	CIPOLD (Confidential Inquiry into Premature Deaths of People with Learning Disabilities)		
2014	The Care Act 2014 (England)		
2019	The Long-Term Plan (England)		
2022	Health and Care Act 2022 (England)		

Table 9.1 Community care policy development timeline in the United Kingdom and the Republic of Ireland

Several initiatives relevant to policy implementation and community nursing roles of intellectual disability nurses were proposed in *Valuing People* (DH, 2001). To improve the implementation of health policy initiatives and access to services for people with intellectual disabilities, health action planning was introduced (DH, 2002, 2009). Health facilitation and health liaison were also introduced (DH, 2001). These policy initiatives affected the community nursing roles of community intellectual disability nurses.

Strengthening the Commitment (DH, 2012a) and *Shaping the future of Intellectual Disability Nursing in Ireland* (McCarron *et al.*, 2018) gave voice to intellectual disability nurses advocating a refocus of the role to support and promote the broad range of health needs of people with an intellectual disability in a variety of settings.

These reports support the recommendations from *Transforming Care: A national response to Winterbourne View Hospital* (DH, 2012b) which called for the reduction on inpatient provision for people with an intellectual disability and/or autism with a coexisting mental health condition. In addition, the *Confidential Inquiry into the Premature Deaths of People with a Learning Disability (CIPOLD)* (Heslop *et al.*, 2013) again highlighted the inequalities in health experienced by people with an intellectual disability calling for the improved support for physical healthcare for people with an intellectual disability to prevent avoidable deaths.

The NHS England *Long Term Plan* (NHS England, 2019) sets out a vision for the twenty-first century, identifying the tackling of health inequalities for people with an intellectual disability as a key priority, alongside offering a commitment to boost community services through the integration of health and social care. These measures affirm the role of the community intellectual disability nurse to drive a responsive and holistic model of care for people in their own home.

Community intellectual disability nursing practice

Models of community care

Community nursing is at the heart of this model of care and in response community nursing services have developed into complex, multi-disciplinary teams. The work of nurses in the community encompasses the promotion of health, healing, growth and development, as well as the prevention and treatment of disease, illness, injury and disability.

(RCN, 2012, p. 1)

The future of community intellectual disability nursing

The structures of community health and healthcare services in the United Kingdom and Ireland are complex and present significant challenges on how community intellectual disability nurses meet the health and healthcare needs of the people they care for. The population of people with intellectual disabilities is increasing in number and is ageing and this changing demographic has led to changes in the health needs of this population. The fragmentation of health services for people with intellectual disabilities between primary care and specialist intellectual disability services leads to unnecessary philosophical and inter-agency tensions. Publications such as Heslop *et al.* (2013) and the Learning Disabilities Mortality Review (LeDER, 2018) continue to highlight the need for preventive health in the United Kingdom. This in turn emphasises the need for the public health roles of community intellectual disability nurses to be made more explicit in the organisations in which they work. Clarity about, and development of new models of how community intellectual disability nurses will enact their community nursing roles in the future need to have a strategic impetus.

Understanding the distribution of the population and morbidity rates of people with intellectual disabilities is increasingly important to ensure community intellectual disability nurses continue to deliver targeted and appropriate community services for people with intellectual disabilities. The importance of the accuracy of demographic information on the roles of community intellectual disability nurses in the future cannot be over-emphasised. Demographic intelligence is important in the investigation and diagnosis of the epidemiological problems that affect people with intellectual disabilities. In addition, this would be useful in facilitating prioritisation of health programmes for people with intellectual disabilities. Furthermore, this would enable better targeting of community health initiatives. Demographic intelligence would also be useful in monitoring and evaluating the impact of health programmes and strategies targeted at the population of people with intellectual disabilities. Finally, demographic intelligence is likely to be key to ensuring that health programmes and strategies for people with intellectual disabilities are evidence-based.

BOX 9.4
CASE STUDY 9.2

John is a 34-year-old male with moderate intellectual disabilities. He was observed experiencing full body convulsive movements whilst at his work placement. An ambulance was called, because the day care workers had not previously witnessed him having a tonic-clonic seizure. No medication was administered, as the seizure had ended by the time paramedics arrived. John has a diagnosis of epilepsy and is known to experience tonic-clonic seizures. On average, he has one seizure every three months with a duration of approximately 30 seconds to 1 minute, usually late in the day just prior to going to bed at 10:30 p.m. John's epilepsy was diagnosed when he was a child and his seizures have been well managed on sodium valproate 500 mg twice daily and carbamazepine 200 mg thrice daily for the past five years. This has been assessed as providing him with the best seizure control. Since his father died three months ago from a myocardial infarction, John now lives with his mother. He can communicate verbally and generally demonstrates an ability to understand information given to him. Information needs to be explained appropriately, and he needs to be given time to consider it. He also needs to be given an opportunity to ask any questions. He is unable to read or write. Since his referral to the Community Intellectual Disability Team (CTLD) his mother reports that he has been very confused and agitated and keeps saying he 'does not know what is happening' and this is 'just like what happened to Dad'. He is reported to have been displaying a lack of motivation, disengagement with usual company, general restlessness, and a disturbed sleep pattern over the last four to six weeks. John is prescribed no other medication other than anticonvulsants.

■ Explore the role of the community intellectual disability nurse in meeting John's health and healthcare needs.

■ Explore and justify any assessment you might need to carry out, using a recognised assessment tool(s). You will need to consider and highlight the role(s) of other professionals in the assessment process.

■ Using the information obtained during the assessment process, draw up a health action plan. You will need to clearly provide a rationale for your approach to health action planning (see Chapter 4). You will need to clearly identify John's needs, proposed interventions, and expected outcomes. You will need to clearly identify the role of the multi-disciplinary team.

■ Identify relevant NMC/NMBI competencies that are applicable in this case.

The *'health liaison'* role of community intellectual disability nurses in the delivery of health services for people with intellectual disabilities is important as an expert in adjusting to the needs of the individual with intellectual disabilities has much to offer in this liaison role and there is evidence indicating that this role is increasingly being based in acute services (Brown *et al.*, 2011) (see Figure 9.3). There is need for this role to be more prominent in the delivery of health services for people with intellectual disabilities by community intellectual disability nurses.

Community intellectual disability nurses' roles in meeting the health and healthcare needs of people with intellectual disabilities are complex and include healthcare delivery, health protection, health prevention, health surveillance, research, and leadership, in addition to the public health roles identified in previous studies (Mafuba, 2013). However, the role of the community intellectual disability nurse continues to lack clarity in how best to meet the health and healthcare needs of people with intellectual disabilities. This lack of role clarity for community intellectual disability nurses may lead to role confusion and ineffective implementation of health services for people with intellectual disabilities (Fyson, 2002; Ross, 2001). Ensuring strategic role clarity of community intellectual disability nurses could result in improved flexibility and responsiveness to the health and healthcare needs of people with intellectual disabilities in both primary and acute services.

There is an increasing acceptance of the importance of the health facilitation role of community intellectual disability nurses among other professionals within primary and acute healthcare settings. This development has evidently enhanced the roles of community intellectual disability nurses. The increasing genericisation of the delivery of healthcare for people with intellectual disabilities and the shift from treatment to preventive health indicates a need for community intellectual disability nurses to focus on enhancing their health facilitation knowledge and skills. This change in roles has been noted before (Barr, 2006), and is inevitable and unavoidable. Supporting people with

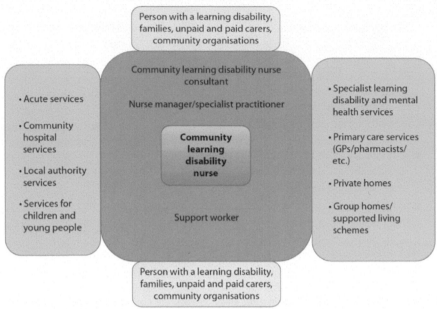

Figure 9.3 *Source:* Adapted from Elliott *et al.* (2012) *Study of the Implementation of a New Community Health Nurse Role in Scotland*. Edinburgh: Scottish Government Social Research, p. 12

Model of community care.

intellectual disabilities access acute and other mainstream services is an important role for community intellectual disability nurses.

Community intellectual disability nurses must work collaboratively with other primary health and social care agencies to reduce health inequalities by facilitating access to health services, including public health services. This will require community intellectual disability nurses to establish partnerships working with local primary care services and work in collaboration with various primary care agencies to mitigate the impact of health inequalities on people with intellectual disabilities. However, to be effective in working in partnership and in collaboration with other agencies, community intellectual disability nurses need to be aware that the health needs of people with intellectual disabilities may not necessarily be a priority for other agencies. In addition, this will require that community intellectual disability nurses provide leadership in enhancing and improving access to generic health services, promoting inclusion in generic public health services, preventing ill health, promoting equality of access, improving the quality of life of people with intellectual disabilities, and working to reduce the adverse impacts of the circumstances of individuals with intellectual disabilities.

For *'effective collaboration'*, community intellectual disability nurses need to engage with health action planning, health facilitation, and health liaison. Castledine (2002) has noted that community intellectual disability nurses could play a significant role in the development of coordinated approaches to delivering health services for people with intellectual disabilities. Twenty years on this is supported in more recent literature, as community intellectual disabilities nurses adapt to the changing dynamics of their role to encompass health issues associated with older age such as dementia and supporting the people they care for at the end of life (Chapman, Lacey and Jervis, 2018; Arrey, Kirshbaum and Finn, 2019). In addition, this literature has demonstrated that community intellectual disability nurses could be key in developing appropriate pathways and protocols for access to health and healthcare for people with intellectual disabilities. These roles need to focus on the development of health action plans, effective systems of liaison, and the development of intellectual environments for other professionals, agencies, and people with intellectual disabilities and their carers.

Conclusion

The variation of the public health roles discussed here demonstrates the intricacies of how public health services are organised, and the challenges that people with intellectual disabilities face when accessing these services. The health facilitation and professional advocacy roles of community intellectual disability nurses highlight their responsibility to challenge public health services to improve accessibility for people with intellectual disabilities. In addition, community intellectual disability nurses need to collaborate and work in partnership with others to fulfil these roles (Broughton and Thomson, 2008). To work effectively as agents of change, community intellectual disability nurses need to have *'leadership'* skills at all levels. Community intellectual disability nurses will need to assume *'leadership roles'* in implementing preventive health programs, developing appropriate services, planning, and develop shared care with primary and secondary health services. These leadership skills are important to influence others and facilitate the collaboration that is essential to developing appropriate public health pathways and implementation of public health policies for people with intellectual disabilities. The importance of the leadership roles of community intellectual disability nurses in the development of appropriate services for people with intellectual disabilities have been highlighted previously and align with NMC Code (NMC, 2018a), and NMC standards (NMC, 2018b).

References

Aikaterini Malli, M., *et al.* (2018) Austerity and the lives of people with learning disabilities: A thematic synthesis of current literature. *Disability & Society*, 33(9), pp. 1412–1435.

Arrey, S.K., Kirshbaum, M.N. and Finn, V. (2019) In search of care strategies for distressed people with communication difficulties and a learning disability in palliative care settings: The lived experiences of registered learning disability nurses and palliative care professionals. *Journal of Research in Nursing*, 24(6), pp. 386–400.

Barr, O. (2006) The evolving role of community nurses for people with learning disabilities: Changes over an 11-year period. *Journal of Clinical Nursing*, 15, pp. 72–82.

Barr, O. (2009) Community learning disability nursing. In Sines, D., Saunders, M. and Forbes-Burford, J. (Eds.), *Community health care nursing* (4th edition). Chichester: Wiley-Blackwell.

Barr, O., *et al.* (1999) Health screening for people with learning disabilities by a community learning disabilities nursing service in Northern Ireland. *Journal of Advanced Nursing*, 29(6), pp. 1482–1491.

Boarder, J.H. (2002) The perceptions of experienced community learning disability nurses of their roles and ways of working. *Journal of Learning Disabilities*, 6(3), pp. 281–296.

Bollard, M. (2002) Health promotion and learning disabilities. *Health Education*, 16(27), pp. 47–55.

Broughton, S. and Thomson, K. (2008) Women with learning disabilities: Risk behaviours and experiences of the cervical smear test. *Journal of Advanced Nursing*, 32(4), pp. 905–912.

Brown, M., *et al.* (2011) Learning disability liaison nursing services in south-east Scotland: A mixed-methods impact and outcome study. *Journal of Intellectual Disability Research*, 56(12), pp. 1161–1174.

Buchan, J., *et al.* (2019) *A critical moment: NHS staffing trends, retention and attrition.* London: The Health Foundation.

Castledine, G. (2002) The important aspects of nurse specialist roles. *British Journal of Nursing*, 11(5), p. 350.

Chapman, M., Lacey, H. and Jervis, N. (2018) Improving services for people with intellectual disabilities and dementia: Findings from a service evaluation exploring the perspectives of health and social care professionals. *British Journal of Intellectual Disabilities*, 46(1), pp. 33–44.

Chilton, S. (2012) Nursing in a community environment. In Chilton, S., Bain, H., Clarridge, A. and Melling, K. (Eds.), *A textbook of community nursing.* London: Hodder & Stoughton.

Department of Health and Social Security (1969) *Report of the committee of inquiry into allegations of Ill-treatment of patients and other irregularities at the Ely Hospital, Cardiff.* Cmnd 3975. London: HMSO.

Department of Health and Social Security (1971) *Better services for the mentally handicapped.* Cmnd 4683. London: HMSO.

DH (1990) *NHS and community care act.* London: HMSO.

DH (1999) *Agenda for change: Modernising the NHS pay system.* London: Department of Health.

DH (2001) *Valuing people: A new strategy for the 21st century.* London: TSO.

DH (2002) *Action for health: Health action plans and health facilitation.* London: Department of Health.

DH (2004) *The NHS knowledge and skills framework (NHS KSF) and the development review process.* London: Department of Health.

DH (2009) *Health action planning and health facilitation for people with disabilities: Good practice guidance.* London: Department of Health.

DH (2012a) *Strengthening the commitment: The report of the UK modernising learning disabilities nursing review.* Edinburgh: The Scottish Government.

DH (2012b) *Transforming care: A national response to Winterbourne view hospital.* London: Department of Health.

DH (2016) *Health and wellbeing 2026 delivering together.* London: Department of Health.

Elliott, L., *et al.* (2012) *Study of the implementation of a new community health nurse role in Scotland.* Edinburgh: Scottish Government Social Research.

Fyson, R.E. (2002) *Defining the boundaries: The implementation of health and social care policies for adults with learning disabilities.* Unpublished PhD thesis. Nottingham: University of Nottingham.

Griffiths, R. (1988) *Community care: Agenda for action. Report for the secretary of state for social services.* London: HMSO.

Hames, A. and Carlson, T. (2006) Are primary care staff aware of the role of community teams in relation to health promotion and health facilitation? *British Journal of Learning Disabilities,* 34(1), pp. 6–10.

Heslop, P., *et al.* (2013) *Confidential inquiry into premature deaths of people with disabilities (CIPOLD).* Bristol: Norah Fry Research Centre.

Jay Committee (1979) *Report of the committee of enquiry into mental handicap nursing and care.* Cmnd 7468. London: HMSO.

Jukes, M. (1994) Development of the community nurse in disability. *British Journal of Nursing,* 3(15), pp. 779–783.

Kelly, A. and Symonds, A. (2017) *The social construction of community nursing* (2nd edition). Basingstoke: Palgrave Macmillan.

Laverack, G. (2009) *Public health: Power, empowerment and professional practice* (2nd edition). Basingstoke: Palgrave Macmillan.

LeDer (2018) *Learning disabilities mortality review programme: Annual report 2018.* Bristol: Norah Fry Research Centre, University of Bristol.

Local authorities social services act 1970. London: HMSO.

Mackay, T. (1989) A community nursing service analysis. *Journal of Intellectual Disability Research,* 40(4), pp. 336–347.

Mafuba, K. (2013) *Public health: Community learning disability nurses' perception and experience of their role.* Unpublished PhD thesis. London: University of West London.

Mafuba, K. and Gates, B. (2013) An investigation into the public health roles of community learning disability nurses. *British Journal Learning Disability,* 43(1), pp. 1–7.

Mafuba, K., *et al.* (2018) *Mixed methods literature review on improving the health of people with a learning disability – a public health nursing approach. Final report.* London: University of West London, Public Health England.

Mafuba, K., *et al.* (2021a) *Understanding the contribution of learning disability nurses: Scoping research. Volume 1 of 3 – Scoping literature review report.* London: University of West London, RCN Foundation.

Mafuba, K., *et al.* (2021b) *Understanding the contribution of learning disability nurses: Scoping research. Volume 2 of 3 – scoping survey research report.* London: University of West London, RCN Foundation.

Mansell, I. and Harris, P. (1998) Role of the registered nurse *learning* disability within community support teams for people with *learning* disabilities. *Journal of Learning Disabilities for Nursing, Health and Social Care,* 2(4), pp. 190–194.

Marshall, D. and Moore, G. (2003) Obesity in people with intellectual disabilities: The impact of nurse-led health screenings and health promotion activities. *Journal of Advanced Nursing,* 41(2), pp. 147–153.

McCarron, M., *et al.* (2018) *Shaping the future of intellectual disability nursing in Ireland.* Dublin: HSE.

McConkey, R. and Truesdale, M. (2001) Reactions of nurses and therapists in mainstream health services to contact with people who have learning disabilities. *Journal of Advanced Nursing,* 32(1), pp. 158–163.

McGarry, J. and Arthur, A. (2001) Informal caring in late life: A qualitative study of the experiences of older carers. *Journal of Advanced Nursing,* 33(2), pp. 182–189.

Mental deficiency act 1913. London: HMSO.

Mental health act 1959. London: HMSO.

Mobbs, C., *et al.* (2002) An exploration of the role of the community nurse, learning disability, in England. *British Journal of Learning Disabilities*, 30(1), pp. 13–18.

Morris, P. (1969) *Put away.* London: Routledge and Kegan Paul.

NHS Digital (2020) *NHS HCHS monthly workforce statistics – June 2020.* Available at: https://digital.nhs.uk/data-and-information/publications/statistical/nhs-workforce-statistics/june-2020 (Accessed 5 August 2022).

NHS England (2019) *The NHS long term plan.* Available at: www.longtermplan.nhs.uk (Accessed 5 August 2022).

NHS Executive (1992) *Health services for people with learning disabilities (mental handicap).* London: Department of Health.

NHS Executive (1998) *Signposts for success in commissioning and providing health services for people with learning disabilities.* London: DH.

NHS Health Scotland (2004) *Health needs assessment report: People with learning disability in Scotland.* Glasgow: NHS Health Scotland.

NHS Scotland (2019) *An integrated health and social care workforce plan for Scotland.* Available at: www. gov.scot/publications/national-health-social-care-integrated-workforce-plan/.

NMC (2018a) *The code: Professional standards of practice and behaviour for nurses, midwives and nursing associates.* London: Nursing and Midwifery Council.

NMC (2018b) *Future nurse: Standards of proficiency for registered nurses.* London: NMC.

Nursing and Midwifery Board of Ireland (2016) *Nurse registration programmes standards and requirements* (4th edition). Dublin: Nursing and Midwifery Board of Ireland.

O'Brien, J. and Tyne, A. (1981) *The principle of normalisation: A foundation for effective services.* London: CMH.

Parahoo, K. and Barr, O. (1994) Job satisfaction of community nurses working with people with a mental handicap. *Journal of Advanced Nursing*, 20(6), pp. 1046–1055.

Parahoo, K. and Barr, O. (1996) Community mental handicap nursing services in Northern Ireland: A profile of clients and selected working practices. *Journal of Clinical Nursing*, 5(4), pp. 221–228.

Powell, H., Murray, G. and McKenzie, K. (2004) Staff perceptions of community learning disability nurses' role. *Nursing Times*, 100(19), pp. 40–42.

RCN (1985) *The role and function of the domiciliary nurse in mental handicap.* London: Royal College of Nursing.

RCN (1992) *The role and function of the domiciliary community nursing for people with a learning disability.* London: Royal College of Nursing.

RCN (2012) *The community nursing workforce in England.* London: Royal College of Nursing.

RCN (2021) *Connecting for change: For the future of learning disability nursing.* London: Royal College of Nursing.

Rees, S. (2021) *Do community learning disability nurses (CNLDs) support adults with learning disabilities in Wales to access secondary healthcare: An exploratory study within the social model of disability.* Unpublished PhD thesis. Wales: University of South Wales.

Ross, J. (2001) *Role identification: An impediment to effective core primary healthcare teamwork.* Unpublished MA thesis. Wellington: Victoria University of Wellington.

Scottish Executive (2000) *The same as you.* Edinburgh: Scottish Executive.

Stewart, D. and Todd, M. (2001) Role and contribution of nurses for learning disabilities: A local study in a county of Oxford-Anglia region. *British Journal of Learning Disabilities*, 29(4), pp. 145–150.

Taylor, J.C. (1996) Systems thinking boundaries and role clarity. *Clinical Performance and Quality Healthcare*, 4(4), pp. 198–199.

The Queen's Nursing Institute (2021) *The QNI/QNIS voluntary standards for community learning disability nurse education and practice*. Available at: https://qni.org.uk/wp-content/uploads/2021/06/QNI-and-QNIS-Voluntary-Standards-for-Community-Learning-Disability-Nurse-Education-and-Practice.pdf (Accessed 10 June 2022).

Further Reading

Chilton, S. and Bain, H. (2017) *A textbook of community nursing* (2nd edition). London: Hodder & Stoughton.
Evans, D., Coutsaftiki, D. and Fathers, C.P. (2017) *Health promotion and public health for nursing students* (3rd edition). Exeter: Learning Matters Ltd.
Hubley, J., Copeman, J. and Woodall, J. (2020) *Practical health promotion* (3rd edition). Cambridge: Polity Press.
Jukes, M. (Ed.). (2009) *Learning disability nursing practice – origins, perspectives and practice*. London: Quay Books.
Kelly, A. and Symonds, A. (2017) *The social construction of community nursing* (2nd edition). Basingstoke: Palgrave Macmillan.
Sines, D., Saunders, M. and Forbes-Burford, J. (Eds.). (2013) *Community health care nursing* (4th edition). Chichester: Wiley-Blackwell.

Useful Resources

NMBI: www.nursingboard.ie/en/reqs_stds_reg.aspx
BILD: www.bild.org.uk/
Contact for families with disabled children: https://contact.org.uk/help-for-families/information-advice-services/health-medical-information/
Enable Scotland: www.enable.org.uk/Pages/Enable_Home.aspx
Foundation for People with Learning Disabilities: www.learningdisabilities.org.uk/
General Medical Council: www.gmc-uk.org/learningdisabilities/
Inclusion Ireland: www.inclusionireland.ie/
Intellectual Disability Info Web Pages: www.intellectualdisability.info/
The Improving Health and Lives Learning Disabilities Observatory: www.improvinghealthandlives.org.uk/publications
Mencap: www.mencap.org.uk/
Mencap Northern Ireland: www.mencap.org.uk/northern-ireland
Mencap Wales: http://wales.mencap.org.uk
Nursing and Midwifery Council: http://standards.nmc-uk.org/Pages/Welcome.aspx

CHAPTER 10

Dorothy Kupara and Michael Brown

Intellectual disabilities liaison nursing

Introduction

The population of people with intellectual disabilities is changing with overall increase over the years. They are growing into older age due to several factors. They have significant healthcare needs compared to the general population; therefore, they are frequent users of acute healthcare services. People with intellectual disabilities and their carers experience difficulties when accessing or using acute healthcare services, hence they will require additional support. The acute liaison nurse role has been established in response to the identified difficulties to support to improve their health outcomes. This chapter will explore the current role of the acute liaison nurse for people with intellectual disabilities in achieving person-centred outcomes in acute healthcare services. It will reflect on some of the key developments, guidelines and recommendations that have influenced the acute liaison nursing role.

Therefore, this chapter focuses on the knowledge and practical skills that acute liaison nurses for people with intellectual disabilities will need to meet their needs. This will be contextualised within the Nursing and Midwifery Council for the United Kingdom's *Future nurse: Standards for pre-registration nursing* (NMC, 2018a) and Nursing and Midwifery Board of Ireland (2016) standards and requirements for competence. The role of acute liaison nursing is discussed as an emerging role, as well as intellectual disabilities nurses' ability as individuals and as a profession to adapt and work effectively in acute healthcare settings.

DOI: 10.4324/9781003296461-10

Box 10.1 This chapter will focus on the following issues:

- Background on intellectual disabilities

- Exploration of liaison nursing history

- Development of the acute liaison nurse role for people with intellectual disabilities

- Outline some key policies, national frameworks, reports, and guidelines that have influenced liaison nursing

- Discuss the essential role of the acute liaison nursing for people with intellectual disabilities

    - Raising awareness

    - Health advocacy

    - Reasonable adjustments

    - Mental Capacity

    - Supporting carers

    - Care coordination

    - Policy development

    - Managing change

- Challenges and barriers in intellectual disabilities liaison nursing

Box 10.2 Competences and Proficiencies

NMC Future Nurse: Standards of Proficiency for Registered Nurses (NMC, 2018a)

Platform 1: Being an accountable professional – 1.1, 1.9, 1.11, 1.12, 1.13, 1.14, 1.15, 1.18, 1.20

Platform 2: Promoting health and preventing ill health – 2.2, 2.4, 2.12

Platform 3: Assessing needs and planning care – 3.1, 3.2, 3.3, 3.4, 3.5, 3.6, 3.7 3.8, 3.9 3.10 3.11, 3.12, 3.13, 3.14, 3.15, 3.16

Platform 4: Providing and evaluating care – 4.1, 4.8, 4.10, 4.13, 4.14, 4.15, 4.18

Nursing and Midwifery Board of Ireland (2016) Competences

Domain 2: Nursing practice and clinical decision-making competences – 2.1, 2.2, 2.3, 2.4, 2.5

Domain 3: Knowledge and cognitive competences – 3.2

Domain 5: Management and team competences – 5.1, 5.2

Domain 6: Leadership potential and professional scholarship competences – 6.1

Background

There are approximately 1.5 million people with intellectual disabilities in the UK (Public Health England, 2016; Office of National Statistics (ONS), 2020) and they comprise some 2% of the population (Emerson and Hatton, 2009). It is predicted that the number of people with intellectual disabilities will increase by 14% between 2001 and 2021 (Emerson and Hatton, 2009). Many are growing into old age due to a range of factors which include improved diagnosis, advances in medical technology, an increased awareness of their health needs, and improved monitoring of mortality figures (Brown, Cooper and Diebel, 2012; The Regulation and Quality Improvement Authority, 2016; NHS, 2021a). Increase in life expectancy for people with intellectual disabilities has followed similar trends to those of the general population (Coppus, 2013) though it is 15–20 years shorter than the wider population (Public Health England, 2018).

People with intellectual disabilities experience health inequalities or disparities (Mencap, 2004, 2007, 2012; Michael, 2008; Heslop *et al.*, 2013; Public Health England, 2016; LeDeR, 2020, Care Quality Commission (CQC), 2021). They have poorer health than the general population due to poor communications skills and limited health literacy and these health inequalities can be reduced (Department of Health and Social Care, 2019). The significant health needs are associated with a wide range of complex needs making them use healthcare services more frequently than the general population (Brown *et al.*, 2016). They encounter difficulties when accessing acute healthcare services and have much poorer experiences and outcomes than the general population (NHS Improvement, 2018). People with intellectual disabilities are likely to have extended hospital stay whilst requiring additional support from their families and carers (Drozd and Clinch, 2016). As a response to these difficulties, the acute liaison nursing role has been recommended and developed as a reasonable adjustment to ensure people with intellectual disabilities and their carers have improved hospital experience and patient outcomes.

Attending hospital for medical attention can be stressful and a time of anxiety for anyone (Regulation and Quality Improvement Authority, 2018) and it can be more frightening, complicated, and confusing for people with intellectual disabilities as they may have difficulties adjusting to hospital environments and routines (Giraud-Saunders *et al.*, 2014). The communication difficulties and reduced health literacy they experience make it difficult for them to report and seek medical attention effectively (Robertson *et al.*, 2014) hence the need of acute liaison nurses as a reasonable adjustment. Mencap, a leading UK charity, called for health services to appoint acute intellectual liaison nurses in all acute hospitals in the *Getting it right* charter (Mencap, 2010). The concept of the acute liaison nurse for people with intellectual disabilities was recommended in the *Healthcare for All* report in England (Michael, 2008), and Heslop *et al.* (2013) suggested a care coordinator in hospitals.

Liaison nursing

Until recently, there were no dedicated acute liaison nurses in intellectual disabilities nursing practice, so it is important to give a brief overview of liaison nursing to put this role into context. Whilst the role of the acute liaison nurse for people with intellectual disabilities is a recent development and emerging role in practice, liaison nursing is not entirely a new concept; it was developed in the post-World War 1 period (Robinson, 1987).

History or origins of liaison nursing

The concept of liaison nursing originated from the United State of America (USA) in psychiatry or mental health nursing in the 1950s (Robinson, 1987), but this was slow to develop in the UK and only started in the late 1970s (Aitken *et al.*, 2016). The liaison nurse role evolved from nurses and doctors who developed a care management plan at a general hospital after they realised they were providing different types of medical services which were disjointed. They wanted to provide care throughout all phases of a patient's illness with a team approach, but it was challenging to ensure continuity and comprehensive care for the patient. In response to this challenge, they devised a plan to have a nurse assigned to each medical team and created a professional classification called liaison nurse (O'Connor and Hagan, 1964). Liaison nursing was provided to patients admitted to a general hospital for non-psychiatric conditions but whose hospital experience could be improved by the expertise of health workers with mental healthcare training (Victorian Government Department of Health and Community Services, 1996). Their scope of practice was later extended to emergency departments (Robinson, 1987). 'A liaison nurse is a go-between for nursing and other health professionals concerned with patient care' (O'Connor and Hagan, 1964, p. 101). They were appointed to help bridge the divide between general hospital services and psychiatric services (Ryan, Clemmett and Snelson, 1997).

The core functions of the liaison nurse were to influence patient care through persuasion, nondirective guidance and teaching of nursing staff who carried out direct responsibility of care. The liaison nurse would follow the patient throughout the hospital. Their responsibility was to assist healthcare staff to maintain continuity of care, facilitate communication among all departments in the hospital until the patient was discharged back into the community. Liaison nursing was seen as good practice that ensured the patient was well supported at home and when in hospital and ensured good quality and continuity of care (Roberts, 1997; Sharrock and Happell, 2000; Lloyd and Guthrie, 2012). Liaison nursing in psychiatry became an essential subspecialty and it was the only visible part of psychiatry service.

Traditionally, liaison nurses came to the role without preparation or specific education and only relied on the practical knowledge of staffing and patient needs (Clemence, 1981). The American Nursing Association (ANA) later developed standards of practice for liaison nursing (ANA, 1990) and some academic courses about the role were introduced.

Acute Liaison Nursing for people with intellectual disabilities

In the UK, the needs of people with intellectual disabilities when attending acute hospital care and the role of the liaison nurse is a focus within pre-registration nurse education programmes. There is no post-registration education course to prepare intellectual disabilities nurses to become acute liaison nurses, though there is some sort of preparation in other liaison nursing roles. Therefore, the acute liaison nurse is an expert by virtue of their knowledge and skills of the distinct needs of people with intellectual disabilities, gained through experience and thereby an advanced practitioner by default (Morton-Nance, 2015). In the UK the first acute liaison nursing service for people with Intellectual Disabilities was established in 1997 at the Western General Hospital, Edinburgh (Brown *et al.*, 2016).

The liaison nurse for people with intellectual disabilities is described as highly experienced registered intellectual disability nurses (RIDNs) working exclusively in general hospitals to support people with intellectual disabilities and their families throughout pre-attendance, attendance, admission, and discharge (MacArthur *et al.*, 2015). The core function of the acute liaison nurse for people with intellectual disabilities is diverse and wide-ranging, and the role is collaborative in that they work across primary, secondary, and tertiary service (Morton-Nance, 2015). The acute liaison nurses are expected to develop deeper knowledge and understanding of complex medical procedures through experience when they are enacting their liaison role. The key element of the acute liaison nursing service is to enable compassionate and person-centred care for people with intellectual disabilities by advocating for them and their carers (Brown, Cooper and Diebel, 2012; Brown *et al.*, 2016).

Development of acute liaison nursing

Key developments in intellectual disabilities Liaison Nursing

Government policies and reports have focused on improving health of people with intellectual disabilities, and the support required to enable them to have better access to healthcare. The improvements of care for people with intellectual disabilities have shifted from delivery of healthcare services in hospitals to community settings where they live independently or in supported living (Morton-Nance, 2015). Over the past 50 years there has been a shift away from institutional medical models of care when supporting people with intellectual disabilities (MacArthur *et al.*, 2015) and as they live in the community, they are expected to access acute healthcare services as with the general population, yet they continue to experience barriers when accessing acute healthcare services.

There have been reports evidencing the difficulties and the neglect experienced by people with intellectual disabilities and intellectual disabilities when using hospital services (Mencap, 2004, 2007; Disability Rights Commission (DRC), 2006; Michael, 2008; Parliamentary and Health Service Ombudsman,

2009; Heslop *et al.*, 2013; Public Health England, 2018; LeDeR, 2020; Care Quality Commission (CQC), 2021). These reports have called for the improvement of access to acute healthcare for people with intellectual disabilities.

In 2004, Mencap launched the *Treat me right!* report and campaign which exposed the unequal healthcare that people with intellectual disabilities often receive from healthcare services and professionals. The report called for more work to be done in the National Health Service (NHS) to ensure that people with intellectual disabilities are treated fairly and equally. Subsequently, Mencap highlighted six cases of people who died under NHS care in England in *Death by Indifference* report (Mencap, 2007). These cases highlighted the need for reasonable adjustments to be made for people with intellectual disabilities when accessing acute healthcare services.

Mencap (2007) argued that the six people died unnecessarily because of receiving poor healthcare. The *Death by Indifference* report (Mencap, 2007) exposed what it considered to be a *'national disgrace'* and suggested this to be the result of *'institutional discrimination'* by healthcare services towards people with intellectual disabilities and their carers. The *Death by Indifference* report (Mencap, 2007) raised serious concerns about how people with intellectual disabilities were being treated in the healthcare system and how the government had failed to act to previous calls for changes in the NHS. The report also highlighted that practice, policy, procedures, and systems followed by the acute healthcare staff were not grounded in proper knowledge of the needs of people with intellectual disabilities (Mencap, 2007).

In 2006, the Disability Rights Commission (DRC) conducted an 18-month investigation into the health inequalities experienced by people with mental health problems and/or intellectual disabilities in England and Wales. It produced the *Closing the Gap* report (DRC, 2006) which stated that there was worryingly little or nothing that had been done to implement the recommendations of the *Treat me right!* report (Mencap, 2004). *Closing the Gap* report (DRC, 2006) called the government to make urgent improvements in closing the gaps of inequality that resulted in poor health outcomes for people with intellectual disabilities. *Closing the Gap* (DRC, 2006) showed people with intellectual disabilities and mental health problems were continuing to experience difficulties when accessing healthcare services and reasonable adjustments were not being consistently implemented.

Following *Closing the Gap* report (DRC, 2006) and *Death by Indifference* report (Mencap, 2007), the Department of Health in England commissioned an independent inquiry to learn lessons from the six cases highlighted in the *Death by Indifference* report. Sir Jonathan Michael chaired the inquiry into the healthcare for people with intellectual disabilities to identify the action needed to ensure they receive appropriate medical treatment in the NHS. The inquiry's report, *Healthcare for All*, was published in July 2008 and made 10 key recommendations for the standards of care that people with intellectual disabilities should expect.

The Michael (2008) inquiry found that there was a need to overcome the barriers to delivering effective healthcare for people with intellectual disabilities by implementing reasonable adjustments and recommended the appointment of 'acute liaison nurses'. Phillips (2019) concluded that reasonable adjustments for people with intellectual disabilities involved improving access to the healthcare services amongst other initiatives. Michael (2008) concluded that when peo-ple with intellectual disabilities access acute healthcare services there was poor understanding of their health needs and the risks they present as general health-care staff training was very limited; health risks are complicated, and the behav-iour of people with intellectual disabilities may be challenging and difficult to interpret. It was envisioned that the appointment of 'acute liaison nurses' to provide health facilitation or link working between and across primary and secondary specialised care would give a better hospital experience for people with intellectual disabilities. Whilst the *Healthcare for All* report (Michael, 2008) pointed out poor practice in healthcare it also acknowledged some areas of good practice, but it was patchy and could not be generalised.

In 2008, the Parliamentary Health Service Ombudsman and Local Govern-ment Ombudsman investigated the deaths of the six people highlighted in the *Death by Indifference* report (Mencap, 2007). The Ombudsman published the *Six Lives: The Provision of Public Services to People with Learning Disabilities* report in 2009. The investigation showed some significant and disturbing failures in services across both health and social care (Parliamentary and Health Service Ombudsman, 2009). The report revealed the devastating impact of the behav-iour of the NHS which failed to respond to the needs of individuals in a person-centred way and treated people with intellectual disabilities unfavourably. The Ombudsman emphasised the urgent need to change the NHS's way of provid-ing healthcare services to people with intellectual disabilities. The Parliamen-tary Health Service Ombudsman and Local Government Ombudsman (2009) endorsed the recommendations made in the *Healthcare for All* report (Michael, 2008) and welcomed the English White Paper, *Valuing People Now: A new three-year strategy for people with learning disabilities* (DH, 2009). The Ombudsman went on further to recommend that the leaders in health and social care organ-isations needed to review the effectiveness of their systems to enable them to understand and plan to meet the full range of needs of people with intellectual disabilities in their areas. The report stressed that health and social care services needed to make systematic changes to meet the additional and repeatedly com-plex needs of people with intellectual disabilities. Healthcare services had to adjust and think strategically how they would meet the needs of people with intellectual disabilities when using their services.

The *Valuing People Now: A new three-year strategy for people with learning dis-abilities* (DH, 2009) was the plan for intellectual disabilities services in England until 2011. *Valuing People Now* (DH, 2009) accepted all of Michael (2008)'s rec-ommendations and built them into legislation and policy but this time they were observed to be stronger and more specific compared to aims of *Valuing People* (DH, 2001). The *Death by indifference: 74 deaths and counting A progress report 5 years on* report (Mencap, 2012) highlighted continued failings in the NHS where practices showed disregard of Equality Act 2010 and Mental Capac-ity Act 2005. This report showed changes made were neither wide enough nor deep enough for change to happen in the hospitals.

The *Healthcare for All* report (Michael, 2008) also recommended that the Department of Health in England should establish an intellectual disabilities Public Health Observatory which should be supplemented by a time lim-ited Confidential Inquiry into premature deaths in people with intellectual disabilities. This was required to provide evidence for clinical and professional staff of the extent of the problem and guidance on prevention. The Confidential Inquiry reviewed the patterns of care that people with intellectual disabilities received in health services in England in the period leading up to their deaths, identified errors or omissions contributing to these deaths, illustrated evidence of good practice, and provided improved evidence on avoiding premature death, and it was completed in 2013 (Heslop *et al.*, 2013). The *Confidential Inquiry into Premature Deaths of People with Learning Disabilities (CIPOLD)* report (Heslop *et al.*, 2013) was published. CIPOLD found that the quality and effectiveness of health and social care given to people with intellectual disabilities in England was deficient and reiterated the need to implement reasonable adjustments. Heslop *et al.* (2013) recommended a named healthcare coordinator to be allocated to people with intellectual disabilities with complex or multiple health needs, or two or more long-term conditions when accessing hospital services. CIPOLD again highlighted the need to improve access to acute healthcare services for people with intellectual disabilities.

CIPOLD (Heslop *et al.*, 2013) recommended the setting up of a National Learning Disability Mortality Review Body in England. The Department of Health and NHS England identified the need for better information to enable accurate assessment of the causes of death of people with intellectual disabilities (NHS Digital, 2013). The Learning Disabilities Mortality Review (LeDeR) Programme was set up and was funded by NHS England and NHS Improvement and commissioned by the Healthcare Quality Improvement Partnership (HQIP) (University of Bristol, 2021). It is a service improvement programme which aims to improve care, reduce health inequalities, and prevent premature mortality of people with intellectual disabilities and autistic people by reviewing information about the health and social care support people received (NHS, 2021a). The NHS Long Term Plan 2019 in England made a continuing commitment to the LeDeR programme. The findings from the LeDeR programme confirms that there are many and continuing challenges faced by people with intellectual disabilities in relation to their health.

Roles of acute liaison nurses for people with intellectual disabilities

Acute liaison nurses provide a valuable service to overcome the barriers faced by people with intellectual disabilities and their carers when accessing acute healthcare services. People with intellectual disabilities face increased challenges in accessing and receiving high quality care and the Covid-19 pandemic has further exposed and exacerbated these inequalities (Care Quality Commission, 2021). The barriers occur at patient level, healthcare professional level, and organisational level. The aim of the acute liaison nurse is to improve the patient outcomes and quality of life of people with intellectual disabilities and enhance their patient journey. The roles of acute liaison nurses for people with intellectual disabilities are not exhaustive; this section highlights some of the essential roles.

Raising awareness

The goal of the acute liaison nurse is to ensure person-centred care is provided for the patient with intellectual disabilities. It was established that some health-care professionals lack knowledge or skills to meet the multiple and complex needs of people with intellectual disabilities (Backer, Chapman and Mitchell, 2009; Heslop *et al.*, 2013). This deficit in knowledge and skills leads to poor quality of care and increases safety risks for people with intellectual disabilities. Often health professionals may not be well equipped to meet the needs to people with intellectual disabilities (Doody, Hennessy and Bright, 2022). The acute liaison nurses provide access to training and practice development for healthcare professionals to raise their awareness of the needs of this group (Castles *et al.*, 2013). Training allows the healthcare professionals to respond to the needs and ensures a good patient experience and improved health outcomes (Howieson, 2015). Acute liaison nurses working in different healthcare settings reported that training other healthcare staff was one of their key roles (Health Education England (HEE), 2020).

Health advocacy

The acute liaison nurse ensures a positive hospital experience for people with intellectual disabilities and their carers by advocating for them through pro-fessional advocacy supporting self-advocacy, and promoting rights, choice, and empowerment (Castles *et al.*, 2013; MacArthur *et al.*, 2015; Northway *et al.*, 2017). Health advocacy involves different issues at different levels. The *NMC Code* specifically requires nurses to act as an advocate for the vulnerable, chal-lenging poor practice and discriminatory attitudes and behaviour relating to their care (NMC, 2018b).

Do Not Resuscitate (DNR) orders are instructions which determine if cardio-pulmonary resuscitation (CPR) needs to be administered in the event a person's breathing stops or their heart stops, it tries to get the breathing and heart going again (NHS, 2021b). There is evidence to suggest that more DNR orders have been placed on people with intellectual disabilities when in hospital, even more so during the recent Covid-19 pandemic (Alexander *et al.*, 2020; LeDeR, 2020; NICE, 2021). This raises concerns regarding the human rights of people with intellectual disabilities, therefore there is an essential need to ensure full compli-ance with existing frameworks when DNR orders are being considered (Taggart *et al.*, 2022). The acute liaison nurses advocate on DNR orders to ensure these are not automatically applied to patients with intellectual disabilities without appropriate assessment and understanding of the circumstances of the individ-ual, with decisions based solely on medical evidence and likely outcomes.

An important area of activity for acute liaison nurses includes advising on mental capacity issues (Castles *et al.*, 2013). The acute liaison nurses advocate to ensure the mental capacity is appropriately assessed and the patients with intellectual disabilities are involved in decision making about their care and treatment. The health advocacy role entails supporting the healthcare professional to give accessible information about patients with intellectual disabilities' diagnosis and treatment plans to ensure they receive person-centred care. The acute liaison nurses may also advocate for the family involvement in planning treatment and making key decisions. The acute liaison nurses can advocate by supporting the healthcare professionals to acknowledge the people with intellectual disabilities and their carers as experts in their care, thereby promoting their involvement throughout (Blair, 2011).

Health advocacy also entails advocating for hospital or patient passports of patients with intellectual disabilities to be used by all healthcare professionals. It has been highlighted that pain experienced by people with intellectual disabilities is often poorly recognised and managed by healthcare staff, subsequently affecting their health and quality of life (Public Health England, 2018). Due to the communication difficulties many may have, people with intellectual disabilities find it difficult to explain how they are experiencing the pain, location of the pain, and the impact on their life. To address this health inequality the acute liaison nurse advocates the use of alternative assessment tools as a reasonable adjustment for people who rely on others to assess and identify pain. These situations require the making of reasonable adjustments for people with intellectual disabilities to ensure a positive patient experience and equality in care. In a scoping review of the literature conducted by Mafuba *et al.* (2021) regarding interventions undertaken by intellectual disabilities nurses, health advocacy was identified as one of the key interventions done to enhance the quality of life of people with intellectual disabilities. This highlights that acute liaison nurses' need to develop effective health advocacy in acute healthcare settings to improve the health and healthcare outcomes for people with intellectual disabilities (Northway *et al.*, 2017).

Reasonable adjustments

People with intellectual disabilities can receive person-centred and non-discriminatory care in acute healthcare settings through support of acute liaison nurses by ensuring reasonable adjustments are implemented. Reasonable adjustments are changes that organisations and people providing services or public functions must make for disabled people if the disability puts them at a disadvantage compared with non-disabled peers (Mind, 2018). They are a legal obligation under the Equality Act 2010 to ensure services, including health services, are accessible for people who are disabled, and all people are treated fairly and equitably. They are usually small, yet often significant changes intended to overcome the disadvantage experienced by people with intellectual disabilities in accessing acute healthcare services. Reasonable adjustments can make a significant difference for people with intellectual disabilities and ensure they receive equitable care and treatment (Royal College of Nursing (RCN), 2022). See Box 10.1 for the three requirements for duty to provide reasonable adjustments under the Equality Act 2010.

Box 10.3 Reasonable adjustments in the Equality Act 2010, Section 20

- The first requirement is a requirement, where a provision, criterion or practice of A's puts a disabled person at a substantial disadvantage in relation to a relevant matter in comparison with persons who are not disabled, to take such steps as it is reasonable to have to take to avoid the disadvantage.
- The second requirement is a requirement, where a physical feature puts a disabled person at a substantial disadvantage in relation to a relevant matter in comparison with persons who are not disabled, to take such steps as it is reasonable to have to take to avoid the disadvantage.
- The third requirement is a requirement, where a disabled person would, but for the provision of an auxiliary aid, be put at a substantial disadvantage in relation to a relevant matter in comparison with persons who are not disabled, to take such steps as it is reasonable to have to take to provide the auxiliary aid.

The English *Health and Care Act 2022* places a legal duty on NHS England and Integrated Care Systems (ICSss) to reduce health inequalities for people with disabilities when accessing health and social care to improve their health outcomes. In England, the Care Quality Commission (CQC) monitors all NHS and independent hospitals, to ensure they meet basic requirements of quality and safety. The CQC's monitoring process looks at the hospital's service to see if they are acting on people's needs by making reasonable adjustments as outlined in the Equality Act 2010 (CQC, 2017). Similar healthcare regulators exist in other countries; Healthcare Improvement Scotland (Scotland), Healthcare Inspectorate Wales (Wales), The Regulation and Quality Improvement Authority (Northern Ireland), and the Health Information and Quality Authority (Republic of Ireland).

Reasonable adjustments can occur at two different levels, system and individual (Moloney, Hennessy and Doody, 2021). System level reasonable adjustments involve strategic strategies for addressing barriers that prevent people with intellectual disabilities from accessing a service. Individual level reasonable adjustments are to do with the person with intellectual disabilities and they are usually identified after an assessment. Acute liaison nurses understand what reasonable adjustments are but there is reduced knowledge and understanding of these amongst other healthcare professionals in hospital settings (HEE, 2020).

At system level the acute liaison nurses can support acute healthcare services to implement reasonable adjustments for people with intellectual disabilities by considering in advance the type of adjustments required (Heslop *et al.*, 2019). System level reasonable adjustments are available to all people with disabilities and are embedded in the hospital's care pathways. They include altering policies and procedures by considering the needs of people with intellectual disabilities (Phillips, 2019). Examples of system level adjustments include availability of accessible toilets, wheelchair accessible reception desks, changing places, easy read information like menus or patient information leaflets, effective signposting that is colour coded, flagging up system or alerts of patients who need reasonable adjustments, use of patient or hospital passports, policy that supports people with intellectual disabilities, screening programmes and care pathways that are specifically tailored for people with intellectual disabilities, and many others.

At individual level, the acute liaison nurse would ensure a patient with intellectual disabilities is appropriately assessed to establish the reasonable adjustments needed for them at that time. Acute liaison nurses must establish if the individual level reasonable adjustments are anticipatory, responsive, and flexible (Phillips, 2019) to ensure appropriate interventions are done. Examples of individual level reasonable adjustments that could be facilitated include giving extended time for appointments, ensuring the patient's mental capacity is appropriately assessed using the Mental Capacity Act 2005 legal framework, where a person lacks the mental capacity regarding a specific decision a best interests process of decision-making is followed, coordinated interagency working where there are different professionals involved in the care of the individual, allowing carers to stay with the patient, and many more.

The acute liaison nurse has a role in ensuring reasonable adjustments are implemented in acute healthcare services at both system and individual levels (MacArthur *et al.*, 2015). Staff in general hospital need to be supported and reminded by acute liaison nurses about the need to consider reasonable adjustments (HEE, 2020). Acute liaison nurses advise on reasonable adjustments (Morton-Nance, 2015). They share information across primary, secondary and specialist care services to identify people with intellectual disabilities and the reasonable adjustments needed to ensure good hospital experience (Tuffrey-Wijine *et al.*, 2013; Gray and Watson, 2017). It is necessary to make reasonable adjustments in healthcare services to ensure safe and effective person-centred care and prevent further avoidable deaths (MacArthur *et al.*, 2015; LeDeR, 2020). People with intellectual disabilities need additional and alternative support approaches to achieve positive health outcomes and reasonable adjustments can be used to ensure this happens. It is the acute liaison nurse's responsibility to ensure reasonable adjustments are made (Phillips, 2019) and implementing them brings value to healthcare services and improves the quality of life of people with intellectual disabilities.

Mental capacity

In Scotland the Adults with Incapacity Act came into force in 2000 to protect people aged 16 and over lacking capacity to make some or all decisions regarding their welfare, including care, treatment, and finances (Adults with Incapacity Act, 2000). The Mental Capacity Act (MCA) 2005 in England and Wales came into force towards the end of 2007 and was supported by the Mental Capacity Act Code of Practice (Department of Constitutional Affairs, 2007). The Mental Capacity (Northern Ireland) Act came into force in 2016 and provides the legal framework to enable decision-making for people who lack capacity. Collectively, mental capacity legislation helps to ensure that individuals who may lack capacity to make decisions on their own get appropriate support to make those decisions. When a mental capacity assessment finds that a person lacks capacity, healthcare professionals need to collaborate with the person and their significant others to decide in the individual's best interests (Jayes *et al.*, 2022). Any decision made for a person lacking the relevant mental capacity should be made in accordance with the key principles of the MCA, in line with the best interests process and less restrictive principle (CQC, 2021). Acute liaison nurses support other healthcare professionals and people with intellectual disabilities with the mental capacity assessment process. Advising and training on mental capacity assessments is an important area of activity for acute liaison nurses (Castles *et al.*, 2013; HEE, 2020).

Box 10.4 Mental capacity assessment process

To determine if an individual has capacity involves a two-test stage test. Stage 1 asks the question '*Is the person unable to make a particular decision (the functional test)?*'. Stage 2 asks '*Is the inability to make a decision caused by an impairment of, or disturbance in the functioning of, a person's mind or brain?*'. The MCA says that a person is unable to make their own decision if they cannot do one or more of the following four things:

1. Understand information given to them
2. Retain that information long enough to be able to make the decision

3. Weigh up the information available to make the decision
4. Communicate their decision – this could be by talking, using sign language or even simple muscle movements such as blinking an eye or squeezing a hand.

Supporting carers

Acute liaison nurses provide support for the family or carers of patients with intellectual disabilities when accessing acute healthcare services as some attend hospital with their families or carers. The family or carers have a long history of the needs of the person they are supporting and are experts in their care (Phillips, 2019). The family or carers are important and valuable that they need to be supported and listened to as they navigate the hospital services with the patient with intellectual disabilities. Family or carers of patients often find their opinions ignored by healthcare staff and struggle to be accepted as equal partners in the care of the patient with intellectual disabilities (RQIA, 2018). Acute liaison nurses support the family or carers to enable them to contribute to the effective care and treatment of their relative. Informal carers also need to be supported, but the nurse needs to seek the patient's consent before sharing information with them. As a reasonable adjustment, some carers might need overnight accommodations and meals during the patient with intellectual disabilities' stay in hospital.

Care coordination

When a patient with intellectual disabilities attends hospital for medical assessment, treatment, or review they are likely to have different healthcare professionals involved. As some patients will have long-term and multiple conditions, they can find it difficult to navigate the hospital system to ensure all their needs are met. Lack of care coordination can contribute to premature death (LeDeR, 2020). Acute liaison nurses have a duty to coordinate the care of patients with intellectual disabilities to improve their health outcomes, quality of life and prevent risk of neglect and avoidable deaths. When patients with intellectual disabilities are using different care pathways in the hospital there is a need for the acute liaison nurse to coordinate the care to avoid miscommunication, care that is not compassionate, and not person-centred (Brown *et al.*, 2016). If the care is not effectively coordinated it can leave the patient at risk of harm and neglect within the complex healthcare system.

Policy development and leading change

The organisation and delivery of care to people with intellectual disabilities still need improvement (LeDeR, 2021; King and Duffy, 2022). Acute liaison nurses can be involved in policy development in acute healthcare services and see to it that policies that recognise the needs of people with intellectual disabilities are developed. Job descriptions of acute liaison nurses show that they are expected to be involved in the development and implementation of policy in acute hospitals (Kupara, 2022). The acute liaison nurses bring about change in acute healthcare services to ensure they respond to the needs of people with intellectual disabilities more effectively. Intellectual disabilities nurses working with greater autonomy and flexibility afforded by developments in practice need to influence not only their own practice but that of others (Mafuba, 2013). Acute liaison nurses need to be politically sensitised to the health policy processes in acute healthcare services to influence and contribute to its development, implementation, and evaluation.

Clinical leadership is needed in healthcare services to ensure service development (King and Duffy, 2022). Acute liaison nurses provide clinical leadership by being the link between primary and secondary healthcare and specialist intellectual disability services. They can set up champions for people with intellectual disabilities across clinical areas to ensure the health inequalities are reduced by ensuring reasonable adjustments are made and advocating for them. Under the leadership of acute liaison nurses, the champions for people with intellectual disabilities can support change in clinical areas by ensuring that policy changes are being followed and provide person-centred care that is delivered effectively (Jennings, 2019). Care pathways specifically tailored for people with intellectual disabilities are developed, implemented, used appropriately, and evaluated. Acute liaison nurses need to be effective change agents to ensure policies that enhance and improve the hospital experience for people with intellectual disabilities and their carers. They need to possess effective leadership skills as they are expected to provide a model for leadership for others to aspire to (NMC, 2018b), they need to lead as part of their role.

Acute intellectual disabilities nurses need political astuteness and awareness to be effective agents of change. They need to develop effective local, national, and international networks that will enhance their effectiveness as agents of change (Mafuba, 2013). The nurses need to think and act strategically to influence the direction and pace of change in the hospitals.

Research

Senior acute liaison nurses may contribute research initiatives as part of their role as outlined in their job descriptions (Kupara, 2022). The acute liaison nurses will also contribute to service audit, enquire, and use the findings to improve practice and patient outcomes, and disseminate good practice within and beyond the acute healthcare organisation. They use the research evidence to support and enable changes to practice and service delivery and contribute to local policy in response. Research is vital in improving patient care and treatment options (Royal College of Physicians, 2018) and liaison nurses can lead on this in the acute healthcare settings. Intellectual disabilities nurses engage in research initiatives and professional development (Doody et al., 2022). However, research dimension of the role is the least actioned facet of the clinical specialist nurse role (Doody et al., 2022), possibly due to lack of experience, knowledge, skills, and resources to engage with research or effectively evaluate the impact and outcomes of the role (Bryant-Lukosius et al., 2015).

Box 10.5
Learning Activity 10.1

Having read the background, history, key developments that influenced and core functions of intellectual disabilities liaison nursing, identify and reflect on examples on the experience for people with intellectual disabilities in your own country and elsewhere when they use acute healthcare services. You could consider the following:

- Discuss with members in your team the hospital services in your local area and what has been done to meet the needs of patients with intellectual disabilities and their carers.
- List the essential skills of the acute liaison nurse.
- Identify reasonable adjustments that could be made for a patient with intellectual disabilities and their carers.
- Reflect on your experience of working in collaboration with an acute liaison nurse for people with intellectual disabilities.
- Consider the proficiencies of the NMC Future Nurse: Standards of Proficiency for Registered Nurses (NMC, 2018a), and reflect how they apply to the role of the acute liaison nurse.

■ Identify areas that could be investigated further to improve the acute liaison nursing role.

■ Discuss what acute liaison nurses need to do to manage and lead on change in acute healthcare services that result in the enhancement of their roles and improve patient outcomes.

■ Discuss ways in which acute liaison nurses could contribute to policy development that affect liaison nursing practice or health and health-care outcomes for people with intellectual disabilities in acute health-care services.

■ Identify and reflect on what acute liaison nurses could to improve their advocacy and involvement in mental capacity assessment pro-cesses for patients with intellectual disabilities.

Challenges of Liaison nursing

It has been well established that people with intellectual disabilities experience significant difficulties when using acute healthcare services and acute liaison nursing role is a reasonable adjustment to improve their hospital experience. The acute liaison nurse has been positively evaluated yet there remain challenges and areas in need of development to further enhance the role.

While acute healthcare staff are striving to respond to the needs of people with intellectual disabilities, some failings continue to exist. Some healthcare services are not fully complying with legislation, policy, and best policy guid-ance (McCormick, 2021). This is in relation to a lack of effective communica-tion, respect, and the implementation of reasonable adjustments. There is still lack of consideration of the need for reasonable adjustments to existing policies and processes for people with intellectual disabilities (LeDeR, 2021).

Education to raise awareness of the needs of people with intellectual dis-abilities is one of the key roles of acute liaison nurses but not all healthcare staff have undertaken the training even though the acute liaison nurses have been providing this. It is envisaged that with the *Oliver McGowan Mandatory Training in Learning Disability and Autism* passed into law as part of the Health and Care Act 2022 in May 2022, more healthcare staff will now undertake intellectual dis-abilities training. The *Oliver McGowan Mandatory Training in Learning Disability and Autism* in England aims to educate and train health and social care staff, at the right level for their role, to provide better health and social care outcomes for people with intellectual disabilities and autistic people (Mencap, 2022). Health-care staff will have a better understanding of people's needs, resulting in better services and improved health and well-being outcomes (HEE, 2022).

Acute liaison nurses are involved in supporting the identification and deliv-ery of reasonable adjustments when people with intellectual disabilities access acute hospital services (Castles *et al.*, 2013; MacArthur *et al.*, 2015), however, the availability of acute liaison nurses remains patchy and there is limited availability of acute liaison nursing services (LeDeR, 2021). There is also a need to provide liaison nursing services during out of working (office) hours (Castles *et al.*, 2013; McCormick, 2021).

The understanding and application of the Mental Capacity Acts continues to be a significant problem in the care of people with intellectual disabilities (LeDeR, 2020, 2021). Adherence to this legislation when supporting people with intellectual disabilities remains patchy. With the *Oliver McGowan Mandatory Training in Learning Disability and Autism* in England being implemented, it is anticipated that there will be improvements in understanding and applying the principles of the mental capacity assessment framework.

Acute liaison nurses for people with intellectual disabilities come into the role without further preparation besides their knowledge and experience, yet they are expected to change culture in complex acute healthcare organisations. There is a need to consider advanced courses that prepare the nurses to be more strategic and effective change agents.

BOX 10.6
CASE STUDY 10.1

Example of good practice in intellectual liaison nursing

Ged Jennings is an Acute Intellectual Disability Liaison Nurse employed alongside another RNLD, within the wider safeguarding team, at the Royal Liverpool and Broadgreen University Hospital Trust (RLBUHT), a city centre general hospital. Ged has worked in a wide variety of roles and settings in the health and social care sector for over 20 years, including acute hospitals, specialist inpatient wards, day services and providing community support for people with an intellectual disability, autism, or both. Ged is extremely passionate about intellectual disability awareness training and is a strong advocate for the people and families he supports. He also has a desire to ensure that hospital staff

are aware of and supported to make reasonable adjustments so that the people he supports experience positive outcomes in the care they receive. Ged was tremendously proud to be part of the Acute Intellectual Disability Liaison Team that were shortlisted for an RCNi award in 2018 and who eventually went on to win the 'Team Of The Year' Award in 2019.

The liaison team at RLBUHT was created in 2016 and has two nurses, who work as part of the safeguarding team. The number of patients supported by the liaison team has continually grown since its inception, with an increase of almost 40% between 2017 and 2018. The liaison team created the intellectual disability champions network at RLBUHT in 2017 after it was recognised that the liaison team was not sufficient to bring about cultural change as the commitment of staff in clinical areas was needed. The acute liaison team led by Ged set up the network of intellectual disability champions to promote staff engagement across the trust and improve care for patients with intellectual disabilities. This was an innovation to support the team in their liaison nursing role.

The champions act as a source of support and knowledge for patients, relatives, and staff alike. They are a link between the intellectual disability team and staff/patients in the clinical areas. It was recognised that for the intellectual disability champion role to be effective it needed to be independent of ward managers to allow the champions to make autonomous decisions. The name 'champion' was opted instead of 'link nurse' to highlight that the role was open to all staff, not just certain pay bands or staff.

Intellectual disability champions were recruited through training events, the trust's webpage, and internal communications department. Some staff approached the acute liaison team to express their interest to become champions. When the champion is recruited, they sign a contract to formalise their commitment, and have an outline of their roles and responsibilities. The champions include nurses, healthcare assistants, therapists, students, the CEO of the trust, the director of nursing, medical staff, trust volunteers with intellectual disabilities and/or autism, and volunteers' relatives. The aim was to have two champions per ward, but this is not limited, and some have three. On successful recruitment the champion receives training and certificate of attainment. The training focuses on health inequities in acute hospitals and how clinical staff can improve the care they provide. Additionally, specialist training to further enhance the champions' knowledge is provided and they are invited to quarterly meetings. People with intellectual disabilities and/or autism are regularly invited to speak at these meetings, to explain how it feels to be a patient in an acute hospital. The champions also share best practice, give each other peer support, and discuss service innovations that could be replicated.

The intellectual disability champions advocate for vulnerable patients and their families; act as a source of information and support in their clinical area; and disseminate information from the liaison team in the clinical areas. By doing this they help to continuously improve patient care and ensure that addressing the needs of patients with intellectual disabilities remains a top priority. The champions are expected to create a one-page profile about themselves and set up an intellectual disability noticeboard in their ward or clinical area. The one-page profiles give health and social care professionals and patients and their relatives or families at a glance information about intellectual disabilities information. The one-page profiles are also given to patients and their carers alongside the intellectual disability information pack on admission. Patients will know who and how to contact the intellectual disability liaison team if need arises. The champions are expected to set up intellectual disability noticeboards in their clinical areas with information about how to contact the liaison team and blank health passport. The champions are encouraged to be creative and use accessible information.

The intellectual disability champions have helped improve the experience of hospital care for people with intellectual disabilities. They have helped reduce their average hospital stay. The patients have given feedback that they found the care provided by the ward-based champions to be excellent. On reflection, Ged and his team found that the intellectual disability champion network grew rapidly, whilst it was time consuming and labour intensive to set up, but it has resulted in positive outcomes for patients and hospital staff. The network has promoted the intellectual disability agenda across the trust, increased staff engagement and awareness, and improved practice, notably through a better understanding of reasonable adjustments. There are plans to grow the network regionally.

Tasks

Consider and reflect upon the implications of the acute intellectual disability nursing role for the following

- People with intellectual disabilities when using hospital services
- Families of people with intellectual disabilities

- Formal and informal carers of people with intellectual disabilities
- Hospital staff who provide care and treatment to people with intellectual disabilities
- The healthcare organisations that provide acute care

Source: Adapted from

Jennings, G. (2019) Introducing learning disability champions in an acute hospital. *Nursing Times*, 115(4), pp. 44–47.

Jennings, G. (2018) *A week in the life of an 'acute liaison learning disability nurse.* Available at: https://learningdisabilitynurse.co.uk/real-nurses/a-week-in-the-life-of-an-acute-liaison-learning-disability-nurse (Accessed 10 June 2022).

Conclusion

The demographic changes and increase in the population of people with intellectual disabilities mean the acute liaison nursing role is central to the delivery of safe, effective person-centered care and support in acute healthcare services. The health and healthcare needs of people with intellectual disabilities, and how healthcare is delivered, is complex. Consequently, intellectual disability nurses need to understand the need for their acute liaison nursing roles to extend beyond traditional professional practice and geographical boundaries.

Nationally and internationally, there will be increased need for acute healthcare for people with intellectual disabilities. Consequently, intellectual disability nurses, like other healthcare professionals, will continue to be valuable to acute healthcare services to ensure the health and healthcare needs of people with intellectual disabilities are met, and in hospitals are fully prepared and equipped to meet these needs.

Intellectual disabilities nurses need to develop formal and informal networks at local, national, and international levels to remain relevant. Intellectual disabilities nurses in the United Kingdom and Ireland can and need to be an important force for change of their own practice, health policy, and how acute healthcare is organised and delivered to people with intellectual disabilities. The acute liaison nurses need to continue to be seen as a reasonable adjustment whilst they develop their leadership skills to be effective change agents. They might need to have standards of practice developed and required to undertake some formal preparation for the role to bring up change of culture effectively and in a timely manner. To strengthen the contribution of acute liaison nursing to improve the health outcomes and hospital experience of people with intellectual disabilities there is a need to make the service more available and promote the role through further professional development to be recognised as a clinical specialist role.

References

Adults with incapacity (Scotland) act 2000 Edinburgh: The Stationery Office.
Aitken, P., *et al.* (2016) A history of liaison psychiatry in the UK. *British Journal of Psychiatry Bulletin*, 40(4), pp. 199–203.

Alexander, R., *et al.* (2020) Guidance for the treatment and management of COVID-19 among people with intellectual disabilities. *Journal of Policy and Practice in Intellectual Disabilities*, 17(2), pp. 256–269.

American Nurses Association (1990) *Standards of consultation-liaison nursing practice.* Kansas: ANA Council on Psychiatric and Mental Health Nursing.

Backer, C., Chapman, M. and Mitchell, D. (2009) Access to secondary healthcare for people with learning disabilities: A review of the literature. *Journal of Applied Research in Intellectual Disabilities*, 6(22), pp. 514–525.

Blair, J. (2011) Care adjustments for people with learning disabilities in hospitals. *Nursing Management*, 28(8), pp. 21–24.

Brown, F.J., Cooper, K. and Diebel, T. (2012) Access to mainstream health services: A case study of the difficulties faced by a child with learning disabilities. *British Journal of Learning Disabilities*, 41(2), pp. 128–132.

Brown, M., *et al.* (2016) The perspectives of stakeholders of intellectual disability liaison nurses: A model of compassionate, person-centred care. *Journal of Clinical Nursing*, 25, pp. 972–982.

Bryant-Lukosius, D., *et al.* (2015) The effectiveness and cost-effectiveness of clinical nurse specialist led hospital to home transitional care: A systematic review. *Journal of Evaluation in Clinical Practice*, 21, pp. 763–781.

Care Quality Commission (2017) *The state of health care and adult social care in England.* Available at: www.cqc.org.uk/sites/default/files/20171123_stateofcare1617_report.pdf (Accessed 6 June 2022).

Care Quality Commission (2021) *The state of health care and adult social care in England 2020/21.* Available at: www.cqc.org.uk/publications/major-report/state-care (Accessed 6 June 2022).

Castles, A., *et al.* (2013) Experiences of the implementation of a learning disability nursing liaison service within an acute hospital setting: A service evaluation. *British Journal of Learning Disabilities*, 42(4), pp. 272–281.

Clemence, B.A. (1981) Liaison nurse: What is the role? *Journal of Nursing Education*, 20(7), pp. 42–46.

Coppus, A.M. (2013) People with intellectual disability: What do we know about adulthood and life expectancy? *Developmental Disabilities Research Reviews*, 18(1), pp. 6–16.

Department of Constitutional Affairs (2007) *Mental capacity act 2005 code of practice.* London: The Stationary Office.

Department of Health (2009) *Valuing people now: A new 3-year strategy for people with learning disabilities. Making it happen for everyone.* London: The Stationery Office.

Department of Health and Social Care (2019) *The government's revised mandate to NHS England for 2018–19.* Available at: https://assets.publishing.service.gov.uk/government/uploads/system/uploads/attachment_data/file/803111/revised-mandate-to-nhs-england-2018-to-2019.pdf (Accessed 4 June 2022).

DH (2001) *Valuing people: A new strategy for learning disability for the 21st century.* London: Department of Health.

Disability Rights Commission (2006) *Equal treatment: Closing the gap.* Stratford Upon Avon: Disability Rights Commission.

Doody, O., Hennessy, T. and Bright, A. (2022) The role and key activities of clinical nurse specialists and advanced nurse practitioners in supporting healthcare provision for people with intellectual disability: An integrative review. *International Journal of Nursing Studies*, 129. doi:10.1016/j.ijnurstu.2022.104207.

Drozd, M. and Clinch, C. (2016) The experiences of orthopaedic and trauma nurses who have cared for adults with a learning disability. *International Journal of Orthopedic and Trauma Nursing*, 22, pp. 13–23.

Emerson, E. and Hatton, C. (2009) *Estimating future numbers of adults with profound multiple learning disabilities in England*. Lancaster: Centre for Disability Research, Lancaster University.

Giraud-Saunders, A., *et al.* (2014) *Working together 2: Easy steps to improve support for people with learning disabilities in hospital – guidance for hospitals, families and paid support staff*. London: Public Health England.

Gray, J. and Watson, V. (2017) Evaluation of a learning disability liaison nurse service. *Learning Disability Practice*, 20(5), pp. 35–41.

Health and care act 2022. Available at: www.legislation.gov.uk/ukpga/2022/31/contents/enacted. (Accessed 28 July 2022).

Health Education England (2020) *Project report: Understanding the who, where and what of learning disability liaison nurses*. Available at: https://learningdisabilitynurse.co.uk/real-nurses/gwen-moulster-obe-review-of-liaison-nursing (Accessed 31 May 2022).

Health Education England (2022) *The Oliver McGowan mandatory training in learning disability and autism*. Available at: www.hee.nhs.uk/our-work/learning-disability/oliver-mcgowan-mandatory-training-learning-disability-autism (Accessed 4 June 2022).

Heslop, P., *et al.* (2013) *Confidential inquiry into premature deaths of people with learning disabilities (CIPOLD): Final report*. Bristol: Norah Fry Research Centre.

Heslop, P., *et al.* (2019) Implementing reasonable adjustments for disabled people in healthcare services. *Nursing Standard*. doi:10.7748/ns.2019.e11172.

Howieson, J. (2015) Experiences of acute hospital services among people with mild to moderate learning disabilities. *Learning Disability Practice*, 18(9), pp. 34–38.

Jayes, M., Borrett, S. and Bose, A. (2022) Mental capacity legislation and communication disability: A cross-sectional survey exploring the impact of the COVID-19 pandemic on the provision of specialist decision-making support by UK SLTs. *International Journal of Language & Communication Disorders*, 57, pp. 72–181.

Jennings, G. (2018) *A week in the life of an 'acute liaison learning disability nurse*. Available at: https://learningdisabilitynurse.co.uk/real-nurses/a-week-in-the-life-of-an-acute-liaison-learning-disability-nurse (Accessed 10 June 2022).

Jennings, G. (2019) Introducing learning disability champions in an acute hospital. *Nursing Times*, 115(4), pp. 44–47.

King, T.A. and Duffy, J. (2022) Peri-operative care of elective adult surgical patients with a learning disability. *Anaesthesia*, 77, pp. 674–683.

Kupara, D. (2022) *The roles of learning disabilities acute liaison nurses in acute healthcare settings: An exploratory sequential mixed methods study*. Unpublished Partial MPhil/PhD thesis. London: University of West London.

LeDeR (2020) *LeDeR annual report 2019*. Available at: https://leder.nhs.uk/resources/annual-reports (Accessed 4 June 2022).

LeDeR (2021) *LeDeR annual report 2020*. Available at: https://leder.nhs.uk/resources/annual-reports (Accessed 4 June 2022).

Lloyd, G.G. and Guthrie, E. (2012) *Handbook of Liaison psychiatry*. Cambridge: Cambridge University Press.

MacArthur, J., *et al.* (2015) Making reasonable and achievable adjustments: The contributions of learning disability liaison nurses in 'getting it right' for people with learning disabilities receiving general hospitals care. *Journal of Advanced Nursing*, 71(7), pp. 1552–1563.

Mafuba, K. (2013) *Public health: Community learning disability nurses' perception and experience of their role*. Unpublished PhD thesis. London: University of West London.

Mafuba, K., *et al.* (2021) *Understanding the contribution of intellectual disability nurses: Scoping research. Volume 1 of 3: Scoping literature review report*. London: RCN Foundation.

McCormick, F. (2021) Experiences of adults with intellectual disabilities accessing acute hospital services: A systematic review of the international evidence. *Health Social Care Community*, 29, pp. 1222–1232.

Mencap (2004) *Treat me right! Better health for people with learning disabilities*. London: Mencap.

Mencap (2007) *Death by indifference: Following up the treat me right report*. London: Mencap.

Mencap (2010) *Getting it right charter*. London: Mencap.

Mencap (2012) *Death by indifference: 74 deaths and counting*. London: Mencap.

Mencap (2022) *The Oliver McGowan mandatory training*. London: Mencap.

Michael, J. (2008) *Healthcare for all: Report of the independent inquiry into access to healthcare for people with learning disabilities*. London: Department of Health.

Mind (2018) *Discrimination in everyday life*. Available at: www.mind.org.uk/information-support/legal-rights/discrimination-in-everyday-life/overview/ (Accessed 4 June 2022).

Moloney, M., Hennessy, T. and Doody, O. (2021) Reasonable adjustments for people with intellectual disability in acute care: A scoping review of the evidence. *BMJ Open*, 11(2). doi:10.1136/bmjopen-2020-039647.

Morton-Nance, S. (2015) Unique role of learning disability liaison nurses. *Learning Disability Practice*, 18(7), pp. 30–34.

NHS Digital (2013) *Learning disabilities census report - England, 30th of September 2013*. Available at: https://digital.nhs.uk/data-and-information/publications/statistical/learning-disabilities-census-report/learning-disabilities-census-report-england-30th-of-september-2013 (Accessed 26 November 2022).

NHS England (2021a) *Learning from lives and deaths – people with a learning disability and autistic people (LeDeR) policy 2021*. Available at: www.england.nhs.uk/wp-content/uploads/2021/03/B0428-LeDeR-policy-2021.pdf (Accessed 4 June 2022).

NHS England (2021b) *Do not attempt cardiopulmonary resuscitation (DNACPR) decisions*. Available at: www.nhs.uk/conditions/do-not-attempt-cardiopulmonary-resuscitation-dnacpr-decisions/ (Accessed 6 June 2022).

NHS Improvement (2018) *The learning disability improvement standards for NHS trusts*. Available at: www.england.nhs.uk/learning-disabilities/about/resources/the-learning-disability-improvement-standards-for-nhs-trusts/ (Accessed 8 June 2022).

NICE (2021) *Clinical guide for front line staff to support the management of patients with a learning disability, autism or both during the COVID19 pandemic – relevant to all clinical specialities*. Available at: www.nice.org.uk/media/default/about/covid-19/specialty-guides/management-patients-learning-disability-autism-during-pandemic.pdf (Accessed 6 June 2022).

Northway, R., *et al.* (2017) Supporting people across the lifespan: The role of learning disability nurses. *Learning Disability Practice*, 20(3), pp. 22–27.

Nursing and Midwifery Board of Ireland (2016) *Nurse registration programmes standards and requirements* (4th edition). Dublin: Nursing and Midwifery Board of Ireland.

Nursing and Midwifery Council (2018a) *Future nurse: Standards of proficiency for registered nurses*. London: NMC.

Nursing and Midwifery Council (2018b) *The code: Professional standards of practice and behaviour for nurses, midwives and nursing associates*. London: NMC.

O'Connor, D. and Hagan, F. (1964) Liaison nurse. *American Journal of Nursing*, 64(6), pp. 101–103.

Office for National Statistics (2020) *Estimates of the population for the UK, England and Wales, Scotland and Northern Ireland*. Available at: www.ons.gov.uk/people populationandcommunity/populationandmigration/populationestimates/

datasets/populationestimatesforukenglandandwalesscotlandandnorthernireland (Accessed 1 June 2022).

Parliamentary Health Service Ombudsman and Local Government Ombudsman (2009) *Six lives: The provision of public services to people with learning disabilities.* London: The Stationery Office.

Phillips, L. (2019) Learning disabilities: Making reasonable adjustments in hospital. *Nursing Times*, 115(10), pp. 38–42.

Public Health England (2016) *People with learning disabilities in England 2015: Main report.* Available at: https://assets.publishing.service.gov.uk/government/uploads/system/uploads/attachment_data/file/613182/PWLDIE_2015_main_report_NB090517.pdf (Accessed 4 June 2022).

Public Health England (2018) *Research and analysis: Learning disabilities and CQC inspection reports.* Available at: www.gov.uk/government/publications/learning-disabilities-and-cqc-inspection-reports/learning-disabilities-and-cqc-inspection-reports#contents (Accessed 4 June 2022).

Regulation and Quality Improvement Authority (2018) *Guidelines on caring for people with a learning disability in general hospital settings.* Available at: www.rqia.org.uk/RQIA/files/41/41a812c6-fee8-45ba-81b8-9ed4106cf49a.pdf (Accessed 4 June 2022).

Regulatory Quality Inspection Authority (2016) *Review of adult learning disability community services phase II.* Available at: www.rqia.org.uk/RQIA/files/4a/4a883fbc-92a7-4fda-97b0-ac2e664e5d8d.pdf (Accessed 1 June 2022).

Roberts, D. (1997) Liaison mental health nursing: Origins, definition and prospects. *Journal of Advanced Nursing*, 25, pp. 101–108.

Robertson, J., *et al.* (2014) The impact of health checks for people with intellectual disabilities: An updated systematic review of evidence. *Research in Developmental Disabilities*, 35(10), pp. 2450–2462.

Robinson, L. (1987) Psychiatric consultation liaison nursing and psychiatric consultation liaison doctoring: Similarities and differences. *Archives of Psychiatric Nursing*, 1, pp. 73–80.

Royal College of Nursing (2022) *Learning disabilities: Reasonable adjustments.* Available at: www.rcn.org.uk/clinical-topics/Learning-disabilities/Reasonable-Adjustments (Accessed 4 June 2022).

Royal College of Physicians (2018) *Recognising research: How research improves patient care.* Available at: https://bit.ly/2rOiwQF (Accessed 10 June 2022).

Ryan, J.M., Clemmett, S. and Snelson, A. (1997) Role of a psychiatric liaison nurse in an A & E department. *Accident and Emergency Nursing*, 5, pp. 152–155.

Sharrock, J. and Happell, B. (2000) The psychiatric consultation-liaison nurse: Towards articulating a model for practice. *Australian and New Zealand Journal of Mental Health Nursing*, 9, pp. 19–28.

Taggart, L., *et al.* (2022) Preventing, mitigating, and managing future pandemics for people with an intellectual and developmental disability – learnings from COVID-19: A scoping review. *Journal of Policy and Practice in Intellectual Disabilities*, 19(1), pp. 4–34.

Tuffrey-Wijne, I., *et al.* (2013) Identifying the factors affecting the implementation of strategies to promote a safer environment for patients with learning disabilities in NHS hospitals: A mixed-methods study. *NIHR Journal Library.* doi:10.3310/hsdr01130.

University of Bristol (2021) *The learning disabilities mortality review programme (LeDeR) annual report.* Available at: www.bristol.ac.uk/sps/news/2021/leder-annual-report-2020.html (Accessed 2 August 2022).

Victorian Government Department of Health and Community Services (1996) *Review of consultation-liaison services in Victorian hospitals.* Melbourne: Victorian Government Department of Health and Community Services.

Further Reading

Chapman, A., Dodd, K. and Rogers, L. (2020) Knowledge of mental capacity assessment in staff working with people with learning disabilities. *Advances in Mental Health and Intellectual Disabilities*, 14(1), pp. 14–24. doi:10.1108/AMHID-05-2019-0014.

Useful Resources

Care Quality Commission: www.cqc.org.uk/

Health Information and Quality Authority: www.hiqa.ie/about-us/who-we-work-memorandums-understanding

Healthcare Improvement Scotland: www.healthcareimprovementscotland.org/

Healthcare Inspectorate Wales: https://hiw.org.uk/

NHS Digital Series/Collection Health and Care of People with Learning Disabilities: https://digital.nhs.uk/data-and-information/publications/statistical/health-and-care-of-people-with-learning-disabilities

Nursing and Midwifery Board of Ireland An Bord Altranais: www.nmbi.ie/Home

Nursing and Midwifery Council: www.nmc.org.uk/about-us/

The Regulation and Quality Improvement Authority: www.rqia.org.uk/

CHAPTER 11

Kay Mafuba, Hazel Chapman, Rebecca Chester, Joann Kiernan, Dorothy Kupara and Chiedza Kudita

Current and future roles of intellectual disability nurses

Introduction

Within the arena of an ever-changing context of health and social care that is dictated by political imperatives at policy level, both nationally and internationally, and with the ever-growing move toward citizenship, and the importance of human rights, intellectual disability nursing needs to place itself carefully – within the family of nursing and within a complex landscape of human service organisations, as well as the wider community of intellectual disabilities.

This chapter briefly reflects on the past but most importantly looks at the present and to the future of the modern intellectual disability nurse practitioner. It discusses issues affecting intellectual disability nursing, such as changing professional requirements, policy directions such as *Strengthening the Commitment* (Scottish Government, 2012), and ever-growing opportunities for intellectual disability nurses to assert themselves in a widening practice arena.

Therefore, this chapter focuses on the knowledge and practical skills that intellectual disability nurses will need to meet the needs of people with intellectual disabilities now and in the future, and this will be contextualised within the Nursing and Midwifery Council for the United Kingdom's Future nurse standards (NMC, 2018) and Nursing and Midwifery Board of Ireland (2016) standards and requirements for competence. The future of intellectual disability nursing is discussed in the context of policy directions, emerging roles, and intellectual disability nurses' clinical and other expertise, and their ability as individuals and as a profession to adapt and work effectively in multidisciplinary and interagency settings. In this chapter we present a wide range of research evidence that demonstrates the unique contributions of intellectual disability nurses.

DOI: 10.4324/9781003296461-11

Box 11.1 This chapter will focus on the following issues:

- Challenges for professional identity
- The need for intellectual disability nursing
  - Extent of the health and healthcare needs of people with intellectual disabilities
  - Current healthcare policies and professional requirements
- Current and future spheres of practice
  - Current and future roles of intellectual disability nurses
    - Maternity interventions
    - Interventions across all age groups
    - Interventions for children
    - Interventions for adults
    - Interventions for older adults
    - End-of-life interventions
- Impacts of intellectual disability nursing

Box 11.2 Competences

Nursing and Midwifery Council (2018) Proficiencies

Platform 1 – Being an accountable professional – 1.1, 1.3, 1.6, 1.9, 1.17, 1.19

Platform 2: Promoting health and preventing ill health – 2.4

Platform 3: Assessing needs and planning care – 3.8

Platform 5: Leading and managing nursing care and working in teams – 5.4

Platform 6: Improving safety and quality of care – 6.2, 6.3, 6.8, 6.9, 6.10, 6.11, 6.12

Platform 7: Coordinating care – 7.4, 7.12, 7.13

Nursing and Midwifery Board of Ireland (2016) Competences

Domain 1: Professional values and conduct of the nurse competences – 1.1, 1.3

Domain 2: Nursing practice and clinical decision-making competences – 2.5

Domain 3: Knowledge and cognitive competences – 3.1, 3.2

Domain 6: Leadership potential and professional scholarship competences – 6.1, 6.2

Challenges for professional identity

The United Kingdom and Ireland are now the only countries to provide a specialist pre-registration qualification programme for nurses caring for people with intellectual disabilities. In both countries, intellectual disability nursing developed because of the medicalisation of the colony system for 'mental defectives' into mental deficiency hospitals, which required trained nurses. Since its inception in the early part of the twentieth century, like people with intellectual disabilities, intellectual disability nursing has been largely invisible, and its relevance and position within the nursing profession has been repeatedly questioned. Intellectual disability nursing's origins in large psychiatric institutions in the United Kingdom, and religious orders and mental asylums in Ireland, have resulted in the profession being associated with widely reported malpractice, and poor practice in these institutions. Events of the past few years, such as the abuses at Winterbourne View and the Connor Sparrowhawk case among others, demonstrate that standards of professional practice, competency and integrity need to be high in relation to intellectual disability nurses, who support some of the most vulnerable people in society. Intellectual disability nurses have a collective professional responsibility to ensure that those who fail to safeguard, abuse, or commit criminal offences against vulnerable individuals with intellectual disability have no place in the profession.

Collectively, intellectual disability nurses may not have considered the full implications of such events, which have negatively affected the positive contributions they make to the lives of people with intellectual disabilities. This inability to focus on the positive contribution that intellectual disability nursing has made to the lives of people with intellectual disabilities has perhaps resulted in misunderstanding and confusion of its role among the wider health and social care communities. Perhaps even more significant is the resulting confusion among intellectual disability nurses themselves about what their role involves (Stewart and Todd, 2001). As a professional group, intellectual disability nurses need to take responsibility and a lead in defining and developing their role and be instrumental in shaping the future of their sphere of practice. It could be argued that *The Same as You* (Scottish Government, 2000), *Valuing People* (DH, 2001), *Healthcare for All* (Michael, 2008), *Strengthening the Commitment* (DH *et al.*, 2012), *The Health Equalities Framework* (Atkinson *et al.*, 2013), *Nurse registration programmes standards and requirements* (4th *edition*) (NMBI, 2016), *Future nurse: Standards of proficiency for registered nurse* (NMC, 2018), and other recent policy documents, reports, and service re-organisations have, over the years, provided numerous opportunities for intellectual disability nurses to clarify their positive contributions to the lives of people with intellectual disabilities.

The challenge for intellectual disability nursing is to be proactive in defining its contribution to the lives of people with intellectual disabilities, to develop their skills, and to develop an evidence base that validates their contribution to the health and well-being of people with intellectual disabilities. If intellectual disability nurses are to continue to make a positive difference to the lives of people with intellectual disabilities, such nurses will need to collaborate and be proactive in articulating and validating their contributions to people with intellectual disabilities and the nursing profession.

The need for intellectual disability nursing

Extent of the health and healthcare needs of people with intellectual disabilities

It is estimated that there are currently 1.5 million people with an intellectual disability in the UK and this population is changing and increasing, with approximately 2.16% of adults and 2.5% of children identified as having an intellectual disability (Mencap, 2020). Life expectancy of people living with intellectual disabilities is increasing, as well as the complexity of the health and social care needs and conditions of this population (Truesdale and Brown, 2017). There is a disparity between the health and the healthcare needs of people with intellectual disabilities as compared to that of the general population and these disparities are avoidable (Kerr, 2004; van Schrojenstein Lantman-de Valk *et al.*, 2007). People with intellectual disabilities are known to have much greater health needs than those of comparable age groups who do not have intellectual disabilities (Backer, Chapman and Mitchell, 2009), and experience higher preventable mortality rates (LeDeR, 2020).

Research demonstrates that people with intellectual disabilities are often or more likely to be dependent on others for their health and healthcare outcomes (Campbell and Martin, 2009) and that these outcomes could be improved through appropriate intellectual disability nursing interventions. People with intellectual disabilities are high and frequent users of all health services, including primary care, child health services, acute healthcare services, and specialist intellectual disability services.

The avoidable disparity between the health, and the health needs of people with intellectual disabilities as compared to that of the general population has been acknowledged over many years (Kerr, 2004; Straetmans *et al.*, 2007; Hatton and Emerson, 2015; Kavanagh *et al.*, 2017; LeDer, 2020). These disparities result from poor access to health services, limited options in lifestyle, and poor living standards, but could be improved through appropriate intellectual disability nursing interventions.

People with intellectual disabilities are known to have much greater health needs than those of comparable age groups who do not have intellectual disabilities (Backer, Chapman and Mitchell, 2009; Savage and Emerson, 2016; Emerson *et al.*, 2016a, 2016b; Robertson *et al.*, 2017). For example, they experience higher rates of mental health related disorders as compared to the general population and these health problems are commonly and widely undiagnosed, misdiagnosed, and untreated (Llewellyn, Vaughan and Emerson, 2015; Emerson and Brigham, 2015). In addition, they experience higher rates of visual impairments, higher rates of epilepsy, hypertension and hypothyroidism, and obesity. People with intellectual disabilities are more likely to die from preventable causes (Mencap, 2007; Heslop *et al.*, 2013, 2014; Robertson *et al.*, 2015; Bakker-van Gijssel *et al.*, 2017). The life expectancy of people with intellectual disabilities has increased with that of the wider population in recent years. However, overall life expectancy remains lower, and mortality rates remain significantly higher than those of the wider population (Heslop *et al.*, 2013, 2014; Robertson *et al.*, 2015; Bakker-van Gijssel *et al.*, 2017). Intellectual disability nurses play an important role in minimising the potential consequences of the risks that result in the preventable premature death of people with intellectual disabilities.

International studies have demonstrated widespread concerns about the inequalities in health for people with intellectual disabilities (Melville *et al.*, 2006; Kavanagh *et al.*, 2017), and poor access to healthcare (Brown *et al.*, 2010). These disparities in health, and poorer health outcomes for people with intellectual disabilities have been attributed to service users' conditions, health organisations, and health service systems. Communication difficulties and limited understanding of the diagnostic and treatment issues for people with intellectual disabilities, and mainstream healthcare professionals' limited augmentative communication skills further limits the diagnosis and treatment of people with intellectual disabilities appropriately (Blair, 2013). People with intellectual disabilities have complex health needs, and comorbidity is common. Lifestyle-related comorbidity is a significant contributory factor to disparities in health for people with intellectual disabilities. Cognitive impairments can limit people with intellectual disabilities' ability to health services without appropriate interventions.

People with intellectual disabilities experience unequal access to health services (DRC, 2006). They experience inadequate diagnosis of treatable conditions (Mencap, 2007; DH, 2007; Heslop *et al.*, 2013, 2014; Robertson *et al.*, 2015). A significant proportion of health inequalities experienced by people with intellectual disabilities are linked to poor access to quality healthcare provision (Michael, 2008; Mencap, 2012), and therefore preventable. In recent years, UK government health policy has focused on improving people with intellectual disabilities' access to mainstream services. However, the continuing disparities in health experienced by people with intellectual disabilities suggest that policies alone are not enough.

Barriers to accessing health services experienced by people with intellectual disabilities contribute to health inequalities. The lack of role clarity of the professionals working with people with intellectual disabilities has been consistently identified as one of the most common barriers (Mafuba, 2009, 2013; Mafuba and Gates, 2015; Mafuba *et al.*, 2018b). Primary healthcare services have an important role in meeting the public health needs of people with intellectual disabilities but there is a lack of evidence as to the interventions intellectual disability nurses play in meeting these needs.

Poor uptake of health services amongst the population of people with intellectual disabilities is a longstanding issue (Allerton and Emerson, 2012;

Robertson *et al.*, 2014). Studies have shown that people with intellectual disabilities are likely to be passive participants in their health and healthcare, and that they are dependent on others for their health and healthcare outcomes (Campbell and Martin, 2009). Delivering effective health services for people with intellectual disabilities is challenging. McIlfatrick, Taggart and Truesdale-Kennedy (2011) have observed that the provision of health services for people with intellectual disabilities is opportunistic, despite evidence that point to a need for targeted activities (Chauhan *et al.*, 2010; Robertson *et al.*, 2014). Preventative nursing interventions such as health screening are effective in identifying the health needs of people with intellectual disabilities (Emerson, Copeland and Glover, 2011; Robertson *et al.*, 2014).

The proportion of children with multiple and complex intellectual disabilities who are living into adulthood and the number of people with intellectual disabilities living into older age is also increasing. Because of the increase in the number of children and young people with intellectual disabilities living into adulthood, there will be major implications for education, health, social care and criminal justice and secure services in the future. The population of older people with intellectual disabilities will increase four times faster than the overall adult intellectual disability population (NICE, 2018). By 2030, there will be a 30% increase in the number of adults with intellectual disabilities aged 50+ using social care services (NICE, 2018). As life expectancy has increased, more people with intellectual disabilities are experiencing chronic multi-morbidities. This will create substantial pressure on services, which has not yet been fully quantified (NICE, 2018). This will have significant implications on the interventions undertaken by intellectual disability nurses to support and meet the needs of this population.

Current healthcare policies and professional requirements

Although the shift from treatment to preventive interventions has resulted in questions and anxieties about the future roles of intellectual disability nurses, *The Same as You* (Scottish Government, 2000), *Valuing People* (DH, 2001), *Healthcare for All* (Michael, 2008), *Strengthening the Commitment* (DH et al., 2012), *The Health Equalities Framework* (Atkinson *et al.*, 2013), *Nurse registration programmes standards and requirements* (4th *edition*) (NMBI, 2016), *Future nurse: Standards of proficiency for registered nurse* (NMC, 2018), and the *Mental Health Services for Adults with Intellectual disabilities: National Model of Service* (HSE Mental Health Services, 2021) clearly demonstrate the continued professional need for, and political commitment to, intellectual disability nursing in both the UK and Republic of Ireland. What is perhaps important for intellectual disability nurses is for them to focus on the opportunities individually and collectively for enhancing the contributions they make in meeting the health and healthcare needs of people with intellectual disabilities.

Box 11.3
Intellectual Activity 11.1

Having read the section on the need for intellectual disability nursing in the United Kingdom and Ireland, identify and reflect on examples about how intellectual disability nurses in your own country and elsewhere have done the following

■ Contributed to developing expertise and specialist knowledge in intellectual disability nursing practice

■ Enhanced interprofessional coordination

■ Provided professional leadership that made a significant difference to intellectual disability nursing practice

■ Undertaken research that has affected the intellectual disability nursing profession

■ Managed change that resulted in the enhancement of the roles of intellectual disability nurses at national or international levels

■ Contributed to health policy development that affected intellectual disability nursing practice or health and healthcare outcomes for people with intellectual disabilities

■ Contributed to workforce planning that enhanced intellectual disability nursing roles

■ Acted as a professional health advocate for people with intellectual disabilities, which resulted in improved recognition of intellectual disability nursing at national or international levels

■ Contributed to improved professional recognition and identity for intellectual disability nursing

Current and future spheres of practice

Strengthening the Commitment (DH *et al.*, 2012), *Nurse registration programmes standards and requirements* (4th *edition*) (NMBI, 2016), and *Future nurse: Standards of proficiency for registered nurse* (NMC, 2018) demonstrate professional and political recognition that intellectual disability nurses have much to contribute to current and future healthcare provision and development for people with intellectual disabilities. Intellectual disability nurses will need to take essential roles in initiatives targeted at developing health and healthcare services for people with intellectual disabilities. This is essential to facilitate partnerships with other professionals, organisations, people with intellectual disabilities, their families, carers, and other stakeholders. The complexities of the health and healthcare needs of people with intellectual disabilities, current models of health service provision, and challenges people with intellectual disabilities experience when they access health and healthcare services means that partnership working will be key to improving the health and healthcare outcomes for people with intellectual disabilities.

The population of people with intellectual disabilities is growing. This is characterised by children with intellectual disabilities and complex health and healthcare needs surviving into adulthood. In addition, the population of older adults with intellectual disabilities is increasing in line with overall life expectancy trends. This will have a significant effect on intellectual disability nursing as new health and healthcare challenges emerge and increase with the growing population. Intellectual disability nurses should focus on developing knowledge and skills that will equip them to work more effectively with people with intellectual disabilities across their lifespans. This will require intellectual disability nurses to take on new roles in non-traditional areas of their practice to effectively address the many complex and comorbid health needs of people with intellectual disabilities.

People with intellectual disabilities have a complex health profile that is different from that of the general population. As more people with severe intellectual disabilities and complex health and healthcare needs increases, there is likely to be an increase in complex comorbid health needs. Emerson and Baines (2010) have concluded that mental illness, autism spectrum disorder, behavioural challenges, and dementia are all more common in people with intellectual disabilities. As the population of people with intellectual disabilities increase, so too will the prevalence of these conditions (Torr and Davis, 2007). Intellectual disability nurses need to be cognizant of these population trends so that they can develop new roles in new healthcare settings where services for people with intellectual disabilities with increasingly complex health needs will be delivered in the future.

People with intellectual disabilities experience significant barriers when accessing health services, resulting in poorer health outcomes as compared to people without intellectual disabilities (Cooper *et al.*, 2011). This increasingly complex repertoire of needs will require increased and more frequent use of healthcare services. With mainstream professional healthcare education often lacking emphasis on the needs of people with intellectual disabilities (DH, 2008), intellectual disability nurses need to develop new roles in mainstream health and healthcare services.

Current and future roles of intellectual disability nurses

Current healthcare policies and healthcare professional education in the United Kingdom and Ireland recognise the contributions of and need for specialist intellectual disability health services and intellectual disability nurses. Such services, even considering the significant shift toward the mainstreaming of healthcare for people with intellectual disabilities, particularly in the United Kingdom, mean that intellectual disability nurses now and in the future will continue to be important and have significant roles in assessing, treating, supporting, educating, and coordinating the delivery of care for people with intellectual disabilities across the lifespan. The need for preventive interventions, primary care, and specialist intellectual disability services will remain an essential part of healthcare and professional education systems in both the United Kingdom and Ireland for the foreseeable future. In a study involving intellectual disability nurses from several countries including the United Kingdom and Ireland, Mafuba *et al.* (2021a, 2021b, 2021c) identified 878 interventions undertaken by intellectual disability nurses. These interventions were categorised into five themes, and these are:

- effectuating nursing procedures,
- enhancing impact of ID services,
- enhancing impact of mainstream services,
- enhancing ID nursing practice, and
- enhancing quality of life.

Effectuating nursing procedures interventions are intellectual disability nursing activities that involve performing practical tasks with people with intellectual disabilities. *Enhancing impact of intellectual disability services* incorporates interventions directed at improving the work of organisations that specifically specialise on working with people with intellectual disability such as residential home services. *Enhancing impact of mainstream services* incorporates interventions directed at improving the work of mainstream healthcare organisations. *Enhancing intellectual disability nursing practice* incorporates activities undertaken by intellectual disability nurses to improve their own practice and the intellectual disability nursing profession. *Enhancing quality of life* incorporates interventions undertaken by intellectual disability nurses to promote the health and wellbeing of people with intellectual disabilities. Figure 11.1 illustrates the complex roles undertaken by intellectual disability nurses.

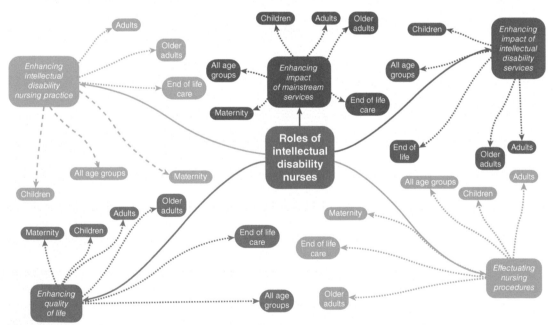

Figure 11.1   *Source:* Adapted from Mafuba *et al.* (2021c)

Roles of intellectual disabilities nurses.

The interventions undertaken by intellectual disability nurses are wide ranging and advanced and complex. Here we discuss the evidence for these according to the lifespan:

- Maternity,
- All age groups, children,
- Adults,
- Older adults, and
- End of life.

Maternity interventions

In their research Mafuba *et al.* (2021a, 2021b, 2021c) reported that intellectual disability nurses played a small but important role in the maternity care of women with intellectual disabilities. Intellectual disability nurses support pregnant women/parents with intellectual disabilities (including through child protection proceedings), assisted others to work with pregnant women with intellectual disabilities, and provided psychological support to expectant parents with intellectual disabilities. There is an important need for intellectual disability nurses to work with women with intellectual disabilities to access maternity and pre-natal screening services (Marriott *et al.*, 2015; McCarron *et al.*, 2018). Also, providing this support is important because without such support it is likely that pregnant women with intellectual disabilities may be unable to access appropriate maternity services. Expectant mothers with intellectual disabilities are likely to face child protection issues and intellectual disability nurses can undertake important interventions to support them through these processes. Going through pregnancy is likely to be a challenging experience for most women, and it could be argued that the challenges are likely to be greater for women with intellectual disabilities. Intellectual disability nurses are well placed to work directly with pregnant women with intellectual disabilities through supporting them psychologically. Such interventions are likely to be complex and varied and will require intellectual disability nurses to develop a complex repertoire of knowledge and skills.

Interventions across all age groups

Intellectual disability nurses undertake *effectuating nursing procedures* interventions across the lifespan and in a wide range of settings (Mafuba *et al.*, 2021a, 2021b, 2021c). These interventions include assessing and managing co-morbidities associated with intellectual disability, autism, and mental health, assessing people for equipment, carrying out diagnostic assessments, and sleep assessments (Mafuba *et al.*, 2021a, 2021b, 2021c; McCarron *et al.*, 2018; Quinn and Smolinski, 2018; Doody, Slevin and Taggart, 2017; Delahunty, 2017; Nelson and Carey, 2016; MacArthur *et al.*, 2015; Morton-Nance, 2015; Chapman, 2015; Bailey, 2014; Brown *et al.*, 2012; Sheerin, 2012; Ng, 2011; Mason and Phipps, 2010; McKeon, 2009; Slevin and Sines, 2005). People with intellectual disabilities live with complex and changing needs that require continuous assessment to maintain and improve their health and well-being. The role of intellectual disability nurses in care planning, implementing care interventions and managing health conditions was widely reported. These are important interventions and they have been reported previously (Taua, Hepworth and Neville, 2012; Dahm and Wadwnsten, 2008).

Intellectual disability nurses undertake interventions to address health inequalities associated with constipation, dysphagia, aspiration, and oral health. The importance of the intellectual disability nurse role in addressing the determinants and health inequalities experienced by people with intellectual disabilities has been previously highlighted (Cope and Shaw, 2019; Sheerin, 2012). The nursing procedures performed by intellectual disability nurses across the lifespan are complex and varied and include facilitating specialist clinics, facilitating communication, monitoring developmental growth, managing pain, providing bereavement counselling, undertaking de-escalation activities to prevent crises and admissions to hospital, carrying out wound care, undertaking airway management (tracheostomy, ventilators). This complexity requires intellectual disability nurses to be adaptable to deliver effective care to people with intellectual disabilities. Intellectual disability nursing interventions to *enhancing impact of intellectual disability services* include; adapting communication for easy understanding, autism support (community), best interest assessments, benchmarking, coaching (quality improvement), writing guidelines and protocols (e.g., preventing falls), bowel management, administering required medication (PRN), training (worldwide), epilepsy awareness and emergency medication training, promoting positive behaviour support (PBS) approaches, intellectual disability awareness training (professionals, carers, primary care) (Oulton *et al.*, 2019; Doody, Slevin and Taggart, 2019; Cleary and Doody, 2017; Marriott *et al.*, 2015; Arrey, 2014; Lovell *et al.*, 2014; Taggart, Truesdale-Kennedy and McIlfatrick, 2011; DH, 2007), and support families (Cope and Shaw, 2019; McCarron *et al.*, 2018; Doody, Slevin and Taggart, 2017; Northway *et al.*, 2017; Bailey, Doody and Lyons, 2014).

Intellectual disability nurses spend a significant amount of time focusing on ensuring that other intellectual disability staff, and voluntary and independent services effectively support people with intellectual disabilities. These interventions are at individual, organisational and strategic levels (Mafuba *et al.*, 2018a). The interventions performed by intellectual disability nurses can contribute to the impact of intellectual disability services when supporting people with intellectual disabilities. Intellectual disability nurses need to support other healthcare and social care professionals who work directly with people with intellectual disabilities in the community across the lifespan.

Intellectual disability nurses undertake a wide range of interventions focused on *enhancing the impact of mainstream services* across the lifespan. These interventions include: assessing effectiveness of interventions (Mafuba *et al.*, 2018a), addressing determinants of health and health inequalities, monitoring effectiveness of medications and treatments (Adams and Shah, 2016), facilitating access to health services (Mafuba *et al.*, 2018a, 2018b; Mafuba and Gates, 2015; Mafuba, 2009, 2013; Brown *et al.*, 2012; DH, 2007), advising acute hospital of individual needs, coordinating care between teams in acute hospital, advising social care services, advocating for intellectual disability inclusion at corporate level, auditing annual health checks, developing national policy and guidance, facilitating the making of and implementation of reasonable adjustments

(Cope and Shaw, 2019; Mafuba *et al.*, 2018a; MacArthur *et al.*, 2015), facilitating transitions (Delahunty, 2017; Northway *et al.*, 2017), undertaking health liaison activities (Northway *et al.*, 2017; Morton-Nance, 2015), facilitating social pre-scribing, educating acute care staff, training GP practice staff, and strategic level implementation of the health initiatives.

Intellectual disability nurses owe it to themselves and the people they support to ensure that they develop and implement interventions that have a positive impact. Intellectual disability nurses undertake a limited number of activities that focus on *enhancing the impact of intellectual disability nursing practice* across the lifespan (Mafuba *et al.*, 2021a, 2021b, 2021c) through producing teaching/training packages, training and educating staff (Oulton *et al.*, 2019; Doody, Slevin and Taggart, 2019; Cleary and Doody, 2017; Marriott *et al.*, 2015; Taggart, Truesdale-Kennedy and McIlfatrick, 2011), undertaking research and writing for publication, providing clinical leadership (local, regional, and national), creating new roles, coaching, facilitating conferences, and providing peer support among other activities.

Intellectual disability nurses play an important role in *enhancing the quality of life*, health, and well-being of people with intellectual disabilities across the lifespan, and these include: enabling and supporting healthy lifestyle choices and diet (Mafuba *et al.*, 2018a), advising and advocating for people with intellectual disabilities and their families (Cope and Shaw, 2019; McCarron *et al.*, 2018; Ring *et al.*, 2018; Doody, Slevin and Taggart, 2017; Brown *et al.*, 2012, 2016; Morton-Nance, 2015; Dalgarno and Riordan, 2014; Taua, Hepworth and Neville, 2012; Llewellyn and Northway, 2007; Llewellyn, 2005), enabling, empowering and educating people with intellectual disabilities to make their own choices (Sheerin, 2012), educating people with intellectual disabilities and their families and carers about health and healthy lifestyles and how to cope with diagnoses and symptoms (Mafuba *et al.*, 2018a; Mafuba, 2009, 2013; Taggart, Truesdale-Kennedy and McIlfatrick, 2011; Cleary and Doody, 2017; Morton-Nance, 2015; MacArthur *et al.*, 2015; Dalgarno and Riordan, 2014; Northway *et al.*, 2017; Brown *et al.*, 2012; Slevin and Sines, 2005), human rights education (service users), supporting social connectedness and community integration (McCarron *et al.*, 2018), supporting individuals to remain in their home (Northway *et al.*, 2017), adapting environments, adapting information for easy read, developing accessible health information, producing hospital passports, and producing Covid-19 passports. The extent of these interventions clearly demonstrate that intellectual disability nurse interventions are wide ranging across the lifespan.

Interventions for children

Intellectual disability nurses undertake a wide range of assessments including ABAS (adaptive behaviour system) assessments for children, communication assessments, ADHD (attention deficit hyperactivity disorder) assessments, ADHD diagnosis, behaviour management assessment, fetal alcohol spectrum disorders (FASD) diagnosis, identifying children requiring further intellectual disability diagnostic assessment, and intellectual disability diagnostic assessments. Intellectual disability nurses need to have skills to undertake complex assessments of children's needs. Other nursing procedures undertaken by intellectual disability nurses when working with children with intellectual disabilities include growth monitoring, management of PEG (percutaneous endoscopic gastrostomy), prescribing, ventilation care, weight monitoring, behaviour family therapy, facilitating ADHD clinics, adapting CBT (cognitive behaviour therapy), desensitisation, dialectal therapies, sex and relationships education/awareness (e.g., classes at local colleges and schools), syndromes and associated health risks education (individuals, families and carers) (Mafuba *et al.*, 2021a, 2021b, 2021c). These interventions illustrate the spectrum and complexity of the interventions undertaken by intellectual disability nurses when working with children.

Intellectual disability nursing interventions that focus on *enhancing impact of intellectual disability services* related to children include adapting CBT for anxiety and depression for children, advising CAMHS (child adolescent mental health service) colleagues, developing epilepsy guidelines, brain injury education, facilitating early discharge from mental health wards, transition liaison and transition planning, (Mafuba *et al.*, 2021a, 2021b, 2021c), providing positive behaviour support training and handling complaints (Oulton *et al.*, 2019), providing dietary advice (Marshall and Foster, 2002), and acting as links between schools and other services (Delahunty, 2017). These interventions are significant to the health and healthcare outcomes of children with intellectual disabilities.

The roles of intellectual disability nurses in *enhancing impact of mainstream services* are wide ranging and include ASD liaison with specialists regarding sensory needs and sensory diets, consultation with CAMHS teams, educating health visitors, SEN (special education needs) school nursing, desensitisation to clinical procedures using visual aids, and school liaison (Mafuba *et al.*, 2021a, 2021b, 2021c), pre-admission support (Oulton *et al.*, 2019), acting as a link between schools and other services (Delahunty, 2017), and providing dietary advice (Marshall and Foster, 2002).

Intellectual disability nurses undertake a wide range of interventions that focus on *enhancing quality of life* of children with intellectual disabilities and these include undertaking child support and protection interventions, advocating for immunisation uptake, undertaking continence training and continence promotion, developing parenting programmes, delivering emotional literacy training, undertaking internet safety promotion and education, facilitating psychological educational groups for parents and children, teaching life skills, teaching distress tolerance skills (Mafuba *et al.*, 2021b), continence promotion (Marshall and Foster, 2002), and provision of informal support and advice (Oulton *et al.*, 2019). These interventions are significant, and important given the growing population of children with intellectual disabilities, who often have complex and enduring health needs which may impact on their ability to lead healthy and active lifestyles. The emergent new interventions undertaken by intellectual disability nurses demonstrate that they are taking on new roles and developing new and often advanced skills and knowledge not previously associated with intellectual disability nursing practice.

Interventions for adults

Intellectual disability nursing roles in *effectuating nursing procedures* include NEWS (national early warning score) assessment of deterioration, mental capacity assessments, anxiety assessments, assessment of mental health, assessment of people's understanding of their needs, ASD (autism spectrum disorder) diagnosis, behaviour management assessment, blood tests, bowel screening, cardiometabolic assessments, dementia care assessments, developing assessments for the prison service, dysphagia assessments, forensic assessments, physical health assessments (abdominal, respiratory, and cardiovascular auscultation, percussion and palpitation), pressure sore risk assessment, psychosocial crisis assessments, sensory assessments, sex and relationships assessments, assessments in A&E (accident and emergency), triage in dementia clinics, and triage psychiatry clinics (Mafuba *et al.*, 2021a, 2021b, 2021c; Pennington *et al.*, 2019; Dalgarno and Riordan, 2014; Mason and Phipps, 2010; Taua, Neville and Scot, 2017; Doody, Slevin and Taggart, 2019; Quinn and Smolinski, 2018; Barr *et al.*,1999; Drozd and Clinch, 2016). These interventions demonstrate that intellectual disability nurses assess adults with diverse and complex needs. Intellectual disability nurses require knowledge and competence to use a wide range of assessment tools, as well as knowledge of different and often unrelated healthcare needs. For example: behaviour family therapy, catheterisation, chest physiotherapy, deprescribe psychotropic medication, manage self-harm, monitor effectiveness of medications and treatments, run nurse-led clinics, order and interpret investigation, tracheostomy care, talking therapy, venipuncture, and well-being sessions for men (develop and deliver).

Intellectual disability nurses manage a wide range of complex health and healthcare needs in a wide range of contexts and settings (Brown *et al.*, 2012, 2016; Pennington *et al.*, 2019; Marsham, 2012; Drozd and Clinch, 2016; Dalgarno and Riordan, 2014; Taua, Hepworth and Neville, 2012; Mason and Phipps, 2010; Ring *et al.*, 2018; Northway *et al.*, 2017; Adams and Shah, 2016; Lloyd and Coulson, 2014; Barr *et al.*, 1999; Cleary and Doody, 2017; Arrey, 2014; Lee and Kiemle, 2014; Lovell *et al.*, 2014; Doody, Slevin and Taggart, 2019). Given this complexity, intellectual disability nurses need to constantly learn and develop new knowledge and skills essential for engaging in advanced intellectual disability nursing practice. Intellectual disability nurses may have to switch between a wide range of activities in a day's work and are likely to require well advanced multi-tasking skills.

Intellectual disability nursing roles in *enhancing impact of intellectual disability services* include annual medication monitoring, anti-psychotic medication review and monitoring, chairing care program approach (CPA) meetings, develop epilepsy guidelines, organising and facilitating hospital discharge follow up review meetings, formulating service improvement plans, overseeing packages of care, sourcing care providers, supporting service providers/carers, training, and troubleshooting (Mafuba *et al.*, 2021a, 2021b, 2021c). The importance of the roles of intellectual disability nurses in supporting intellectual disability services and developing appropriate guidelines for intellectual disability services to support people with intellectual disabilities better cannot be overemphasised. Intellectual disability nurses practice in complex environments which are often multi-disciplinary and with multiple agencies. This requires them to engage in creative communication to enable things to happen. There is therefore a need for intellectual disability nurses to provide leadership in improving intellectual disability services through troubleshooting and other interventions.

Intellectual disability nurse roles in *enhancing impact of mainstream services* entail an increasingly complex catalogue of activities that include coordinating the assessment process in multiagency contexts, annual health checks monitoring, auditing annual health checks, chairing best interest meetings, dentistry liaison, developing audit tools for intellectual disability services within prison settings, supporting DNACPR (do not attempt cardiopulmonary resuscitation) decisions, forensic support liaison, gatekeeping mental health assessments for admission to hospital, involvement in quality improvement processes, pharmacy liaison, providing pharmacological advice to GPs, reviewing other services, and triaging in A&E (accident and emergency) (Mafuba *et al.*, 2021a, 2021b, 2021c, Northway *et al.*, 2017; Morton-Nance, 2015; Chapman, 2015).

Intellectual disability nurses are undertaking increasingly complex and advanced interventions. For people with intellectual disabilities, these interventions may mean the difference between accessing appropriate mainstream services and support. To improve services and enhance their impact intellectual disability nurses need to work collaboratively to improve access to mainstream services as well as take up direct care roles in mainstream services. The introduction of the *Future nurse* standards (NMC, 2018) places future intellectual disability nurse graduates in the UK in a unique position to assimilate these emerging roles in mainstream services.

There is a dearth of evidence to illustrate activities undertaken by intellectual disability nurses that focus on *enhancing impact of intellectual disability nursing practice*. This is a particular concern in relation to post registration professional development. The activities undertaken by intellectual disability nurses that have been identified include brain injury education, alcohol/substance education, developing and implementing training packages for community nurses, setting standards for intellectual disability nursing practice, and skills training (e.g., skin care, enteral feeding) (Mafuba *et al.*, 2021b, 2021c).

Intellectual disability nurse roles in *enhancing the quality of life* of adults with intellectual disabilities include promoting independence and advocacy, and health promotion activities (Marsham, 2012; Taggart, Truesdale-Kennedy and McIlfatrick, 2011; Cope and Shaw, 2019; Mafuba *et al.*, 2018b; McCarron *et al.*, 2018; Northway *et al.*, 2017; Doody, Slevin and Taggart, 2019, 2017; MacArthur *et al.*, 2015; Wagemans *et al.*, 2015; Morton-Nance, 2015; Bailey, Doody and Lyons, 2014; Brown *et al.*, 2012), hate crime reduction, internet safety promotion and education, neighborhood relations building, support with criminal justice system, anxiety support, behaviour family therapy, dementia support (community), and proactive support in relation to forced marriage (Mafuba *et al.*, 2021b, 2021c).

Interventions for older adults

In *effectuating nursing procedures* for older adults intellectual disability nursing roles include assessing mobility decline, behaviour management assessment, care assessments, carer assessments, cognitive decline assessments, dementia assessment (diagnostic), manual handling risk assessment, physical deterioration assessment (RESTORE2), physical health assessment (abdominal, respiratory, and cardiovascular auscultation, percussion and palpitation), pressure sore risk assessment, catheter care, diet and nutrition management, pain management, pressure care, and stoma care (Drozd and Clinch, 2016; Brown *et al.*, 2012; Arrey, 2014; Nelson and Carey, 2016; Northway *et al.*, 2017; Cleary and Doody, 2017; Wagemans *et al.*, 2015; Mafuba *et al.*, 2021b, 2021c). What must be made clear here is that intellectual disability nurses are involved in increasingly working directly with older adults with intellectual disabilities. This may very well mean that intellectual disability nurses are increasingly taking up new roles in dementia care services and nursing homes where older adults with intellectual disabilities may reside. For intellectual disability nurses working in the community, this may reflect an aging population that require assimilation of new and advanced skills to deliver appropriate interventions.

In *enhancing the impact of intellectual disability services* in relation to older people, intellectual disability nurses deal with a wide range of complex health and social care needs through commissioning changes to service provision, providing dementia support in community, leading multiagency coordination care/meetings, managing hospital discharges, mental capacity assessment, overseeing packages of care, placement breakdown prevention as needs change, supporting making reasonable adjustments, and supporting service providers and carers (Mafuba *et al.*, 2021b). In undertaking these roles intellectual disability nurses work directly with older adults with intellectual disabilities, their families, community service providers, and health and social care staff.

Intellectual disability nursing roles that focus on *enhancing the impact of mainstream services* include coordinating services, reviewing quality of care, social care liaison, supporting and supervising day-care staff, and supporting service providers among other interventions (Cleary and Doody, 2017; Bailey, Doody and Lyons, 2014; Mafuba *et al.*, 2021b). Given the increasing complex landscape of services for older adults in the UK and Ireland, as the population increases, these interventions are vital to healthcare outcomes for older adults with intellectual disabilities. There is a dearth of evidence to illustrate activities undertaken by intellectual disability nurses that focus on *enhancing impact of intellectual disability nursing practice* involving older adults. With the increasing population of older adults with intellectual disabilities, and the need for intellectual disability nurses to assimilate new roles in this area, intellectual disability nurses need to contribute to the development of appropriate interventions for this population.

In addressing the determinants of health to *enhance quality of life* of older adults with intellectual disability nurses are involved in bowel screening promotion, carer assessment, Covid-19 education, dementia support in the community, mental health advocacy, and preparing homes for changed needs (Mafuba *et al.*, 2021b). This is an important area of intellectual disability nursing practice given that older adults often have complex and enduring health needs which may impact on their ability to lead healthy and active lifestyles (Emerson, Copeland and Glover, 2011).

End-of-life interventions

Intellectual disability nurses play important roles in ensuring that people with intellectual disabilities of all ages experience good quality end-of-life care. These roles include assessing changing health conditions and detecting deterioration, interpreting complaints and symptoms, diet and nutrition management, managing end-of-life care, performing last offices, pressure care assessment and care, bereavement counselling, care giving and facilitating communication (Ng, 2011; Wagemans *et al.*, 2015; Bailey, Doody and Lyons, 2014; McCarron *et al.*, 2018; Oulton *et al.*, 2019; Northway *et al.*, 2017; Adams and Shah, 2016; Wagemans *et al.*, 2015; Morton-Nance, 2015; Arrey, 2014; Mafuba *et al.*, 2021b). The range of interventions in this very psychologically difficult and complex area illustrates the uniqueness of the knowledge and skills of intellectual disability nurses who work with people with intellectual disabilities across the lifespan with diverse backgrounds and needs at the most challenging time of their lives. The range of interventions require well developed direct care knowledge and skills, care coordination skills, as well as skills to deliver psychological support.

Intellectual disability nursing roles in *enhancing impact of intellectual disability services* related to end-of-life care include coordinating the assessment process, facilitating communication, undertaking last offices, shaping the nature of end-of-life care, and influencing end-of-life decisions, advance care planning, shaping the nature of end-of-life care and influencing end-of-life decision-making and facilitating reasonable adjustments (Cope and Shaw, 2019; Mafuba *et al.*, 2018a, 2021b; Northway *et al.*, 2017; Cleary and Doody, 2017; Drozd and Clinch, 2016; Wagemans *et al.*, 2015; MacArthur *et al.*, 2015; Marriott *et al.*, 2015; Morton-Nance, 2015). The provision of end-of-life care for people with intellectual disabilities by intellectual disability nurses is increasingly becoming a common occurrence.

The roles of intellectual disability nurses in *enhancing the impact of mainstream services* include facilitating communication, facilitating reasonable adjustments (Mafuba *et al.*, 2021b), facilitating collaborative working (Arrey, 2014), educating healthcare professionals and staff (Cleary and Doody, 2017; Morton-Nance, 2015; MacArthur *et al.*, 2015; Dalgarno and Riordan, 2014; Brown *et al.*, 2012; Slevin and Sines, 2005), providing information (Bailey, Doody and Lyons, 2014), sharing information with other professionals (Mafuba *et al.*, 2018a; Wagemans *et al.*, 2015), and liaising secondary care (McCarron *et al.*, 2018; Marshall and Foster, 2002).

Current palliative care services in the UK are fragmented (Dening, Sates and Lloyd-Williams, 2018), and there is clearly a need for coordination of existing palliative care services for the needs of people with intellectual disabilities to be met. Intellectual disability nurses undertake important interventions to address inequalities in care provision for people with intellectual disabilities who are at the end of their lives. However, there is limited evidence to illustrate activities undertaken by intellectual disability nurses that focus on *enhancing the impact of intellectual disability nursing practice* involving end-of-life care for people with intellectual disabilities across the lifespan. Some of the activities undertaken by intellectual disability nurses in *enhancing the quality of life* of people with intellectual disabilities at the end of their lives include providing psychological support, and training and raising awareness of the needs of people with intellectual disabilities at the end of their lives. End-of-life experiences are likely to be physically and emotionally debilitating for those facing end of life and those around them. Intellectual disability nurses have an important role to play in meeting the palliative care needs of people with intellectual disabilities.

Impact of intellectual disability nursing

The role of the intellectual disability nurse is central to the health and healthcare outcomes for people with intellectual disabilities. The impacts of intellectual disability nursing are wide ranging and complex (see Figure 11.2). Intellectual disability nurses play an important role in problem solving and facilitating access to a wide range of health and social care services on two levels: directly for the services users, and indirectly by advocating for their families or carers. This advocacy ensures that professionals and services make appropriate decisions that result in positive outcomes for people with intellectual disabilities. These decisions resulting from intellectual disability nursing advocacy mean people with intellectual disabilities receive appropriately funded care, adequate levels of support, and equal access to services just like the general population, have their rights respected, and their families and carers receive appropriate support (Mafuba *et al.*, 2021b).

Intellectual disability nurse interventions improve the independence and the ability to make choices by people with intellectual disabilities. The impact of this is that people with intellectual disabilities can make informed decisions about

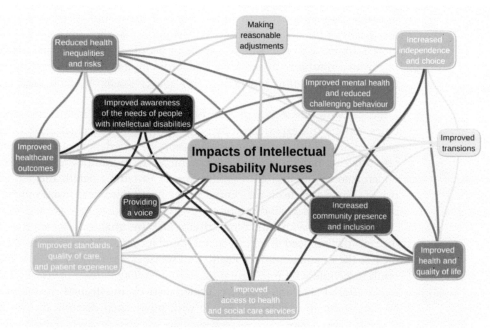

Figure 11.2   *Source:* Adapted from Mafuba *et al.* (2021c)

Impacts of intellectual disability nursing interventions.

their health, healthcare, and lifestyles that result in improved and better quality of life. In addition, the ability to make appropriate and informed decisions is more likely to lead to improved quality of life in the community (Mafuba *et al.*, 2021b).

Preventative intellectual disability nursing interventions are central to improving the health and healthcare outcomes for people with intellectual disabilities. From the evidence from the participants in this survey, these interventions reduce health risks, improve the experience of care, improve physical and mental health, and reduce premature mortality among people with intellectual disabilities (Mafuba *et al.*, 2021b).

The role of intellectual disability nurses in supporting people with intellectual disabilities to access appropriate services is longstanding. What is apparent in the examples of impact provided here is of immense importance and significance to people with intellectual disabilities. The result of this is improved access to services, better assessments and treatments, and person-centred supports resulting in improved healthcare experiences and outcomes.

Standards and quality of care are central to service user experience when people need healthcare interventions. For people with intellectual disabilities this may result in premature mortality. Nursing interventions undertaken by intellectual disability nurses improve patient safety, make mainstream services better informed about the healthcare needs of people with intellectual disabilities, and ensure that they have better experience of care (Mafuba *et al.*, 2021b). The result is that people with intellectual disabilities live longer lives in good health.

The health and healthcare needs of people with intellectual disabilities are complex and many mainstream services lack the awareness of these needs, and in many cases are unable to deliver the care that could be expected. Intellectual disability nursing interventions can support mainstream services to become more responsive to the complex needs of people with intellectual disabilities. Intellectual disability nurses have a key role in ensuring that healthcare staff, managers, and commissioners of healthcare services understand these complex needs.

People with intellectual disabilities experience health inequalities and inequities that are not experienced by people without intellectual disabilities. This more often results in preventable illnesses, poor experiences of health and social care services, and some cases preventable early mortalities. The interventions undertaken by intellectual disability nurses to reduce health inequalities and risk of illness and death are central to the health and healthcare outcomes for people with intellectual disabilities.

Many people with intellectual disabilities are unable to access the services they more often need than the general population. The reasons are multiple and include the fragmentation of health and social care services in the UK that may result in people with intellectual disabilities '*falling through the cracks*' (Mafuba *et al.*, 2021b). The interventions undertaken by intellectual disability nurses are important in preventing people with intellectual disabilities from falling through these cracks.

People with intellectual disabilities often have long term or lifelong care needs. Family life is consequently a significant and important aspect of their lives. Interventions undertaken by intellectual disability nurses result in better supports for the families of people with intellectual disabilities. Improved family lives may lead to improved and better outcomes for people with intellectual disabilities.

Because of complex health needs associated with intellectual disabilities, they are known to need healthcare interventions more often. Healthcare professionals in mainstream services often lack the necessary experience to understand the complexity of the healthcare needs of this population, resulting in diagnostic overshadowing that often results in unintended consequences. Intellectual disability nurses play an important role ensuring appropriate diagnoses and interventions that result in reduced inpatient admissions, improved healthcare outcomes, and reduced suffering and even premature death.

Mental ill-health and challenging behaviours are common among people with intellectual disabilities. The impact of interventions undertaken by intellectual disabilities nurses include reduction in anxiety, reduction in stress and distress, reduction in challenging behaviours, and better mental health and well-being. These impacts are likely to result in improved overall health and quality of life.

BOX 11.4
CASE STUDY 11.1

Non-medical prescribing (epilepsy)

Epilepsy specialist nurses in Northern Ireland and Gloucestershire demonstrated the impact to people with intellectual disabilities of undertaking a non-medical prescribing course. The nurses recognised opportunities to provide advice to people with intellectual disabilities, their families, and their carers about medication changes rather than having them wait for appointments with medical practitioners. This enabled timely and effective treatment, which resulted in the reduction of risks by preventing seizures and adverse effects of medications. The nurses can advise people with intellectual disabilities, their families, and their carers about medication changes promptly, based on assessed need. As is the case with the medical consultant who reviews the client's epilepsy at outpatient clinics, the nurses will be able to recommend medication changes to the GP, enabling a person's medical record to be updated and the necessary medication to be provided for the long term. The nurses also provide expert knowledge about epilepsy in people with intellectual disabilities to support GPs. This reduces the risk of sudden unexpected death in epilepsy and improving the healthcare outcomes for people with intellectual disabilities. Regular appointments, partnership working, and training can lead to improved recording and medication concordance. Reasonable adjustments can be made by strengthening links with other professionals, by providing relevant data to support access to mainstream services.

Tasks

Consider and reflect upon the impact of the non-medical prescribing role for the following

- People with intellectual disabilities who have epilepsy and complex needs

- Families of people with intellectual disabilities who have epilepsy and complex needs

- Formal and informal carers of people with intellectual disabilities who have epilepsy and complex needs

- Intellectual disability nurses (individually and collectively)
- Healthcare organisations

Source: Adapted from *Strengthening the commitment: The report of the UK modernising learning disabilities nursing review.* Edinburgh: Scottish Government, 2012.

Conclusion

The challenges posed by demographic changes to the population of people with intellectual disabilities will necessitate changes to current and future roles of intellectual disability nurses. The health and healthcare needs of people with intellectual disabilities, and how healthcare is delivered, will become increasingly complex. Consequently, intellectual disability nurses need to understand the need for their nursing roles to extend beyond traditional professional practice and geographical boundaries.

Nationally and internationally, health and social care will continue to undergo seismic shifts. Consequently, intellectual disability nurses, like other healthcare professionals, will continue to be exposed to major changes in their roles in meeting the health and healthcare needs of people with intellectual disabilities, and in where they undertake those changing roles.

Intellectual disability nurses need to develop formal and informal collaborations at local, national, and international levels to remain relevant. Intellectual disability nurses in the United Kingdom and Ireland can and need to be an important force for change of their own practice, health policy, and how healthcare is organised and delivered to people with intellectual disabilities. For this potential to be fully realised, intellectual disability nursing needs strong leadership, appropriate pre- and post-registration education, and engagement with workforce planning at local, national, and, to an extent, international levels. This is essential in strengthening efforts to improve the health and healthcare of people with intellectual disabilities.

References

Adams, D. and Shah, C. (2016) Prescribing of psychotropic medicines: The role of learning disabilities nurses. *Learning Disability Practice*, 19(8), pp. 21–25.

Allerton, L. and Emerson, E. (2012) British adults with chronic health conditions or impairments face significant barriers to accessing health services. *Public Health*, 126(11), pp. 920–927.

Arrey, S.K. (2014) *Lived experiences of registered learning disability nurses and palliative care professionals in caring for people with communication difficulties and an intellectual disability experiencing distress in palliative care settings: A hermeneutic phenomenological study*. ProQuest Dissertations Publishing. Available at: https://search.proquest.com/docview/1783893689 (Accessed 24 May 2022).

Atkinson, D., et al. (2013) *The health equalities framework (HEF) – an outcomes framework based on the determinants of health inequalities*. Available at: www.ndti.org.uk/assets/files/The_Health_Equality_Framework_final_word.pdf (Accessed 9 August 2022).

Backer, C., Chapman, M. and Mitchell, D. (2009) Access to secondary healthcare for people with intellectual disabilities: A review of the literature. *Journal of Applied Research in Intellectual Disabilities*, 22(6), pp. 514–525.

Bailey, M., Doody, O. and Lyons, R. (2014) Surveying community nursing support for persons with a learning disability and palliative care needs. *British Journal of Learning Disabilities*, 44(1), pp. 24–34.

Bakker-van Gijssel, E.J., *et al.* (2017) Health assessment instruments for people with intellectual disabilities – a systematic review. *Research in Developmental Disabilities*, 64, pp. 12–24.

Barr, O., *et al.* (1999) Health screening for people with learning disabilities by a community learning disability nursing service in Northern Ireland. *Journal of Advanced Nursing*, 29(6), pp. 1482–1491.

Blair, J. (2013) Everybody's life has worth – getting it right in hospital for people with a learning disability and reducing clinical risks. *Journal of Patient Safety and Risk Management*, 19(3), pp. 58–63.

Brown, M., *et al.* (2010) Equality and access to general healthcare for people with learning disabilities: Reality or rhetoric? *Journal of Research in Nursing*, 15(4), pp. 351–361.

Brown, M., *et al.* (2012) Learning disability liaison nursing services in south-east Scotland: A mixed-methods impact and outcome study. *Journal of Intellectual Disability Research*, 56(12), pp. 1161–1174.

Brown, M., *et al.* (2016) The perspectives of stakeholders of intellectual disability liaison nurses: A model of compassionate, person-centred care. *Journal of Clinical Nursing*, 25(7–8), pp. 972–982.

Campbell, M. and Martin, M. (2009) Reducing health inequalities in Scotland: The involvement of people with learning disabilities as national health service reviewers. *British Journal of Learning Disabilities*, 38(1), pp. 49–58.

Chapman, H.M. (2015) *The health consultation experience for people with learning disabilities: A constructivist grounded theory study based on symbolic interactionism.* Chester: Unpublished PhD thesis. Chester: University of Chester.

Chauhan, U., *et al.* (2010) Health checks in primary care for adults with intellectual disabilities: How extensive should they be? *Journal of Intellectual Disability Research*, 54(6), pp. 479–486.

Cleary, J. and Doody, O. (2017) Nurses' experience of caring for people with intellectual disability and dementia. *Journal of Clinical Nursing*, 26(5–6), pp. 620–631.

Cooper, S.A., *et al.* (2011) Neighbourhood deprivation, health inequalities and service access by adults with intellectual disabilities: A cross-sectional study. *Journal of Intellectual Disability Research*, 55(3), pp. 313–323.

Cope, G. and Shaw, T. (2019) *Capturing the voices of learning disability nurses and people who use services.* London: Foundation of Nursing Studies.

Dahm, M.F. and Wadwnsten, B. (2008) Nurses' experiences of and opinions about using standardised care plans in electronic health records – a questionnaire study. *Journal of Clinical Nursing*, 17(12), pp. 2137–2145.

Dalgarno, M.F. and Riordan, S.A. (2014) Forensic intellectual disability nursing: What's it really like? *Journal of Intellectual Disabilities and Offending Behaviour*, 5(4), pp. 167–177.

Delahunty, L. (2017) Understanding the nurse's role in identifying children with intellectual disability. *Nursing Children and Young People*, 29(6), pp. 33–36.

Dening, K.H., Sates, C. and Lloyd-Williams, M. (2018) Palliative care in dementia: A fragmented pathway? *International Journal of Palliative Nursing*, 24(12), pp. 585–596.

DH (2001) *Valuing people.* London: Department of Health.

DH (2007) *Good practice in intellectual disability nursing*. London: Department of Health.

DH (2008) *Health care for all: Independent inquiry into access to health care for people with learning disabilities*. London: HMSO.

DH, *et al.* (2012) *Strengthening the commitment*. Edinburgh: The Scottish Government.

Doody, O., Slevin, E. and Taggart, L. (2017) Focus group interviews examining the contribution of intellectual disability clinical nurse specialists in Ireland. *Journal of Clinical Nursing*, 26(19–20), pp. 2964–2975.

Doody, O., Slevin, E. and Taggart, L. (2019) A survey of nursing and multidisciplinary team members' perspectives on the perceived contribution of intellectual disability clinical nurse specialists. *Journal of Clinical Nursing*, 28(21), pp. 879–3889.

DRC (2006) *Equal treatment: Closing the gap*. Stratford Upon Avon: Disability Rights Commission.

Drozd, M. and Clinch, C. (2016) The experiences of orthopedic and trauma nurses who have cared for adults with a intellectual disability. *International Journal of Orthopedic Trauma Nursing*, 22, pp. 13–23.

Emerson, E. and Baines, S. (2010) *Health inequalities & people with learning disabilities in the UK*. London: HMSO.

Emerson, E. and Brigham, P. (2015) Exposure of children with developmental delay to social determinants of poor health: Cross-sectional case record review study. *Child Care, Health and Development*, 41(2), pp. 249–257.

Emerson, E., Copeland, A. and Glover, G. (2011) *The uptake of health checks for adults with learning disabilities: 2008/9 to 2010/11*. Available at: www.karentysonspage.org/Emerson%202011%20Health%20Checks%20for%20People%20with%20Intellectual%20Disabilities%202008-9%20%202010-11.pdf (Accessed 6 July 2022).

Emerson, E., *et al.* (2016a) The physical health of British adults with intellectual disability: Cross sectional study. *International Journal for Equity in Health*, 15(1), pp. 1–9.

Emerson, E., *et al.* (2016b) Obesity in British children with and without intellectual disability: Cohort study. *BMC Public Health*, 16(1), pp. 1–10.

Hatton, C. and Emerson, E. (2015) Health disparities, health inequity, and people with intellectual disabilities. *International Review of Research in Developmental Disabilities*, 48, pp. 1–9.

Heslop, P., *et al.* (2013) *Confidential inquiry into premature deaths of people with intellectual disabilities (CIPOLD) – final report*. Bristol: Norah Fry Research Centre.

Heslop, P., *et al.* (2014) The confidential inquiry into premature deaths of people with intellectual disabilities in the UK: A population-based study. *The Lancet*, 383(9920), pp. 889–895.

HSE Mental Health Services (2021) *Mental health services for adults with intellectual disabilities: National model of service*. Dublin: HSE Mental Health Services.

Kavanagh, A., *et al.* (2017) Inequalities in socio-economic characteristics and health and wellbeing of men with and without disabilities: A cross-sectional analysis of the baseline wave of the Australian longitudinal study on male health. *BMC Public Health*, 16(Suppl 3), pp. 23–31.

Kerr, M. (2004) Improving the general health of people with intellectual disabilities. *Advances in Psychiatric Treatment*, 10, pp. 200–206.

LeDeR (2020) *The learning disability mortality review – annual report*. Bristol: University of Bristol Norah Fry Centre for Disability Studies.

Lee, A. and Kiemle, G. (2014) It's one of the hardest jobs in the world: The experience and understanding of unqualified nurses who work with individuals diagnosed with both intellectual disability and personality disorder. *Journal of Applied Research in Intellectual Disabilities*, 28(3), pp. 238–248.

Llewellyn, G., Vaughan, C. and Emerson, E. (2015) Discrimination and the health of people with learning disabilities. *International Review of Research in Developmental Disabilities*, 48, pp. 43–72.

Llewellyn, P. (2005) *An investigation into the advocacy role of the intellectual disability nurse.* Unpublished PhD thesis. Wales: University of Glamorgan.

Llewellyn, P. and Northway, R. (2007) The views and experiences of intellectual disability nurses concerning their advocacy education. *Nurse Education Today*, 27(8), pp. 955–963.

Lloyd, J.L. and Coulson, N.S. (2014) The role of learning disability nurses in promoting cervical screening uptake in women with intellectual disabilities. *Journal of Intellectual Disabilities*, 18(2), pp. 129–145.

Lovell, A., *et al.* (2014) Working with people with learning disabilities in varying degrees of security: Nurses' perceptions of competencies. *Journal of Advanced Nursing*, 70(9), pp. 2041–2050.

MacArthur, J., *et al.* (2015) Making reasonable and achievable adjustments: The contributions of learning disability liaison nurses in 'getting it right' for people with intellectual disabilities receiving general hospitals care. *Journal of Advanced Nursing*, 71(7), pp. 1552–1563.

Mafuba, K. (2009) The public health role of learning disability nurses: A review of the literature. *Learning Disability Practice*, 12(4), pp. 33–37.

Mafuba, K. (2013) *Public health: Community learning disability nurses' perception and experience of their roles: An exploratory sequential multiple methods study.* ProQuest Dissertations Publishing. Available at: https://search.proquest.com/docview/1937411950 (Accessed 27 July 2022).

Mafuba, K. and Gates, B. (2015) An investigation into the public health roles of community learning disability nurses. *British Journal of Learning Disabilities*, 43(1), pp. 1–7.

Mafuba, K., *et al.* (2018a) Community learning disability nurses' public health roles in the United Kingdom: An exploratory documentary analysis. *British Journal of Learning Disabilities*, 22(1), pp. 61–73.

Mafuba, K., *et al.* (2018b) *Mixed methods literature review on improving the health of people with a learning disability – a public health nursing approach. Final report.* London: University of West London, Public Health England.

Mafuba, K., *et al.* (2021a) *Understanding the contribution of learning disability nurses: Scoping research. Volume 1 of 3 – scoping literature review report.* London: University of West London, RCN Foundation.

Mafuba, K., *et al.* (2021b) *Understanding the contribution of intellectual disability nurses: Scoping research. Volume 2 of 3 – scoping survey research report.* London: University of West London, RCN Foundation.

Mafuba, K., *et al.* (2021c) *Understanding the contribution of intellectual disability nurses: Scoping research. Volume 3 of 3 – compendium of intellectual disability nursing interventions.* London: University of West London, RCN Foundation.

Marriott, A., *et al.* (2015) Cancer screening for people with learning disabilities and the role of the screening liaison nurse. *Tizard Learning Disability Review*, 20(4), pp. 239–246.

Marshall, D. and Foster, I. (2002) Providing a healthcare input to children in special schools. *British Journal of Nursing*, 11(1), pp. 28–35.

Marsham, M. (2012) An exploration of community learning disability nurses' therapeutic role. *British Journal of Learning Disabilities*, 40(3), pp. 236–244.

Mason, T. and Phipps, D. (2010) Forensic learning disability nursing skills and competencies: A study of forensic and non-forensic nurses. *Issues in Mental Health Nursing*, 31(11), pp. 708–715.

McCarron, M., *et al.* (2018) *Shaping the future of intellectual disability nursing in Ireland.* Dublin: Health Services Executive.

McIlfatrick, S., Taggart, L. and Truesdale-Kennedy, M. (2011) Supporting women with intellectual disabilities to access breast cancer screening: A healthcare professional perspective. *European Journal of Cancer Care*, 20(3), pp. 412–420.

McKeon, M. (2009) A survey of clinical nursing skills in intellectual disability nursing. *Journal of Intellectual Disabilities*, 13(1), pp. 31–41.

Melville, C.A., *et al.* (2006) The outcomes of an intervention study to reduce the barriers experienced by people with intellectual disabilities accessing primary healthcare services. *Journal of Intellectual Disability Research*, 50(1), pp. 11–17.

Mencap (2007) *Death by indifference: Following up the treat me right report.* London: Mencap.

Mencap (2012) *Death by indifference: 74 deaths and counting.* London: Mencap.

Mencap (2020) *Children – research statistics.* Available at: www.mencap.org.uk/learning-disability-explained/research-and-statistics/children-research-and-statistics (Accessed 24 July 2022).

Michael, J. (2008) *Healthcare for all: Report of the independent inquiry into access to healthcare for people with intellectual disabilities.* London: Department of Health.

Morton-Nance, S. (2015) Unique role of learning disability liaison nurses. *Learning Disability Practice*, 18(7), pp. 30–34.

Nelson, S. and Carey, E. (2016) The role of the nurse in assessing mobility decline in older people with learning disabilities. *Learning Disability Practice*, 19(9), pp. 19–24.

Ng, J.S.W. (2011) *Knowing the patient well: Intellectual disability nurses' experiences of caring for terminally ill people with profound intellectual disabilities in residential care settings.* Unpublished PhD thesis. London: University of Greenwich.

NICE (2018) *Learning disabilities and behaviours that challenges: Service design and delivery.* Available at: www.nice.org.uk/guidance/ng93 (Accessed 27 July 2022).

NMC (2018) *Future nurse: Standards of proficiency for registered nurses.* London: NMC.

Northway, R., *et al.* (2017) Supporting people across the lifespan: The role of learning disability nurses. *Learning Disability Practice*, 20(3), pp. 22–27.

Nursing and Midwifery Board of Ireland (2016) *Nurse registration programmes standards and requirements* (4th edition). Dublin: Nursing and Midwifery Board of Ireland.

Oulton, J., *et al.* (2019) Learning disability nurse provision in children's hospitals: Hospital staff perceptions of whether it makes a difference. *BMC Pediatrics*, 19, p. 192. doi:10.1186/s12887-019-1547-y.

Pennington, M., *et al.* (2019) The impact of an epilepsy nurse competency framework on the costs of supporting adults with epilepsy and intellectual disability: Findings from the EpAID study. *Journal of Intellectual Disability Research*, 63(12), pp. 1391–1400.

Quinn, B.L. and Smolinski, M. (2018) Improving school nurse pain assessment practices for students with intellectual disability. *The Journal of School Nursing*, 34(6), pp. 480–488.

Ring, H., *et al.* (2018) Training nurses in a competency framework tosupport adults with epilepsy and intellectual disability: The EpAID cluster RCT. *Health Technology Assessment*, 22(10). doi:10.3310/hta22100.

Robertson, J., *et al.* (2014) The impact of health checks for people with intellectual disabilities: An updated systematic review of evidence. *Research in Developmental Disabilities*, 35(10), pp. 2450–2462.

Robertson, J., *et al.* (2015) Mortality in people with intellectual disabilities and epilepsy: A systematic review. *Seizure*, 29, pp. 123–133.

Robertson, J., *et al.* (2017) Prevalence of dysphagia in people with intellectual disability: A systematic review. *Intellectual and Developmental Disabilities*, 55(6), pp. 377–391.

Savage, A. and Emerson, E. (2016) Overweight and obesity among children at risk of intellectual disability in 20 low- and middle-income countries. *Journal of Intellectual Disability Research*, 60(11), pp. 1128–1135.

Scottish Government (2000) *The same as you?* Edinburgh: The Scottish Government.

Scottish Government (2012) *Strengthening the commitment: The report of the UK modernising learning disabilities nursing review.* Edinburgh: Scottish Government.

Sheerin, F.K. (2012) Learning disability nursing – responding to health inequity. *British Journal of Learning Disabilities*, 40(4), pp. 266–271.

Slevin, E. and Sines, D. (2005) The role of community nurses for people with intellectual disabilities: Working with people who challenge. *Journal of Nursing Studies*, 42, pp. 415–427.

Stewart, D. and Todd, M. (2001) Role and contribution of nurses for intellectual disabilities: A local study in a county of Oxford-Anglia region. *British Journal of Intellectual Disabilities*, 29(4), pp. 145–150.

Straetmans, J.M.J.A.A., *et al.* (2007) Health problems of people with intellectual disabilities: The impact for general practice. *British Journal of General Practice*, 57(534), pp. 64–66.

Taggart, L., Truesdale-Kennedy, M. and McIlfatrick, S. (2011) The role of community nurses and residential staff in supporting women with intellectual disability to access breast screening services. *Journal of Intellectual Disability Research*, 55(1), pp. 41–52.

Taua, C., Hepworth, J. and Neville, C. (2012) Nurses' role in caring for people with a comorbidity of mental illness and intellectual disability: A literature review. *International Journal of Mental Health Nursing*, 21(2), pp. 163–174.

Taua, C., Neville, C. and Scot, T. (2017) Appreciating the work of nurses caring for adults with intellectual disability and mental health issues. *International Journal of Mental Health Nursing*, 26(6), pp. 629–638.

Torr, J. and Davis, R. (2007) Ageing and mental health problems in people with intellectual disability. *Current Opinion in Psychiatry*, 20(5), pp. 467–471.

Truesdale, M. and Brown, M. (2017) *People with learning disabilities in Scotland: 2017 health needs assessment report.* Edinburgh: NHS Health Scotland.

Van Schrojenstein Lantman-de Valk, H.M.J., *et al.* (2007) Health problems in people with intellectual disability in general practice: A comparative study. *Family Practice*, 17(5), pp. 405–407.

Wagemans, A.M.A., *et al.* (2015) End-of-life decision-making for people with intellectual disability from the perspective of nurses. *Journal of Policy and Practice in Intellectual Disabilities*, 12(4), pp. 294–302.

Further Reading

NMC (2018) *Future nurse: Standards of proficiency for registered nurses.* London: NMC.

Nursing and Midwifery Board of Ireland (2016) *Nurse registration programmes standards and requirements* (4th edition). Dublin: Nursing and Midwifery Board of Ireland.

Useful Resources

Health Education and Improvement Wales: https://heiw.nhs.wales/careers/
roles/nursing/learning-disability-nursing/

HSE Office of the Nursing and Midwifery Service Director: https://healthservice.hse.ie/about-us/onmsd/quality-nursing-and-midwifery-care/shaping-the-future-of-intellectual-disability-nursing-in-ireland.html

Nursing and Midwifery Board of Ireland: www.nmbi.ie/nmbi/media/NMBI/
Publications/nurse-registration-education-programme.pdf?ext=.pdf

NHS Careers: www.nhscareers.nhs.uk/explore-by-career/nursing/careers-in-nursing/
learning-disabilities-nursing/

NHS Scotland Careers: www.careers.nhs.scot/careers/explore-our-careers/nursing/
learning-disability-nurse/

Nursing and Midwifery Council: www.nmc.org.uk/globalassets/sitedocuments/
standards-of-proficiency/nurses/future-nurse-proficiencies.pdf

Skills for Health: www.skillsforhealth.org.uk/workforce-transformation/role-redesign-service/

Appendix A: Nursing and Midwifery Council Standards of proficiency for registered nurses

Box A.1 Platform 1: Being an accountable professional

At the point of registration, the registered nurse will be able to:

1.1 understand and act in accordance with the Code (2015): Professional standards of practice and behaviour for nurses and midwives and fulfil all registration requirements.

1.2 understand and apply relevant legal, regulatory and governance requirements, policies, and ethical frameworks, including any mandatory reporting duties, to all areas of practice, differentiating where appropriate between the devolved legislatures of the United Kingdom

1.3 understand and apply relevant legal, regulatory and governance requirements, policies, and ethical frameworks, including any mandatory reporting duties, to all areas of practice, differentiating where appropriate between the devolved legislatures of the United Kingdom

1.4 understand and apply the principles of courage, transparency and the professional duty of candour, recognising and reporting any situations, behaviours or errors that could result in poor care outcomes

1.5 demonstrate an understanding of, and the ability to challenge, discriminatory behaviour

1.6 understand the demands of professional practice and demonstrate how to recognise signs of vulnerability in themselves or their colleagues and the action required to minimise risks to health

1.7 understand the professional responsibility to adopt a healthy lifestyle to maintain the level of personal fitness and wellbeing required to meet people's needs for mental and physical care

1.8 demonstrate an understanding of research methods, ethics and governance in order to critically analyse, safely use, share and apply research findings to promote and inform best nursing practice

1.9 demonstrate the knowledge, skills and ability to think critically when applying evidence and drawing on experience to make evidence informed decisions in all situations

1.10 understand the need to base all decisions regarding care and interventions on people's needs and preferences, recognising and addressing any personal and external factors that may unduly influence their decisions

1.11 demonstrate resilience and emotional intelligence and be capable of explaining the rationale that influences their judgments and decisions in routine, complex and challenging situations

1.12 communicate effectively using a range of skills and strategies with colleagues and people at all stages of life and with a range of mental, physical, cognitive and behavioural health challenges

1.13 demonstrate the skills and abilities required to support people at all stages of life who are emotionally or physically vulnerable

1.14 demonstrate the skills and abilities required to develop, manage and maintain appropriate relationships with people, their families, carers and colleagues

1.15 provide and promote non-discriminatory, person centred and sensitive care at all times, reflecting on people's values and beliefs, diverse backgrounds, cultural characteristics, language requirements, needs and preferences, taking account of any need for adjustments

1.16 demonstrate the numeracy, literacy, digital and technological skills required to meet the needs of people in their care to ensure safe and effective nursing practice

1.17 demonstrate the ability to keep complete, clear, accurate and timely records

1.18 take responsibility for continuous self-reflection, seeking and responding to support and feedback to develop their professional knowledge and skills

1.19 demonstrate the knowledge and confidence to contribute effectively and proactively in an interdisciplinary team

1.20 act as an ambassador, upholding the reputation of their profession and promoting public confidence in nursing, health and care services

1.21 safely demonstrate evidence-based practice in all skills and procedures stated in Annexes A and B.

Platform 2: Promoting health and preventing ill health

At the point of registration, the registered nurse will be able to:

2.1 understand and apply the aims and principles of health promotion, protection and improvement and the prevention of ill health when engaging with people

2.2 demonstrate knowledge of epidemiology, demography, genomics and the wider determinants of health, illness and wellbeing and apply this to an understanding of global patterns of health and wellbeing outcomes

2.3 understand the factors that may lead to inequalities in health outcomes

2.4 identify and use all appropriate opportunities, making reasonable adjustments when required, to discuss the impact of smoking, substance and alcohol use, sexual behaviours, diet and exercise on mental, physical and behavioural health and wellbeing, in the context of people's individual circumstances

2.5 promote and improve mental, physical, behavioural and other health related outcomes by understanding and explaining the principles, practice and evidence-base for health screening programmes

2.6 understand the importance of early years and childhood experiences and the possible impact on life choices, mental, physical and behavioural health and wellbeing

2.7 understand and explain the contribution of social influences, health literacy, individual circumstances, behaviours and lifestyle choices to mental, physical and behavioural health outcomes

2.8 explain and demonstrate the use of up to date approaches to behaviour change to enable people to use their strengths and expertise and make informed choices when managing their own health and making lifestyle adjustments

2.9 use appropriate communication skills and strength based approaches to support and enable people to make informed choices about their care to manage health challenges in order to have satisfying and fulfilling lives within the limitations caused by reduced capability, ill health and disability

2.10 provide information in accessible ways to help people understand and make decisions about their health, life choices, illness and care

2.11 promote health and prevent ill health by understanding and explaining to people the principles of pathogenesis, immunology and the evidence-base for immunisation, vaccination and herd immunity

2.12 protect health through understanding and applying the principles of infection prevention and control, including communicable disease surveillance and antimicrobial stewardship and resistance.

Platform 3: Assessing needs and planning care

At the point of registration, the registered nurse will be able to:

3.1 demonstrate and apply knowledge of human development from conception to death when undertaking full and accurate person-centred nursing assessments and developing appropriate care plans

3.2 demonstrate and apply knowledge of body systems and homeostasis, human anatomy and physiology, biology, genomics, pharmacology and social and behavioural sciences when undertaking full and accurate person-centred nursing assessments and developing appropriate care plans

3.3 demonstrate and apply knowledge of all commonly encountered mental, physical, behavioural and cognitive health conditions, medication usage and treatments when undertaking full and accurate assessments of nursing care needs and when developing, prioritising and reviewing person centred care plans

3.4 understand and apply a person-centred approach to nursing care, demonstrating shared assessment, planning, decision making and goal setting when working with people, their families, communities and populations of all ages

3.5 demonstrate the ability to accurately process all information gathered during the assessment process to identify needs for individualised nursing care and develop person-centred evidence-based plans for nursing interventions with agreed goals

3.6 effectively assess a person's capacity to make decisions about their own care and to give or withhold consent

3.7 understand and apply the principles and processes for making reasonable adjustments

3.8 understand and apply the relevant laws about mental capacity for the country in which you are practising when making decisions in relation to people who do not have capacity

3.9 recognise and assess people at risk of harm and the situations that may put them at risk, ensuring prompt action is taken to safeguard those who are vulnerable

3.10 demonstrate the skills and abilities required to recognise and assess people who show signs of self-harm and/or suicidal ideation

3.11 undertake routine investigations, interpreting and sharing findings as appropriate

3.12 interpret results from routine investigations, taking prompt action when required by implementing appropriate interventions, requesting additional investigations or escalating to others

3.13 demonstrate an understanding of co-morbidities and the demands of meeting people's complex nursing and social care needs when prioritising care plans

3.14 identify and assess the needs of people and families for care at the end of life, including requirements for palliative care and decision making related to their treatment and care preferences

3.15 demonstrate the ability to work in partnership with people, families and carers to continuously monitor, evaluate and reassess the effectiveness of all agreed nursing care plans and care, sharing decision making and readjusting agreed goals, documenting progress and decisions made

3.16 demonstrate knowledge of when and how to refer people safely to other professionals or services for clinical intervention or support.

Platform 4: Providing and evaluating care

At the point of registration, the registered nurse will be able to:

4.1 demonstrate and apply an understanding of what is important to people and how to use this knowledge to ensure their needs for safety, dignity, privacy, comfort and sleep can be met, acting as a role model for others in providing evidence-based person-centred care

4.2 demonstrate and apply an understanding of what is important to people and how to use this knowledge to ensure their needs for safety, dignity, privacy, comfort and sleep can be met, acting as a role model for others in providing evidence-based person-centred care

4.3 demonstrate the knowledge, communication and relationship management skills required to provide people, families and carers with accurate information that meets their needs before, during and after a range of interventions

4.4 demonstrate the knowledge and skills required to support people with commonly encountered mental health, behavioural, cognitive and learning challenges, and act as a role model for others in providing high quality nursing interventions to meet people's needs

4.5 demonstrate the knowledge and skills required to support people with commonly encountered physical health conditions, their medication usage and treatments, and act as a role model for others in providing high quality nursing interventions when meeting people's needs

4.6 demonstrate the knowledge, skills and ability to act as a role model for others in providing evidence-based nursing care to meet people's needs related to nutrition, hydration and bladder and bowel health

4.7 demonstrate the knowledge, skills and ability to act as a role model for others in providing evidence-based, person-centred nursing care to meet people's needs related to mobility, hygiene, oral care, wound care and skin integrity

4.8 demonstrate the knowledge and skills required to identify and initiate appropriate interventions to support people with commonly encountered symptoms including anxiety, confusion, discomfort and pain

4.9 demonstrate the knowledge and skills required to prioritise what is important to people and their families when providing evidence-based person-centred nursing care at end of life including the care of people who are dying, families, the deceased and the bereaved

4.10 demonstrate the knowledge and ability to respond proactively and promptly to signs of deterioration or distress in mental, physical, cognitive and behavioural health and use this knowledge to make sound clinical decisions

4.11 demonstrate the knowledge and skills required to initiate and evaluate appropriate interventions to support people who show signs of self-harm and/or suicidal ideation

4.12 demonstrate the ability to manage commonly encountered devices and confidently carry out related nursing procedures to meet people's needs for evidence based, person-centred care

4.13 demonstrate the knowledge, skills and confidence to provide first aid procedures and basic life support

4.14 understand the principles of safe and effective administration and optimisation of medicines in accordance with local and national policies and demonstrate proficiency and accuracy when calculating dosages of prescribed medicines

4.15 demonstrate knowledge of pharmacology and the ability to recognise the effects of medicines, allergies, drug sensitivities, side effects, contraindications, incompatibilities, adverse reactions, prescribing errors and the impact of polypharmacy and over the counter medication usage

4.16 demonstrate knowledge of how prescriptions can be generated, the role of generic, unlicensed, and off-label prescribing and an understanding of the potential risks associated with these approaches to prescribing

4.17 apply knowledge of pharmacology to the care of people, demonstrating the ability to progress to a prescribing qualification following registration, and

4.18 demonstrate the ability to coordinate and undertake the processes and procedures involved in routine planning and management of safe discharge home or transfer of people between care settings.

Platform 5: Leading and managing nursing care and working in teams

At the point of registration, the registered nurse will be able to:

5.1 understand the principles of effective leadership, management, group and organisational dynamics and culture and apply these to team working and decision-making

5.2 understand and apply the principles of human factors, environmental factors and strength-based approaches when working in teams

5.3 understand the principles and application of processes for performance management and how these apply to the nursing team

5.4 demonstrate an understanding of the roles, responsibilities and scope of practice of all members of the nursing and interdisciplinary team and how to make best use of the contributions of others involved in providing care

5.5 safely and effectively lead and manage the nursing care of a group of people, demonstrating appropriate prioritisation, delegation and assignment of care responsibilities to others involved in providing care

5.6 exhibit leadership potential by demonstrating an ability to guide, support and motivate individuals and interact confidently with other members of the care team

5.7   demonstrate the ability to monitor and evaluate the quality of care delivered by others in the team and lay carers

5.8   support and supervise students in the delivery of nursing care, promoting reflection and providing constructive feedback, and evaluating and documenting their performance

5.9   demonstrate the ability to challenge and provide constructive feedback about care delivered by others in the team, and support them to identify and agree individual learning needs

5.10   contribute to supervision and team reflection activities to promote improvements in practice and services

5.11   effectively and responsibly use a range of digital technologies to access, input, share and apply information and data within teams and between agencies,

5.12   understand the mechanisms that can be used to influence organisational change and public policy, demonstrating the development of political awareness and skills.

Platform 6: Improving safety and quality of care

At the point of registration, the registered nurse will be able to:

6.1   understand and apply the principles of health and safety legislation and regulations and maintain safe work and care environments

6.2   understand the relationship between safe staffing levels, appropriate skills mix, safety and quality of care, recognising risks to public protection and quality of care, escalating concerns appropriately

6.3   comply with local and national frameworks, legislation and regulations for

assessing, managing and reporting risks, ensuring the appropriate action is taken

6.4   demonstrate an understanding of the principles of improvement methodologies, participate in all stages of audit activity and identify appropriate quality improvement strategies

6.5   demonstrate the ability to accurately undertake risk assessments in a range of care settings, using a range of contemporary assessment and improvement tools

6.6   identify the need to make improvements and proactively respond to potential hazards that may affect the safety of people

6.7   understand how the quality and effectiveness of nursing care can be evaluated in practice, and demonstrate how to use service delivery evaluation and audit findings to bring about continuous improvement

6.8   demonstrate an understanding of how to identify, report and critically reflect on near misses, critical incidents, major incidents and serious adverse events in order to learn from them and influence their future practice

6.9   work with people, their families, carers and colleagues to develop effective improvement strategies for quality and safety, sharing feedback and learning from positive outcomes and experiences, mistakes and adverse outcomes and experiences

6.10   apply an understanding of the differences between risk aversion and risk management and how to avoid compromising quality of care and health outcomes

6.11   acknowledge the need to accept and manage uncertainty, and demonstrate an understanding of strategies that develop resilience in self and others, and

6.12   understand the role of registered nurses and other health and care professionals at different levels of experience and seniority when managing and prioritising actions and care in the event of a major incident.

Platform 7: Coordinating care

At the point of registration, the registered nurse will be able to:

7.1 understand and apply the principles of partnership, collaboration and inter-agency working across all relevant sectors

7.2 understand health legislation and current health and social care policies, and the mechanisms involved in influencing policy development and change, differentiating where appropriate between the devolved legislatures of the United Kingdom

7.3 understand the principles of health economics and their relevance to resource allocation in health and social care organisations and other agencies

7.4 identify the implications of current health policy and future policy changes for nursing and other professions and understand the impact of policy changes on the delivery and coordination of care

7.5 understand and recognise the need to respond to the challenges of providing safe, effective and person-centred nursing care for people who have co-morbidities and complex care needs

7.6 demonstrate an understanding of the complexities of providing mental, cognitive, behavioural and physical care services across a wide range of integrated care settings

7.7 understand how to monitor and evaluate the quality of people's experience of complex care

7.8 understand the principles and processes involved in supporting people and families with a range of care needs to maintain optimal independence and avoid unnecessary interventions and disruptions to their lives

7.9 facilitate equitable access to health-care for people who are vulnerable or have a disability, demonstrate the ability to advocate on their behalf when required, and make necessary reasonable adjustments to the assessment, planning and delivery of their care

7.10 understand the principles and processes involved in planning and facilitating the safe discharge and transition of people between caseloads, settings and services

7.11 demonstrate the ability to identify and manage risks and take proactive measures to improve the quality of care and services when needed

7.12 demonstrate an understanding of the processes involved in developing a basic business case for additional care funding by applying knowledge of finance, resources and safe staffing levels

7.13 demonstrate an understanding of the importance of exercising political awareness throughout their career, to maximise the influence and effect of registered nursing on quality of care, patient safety and cost effectiveness.

Appendix B: Nursing and Midwifery Board of Ireland Competencies for entry to the register of nurses

Box B.1 Domain 1: Professional values and conduct of the nurse competences

Knowledge and appreciation of the virtues of caring, compassion, integrity, honesty, respect and empathy as a basis for upholding the professional values of nursing and identity as a nurse.

1.1 Practise safely
1.2 Practise compassionately (Whilst the elements of empowering a person to maintain dignity and promotion of wellbeing may depend on acquisition and application of knowledge and skills according to the stage of an undergraduate nurse's education, the requirement for showing respect, kindness and compassion is expected of all healthcare staff.
1.3 Practise professionally, responsibly and accountably

Domain 2: Nursing practice and clinical decision-making competences

Knowledge and understanding of the principles of delivering safe and effective nursing care through the adoption of a systematic and problem-solving approach to developing and delivering a person-centred plan of care based on an explicit partnership with the person and his/her primary carer.

In partnership with the person, the primary carer and other health professionals, demonstrates the capacity to:

2.1 Assess nursing and health needs
2.2 Plan and prioritise person-centred nursing care (including selecting interventions based on best evidence and identification of desired goals with the person)
2.3 Deliver person-centred nursing skills, clinical interventions and health activities
2.4 Evaluate person-centred nursing outcomes and undertaking a comprehensive re-assessment
2.5 Utilise clinical judgement

Domain 3: Knowledge and cognitive competences

Knowledge and understanding of the health continuum, life and behavioural sciences and their applied principles that underpin a competent knowledge base for nursing and healthcare practice.

Demonstrates the capacity to:

3.1 Practise from a competent knowledge base

3.2 Use critical thinking and reflection to inform practice

Domain 4: Communication and interpersonal competences

Knowledge, appreciation and development of empathic communication skills and techniques for effective interpersonal relationships with people and other professionals in healthcare settings.

Demonstrates the capacity to:

4.1 Communicate in a person-centred manner

4.2 Communicate effectively with the healthcare team

Domain 5: Management and team competences

Using management and team competences in working for the person's well-being, recovery, independence and safety through recognition of the collaborative partnership between the person, family and multidisciplinary healthcare team.

Demonstrates the capacity to:

5.1 Practise collaboratively

5.2 Manage team, others and self safely

Domain 6: Leadership potential and professional scholarship competences

Developing professional scholarship through self-directed learning skills, critical questioning/reasoning skills and decision-making skills in nursing as the foundation for lifelong professional education, maintaining competency and career development.

Demonstrates the capacity to:

6.1 Develop leadership potential

6.2 Develop professional scholarship

Index

Note: Page numbers in *italics* indicate a figure and page numbers in **bold** indicate a table on the corresponding page.

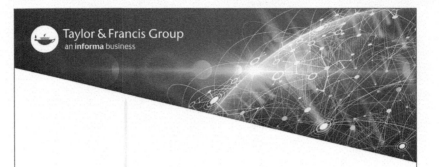